Praise for **Ethical Implications of COVID-19 Management: Evaluating the Aftershock** and **The COVID-19 Pandemic: Ethical Challenges and Considerations**

"The COVID-19 pandemic challenged more than our healthcare system, our community, our supply chains - it challenged the very foundation of the way medical research is conducted, interpreted, and presented to the public. This book highlights the key ethical challenges of the COVID era, from issues of equity in the workplace, to the dissemination of disinformation, to the challenges of vaccine distribution. If we do not learn from the COVID-19 pandemic, we are easy prey for the next virus that will emerge. Think of this book as not only a summation of lessons learned, but as preparation for the future."
F. Perry Wilson, MD MSCE, Associate Professor of Medicine at Yale University, USA, and Author of "How Medicine Works and When it Doesn't"

"One may say that the pandemic has been like a giant Trolley Problem for a global audience. The collection offers a unique space where several authors take up the question whether deontic, consequentialist, or utility ethics best serve action. Other authors mention Gilligan's 'ethics of care', which, for this reader at least, seems like something we could do with a lot more of. In the event, public action was largely driven by politics and the kind of moral intuition that chooses quantity of good over principle – as is illustrated in several chapters. The editors are to be congratulated and thanked for bringing together these timely and valuable essays. They would make salutary reading for the politicians who claim that the pandemic is over when it manifestly is not; that vaccines are a panacea, despite continuing excess deaths and disease; that international initiatives can be wound down because, as one UK politician says, the pandemic is a once-in-a-hundred-years event."
Richard Temperley-Little, Professor of Sustainability Leadership IFLAS, University of Cumbria, UK

"The COVID-19 pandemic had a devastating effect on the education of our children. While school leadership was grappling with making hard decisions to keep communities safe, parents were struggling with changing work and family dynamics. Constant bombardment from social media caused fear and confusion that disrupted the relationship between parents and school leadership. This book provides a balanced approach to understand the effects of the pandemic on our children and communities, creating a starting point for developing a plan to mitigate the social, physical, mental, and instructional effects of the pandemic."
Lynette M. Bryan, Ph.D., Broome-Tioga Board of Cooperative Educational Services (BOCES), Binghamton, New York, USA

"The COVID-19 pandemic and the uncertainty it generated across the world provide myriad opportunities to explore the ethical dilemmas faced and decisions made as a result of those challenges. Through multiple lenses—healthcare, education, language, technology, leadership, law—the contributors to this book provide thoughtful analysis of pandemic responses and consideration of the short and long-term effects and ethical implications of decisions made."
Ruthanne K. Orihuela, Provost and Vice President for Academic Affairs, Community College of Denver, USA

"For a multi-dimensional ethical assessment of the handling of the COVID-19 pandemic, these volumes will prove an essential, perhaps indispensable, but certainly highly instructive source."
Claus Dierksmeier, Professor for Globalization Ethics at the University of Tübingen, Germany

"The COVID-19 pandemic has left the planet now polarized in terms of how to respond to infectious diseases pandemics and with a diminishing trust in public health. The pandemic required nuance and a willingness to look at the risks and benefits of each intervention, but much of that nuance was lost. This book is the definitive resource to bring back nuance to our approach to infectious diseases, through an exploration of ethics, messaging, school closures, the impact of the pandemic on health care workers, global equity, and empathy. This book, written by a variety of experts in the field, has enormous potential to heal our divisiveness around COVID and formulate a roadmap for the next pandemic, and I provide it with my highest endorsement."
Monica Gandhi, MD, Professor of Medicine/Infectious Diseases and Director of the UCSF Center for AIDS Research, University of California San Francisco, USA

"All too often, in times of crisis, ethics are thrown out the window as people strive to deal quickly with the pressures of coping with the emergency. This was all too true during the global pandemic. This book highlights the myriad ethical dilemmas it caused, and suggests ways to keep focused on doing the right things for the right reasons."
Ronald E. Riggio, Ph.D., Professor of Leadership and Organizational Psychology, Kravis Leadership Institute, Claremont McKenna College, Claremont, California, USA

"The COVID 19 pandemic highlighted a myriad of ethical challenges in our public and professional lives, such as the tension between individual rights and collective well-being, the proper role of science and government in society, the appropriate uses of biotechnology, and the disproportionate challenges faced by different groups, among others. But the fundamental issues here are not new; the pandemic merely

forced us to confront them. This book is a much-needed exploration of these issues as we look for a 'new normal' in the post-COVID era, and it will help readers understand and negotiate these ethical dilemmas in a more thoughtful and productive way."
Todd Weaver, Dean, College of Business & Leadership, Point University, Georgia, USA.

"The COVID-19 pandemic of 2019-22 exposed weaknesses in our society's ability to respond to a pandemic threat. This was true not only in terms of public health interventions, but also challenges to our national and global economy, security, and social fabric. These new and important volumes address the ethical dilemmas arising with the many and complex dimensions affected by a serious virus threat."
Peter Hotez, Dean, National School of Tropical Medicine and Professor, Departments of Pediatrics, Molecular Virology & Microbiology, Baylor College of Medicine, Houston, Texas, USA

"These two texts provide a comprehensive and timely account of the many different ethical dilemmas posed by the COVID-19 pandemic. Ranging from a consideration of the long-term effects of on-line schooling for children to the ways in which the pandemic revealed the ugly realities of racial disparities across the globe, these texts are an invaluable resource for anyone wanting to pursue the moral questions raised by the pandemic. Additionally, they reveal the ethical choices faced by governments, businesses, health care providers as well as individual community members both during, and in the aftermath of the novel corona virus."
Donna Ladkin, PhD, Professor of Inclusive Leadership, University of Birmingham, UK

"These two COVID-19 volumes offer a groundbreaking look at the many ethical dilemmas associated with our current pandemic, and with important implications for those future pandemics that will inevitably follow this one. The editors of this collection, Eleftheria Egel and Cheryl Patton, have done a remarkable job, and provided a great service, by curating these diverse writings by scholars from around the world. In so doing, the collection provides a thought-provoking, deep dive into varied ethical considerations associated with this global challenge to human health and societal well-being."
Larry C. Spears, School of Leadership Studies, Gonzaga University, Spokane, USA

"The fallout from COVID-19 has had a wide-ranging impact on diverse social institutions and populations in developing and industrial nations. In many instances, we are still grappling with what its effects will mean for our shared future. This innovative collection provides thoughtful and useful pathways through the myriad ethical issues we face. It raises important questions and proposes valuable solutions while engaging and challenging readers with how best to move forward at this critical historical juncture. Its range is as expansive as the

problems we face. It is essential reading for those who want to navigate through the implications of the pandemic in a more ethical, deliberate, and thoughtful way."
Valerie Palmer-Mehta, Ph.D., Professor of Communication & Communication Internship, and Director, Dept. of Communication, Journalism, & PR, Oakland University, California, USA

"The COVID-19 pandemic has presented enormous ethical and moral challenges. In this collection the authors present their perspectives on these challenges. A very thought-provoking and timely work for our time."
Kathryn M. Edwards M.D., Sarah H. Sell and Cornelius Vanderbilt Chair Professor of Pediatrics, Vanderbilt University Medical Center, Nashville, Tennessee, USA.

Ethical Implications of COVID-19 Management

Evaluating the Aftershock

Edited by

Cheryl Patton and Eleftheria Egel

Ethical Implications of COVID-19 Management: Evaluating the Aftershock

Edited by: Cheryl Patton and Eleftheria Egel

This book first published 2022

Ethics International Press Ltd, UK

British Library Cataloguing in Publication Data

A catalogue record for this book is available from the British Library

Print Book ISBN: 978-1-80441-080-6

eBook ISBN: 978-1-80441-081-3

TABLE OF CONTENTS

PART THREE
SUPPRESSION MEASURES: COSTS AND BENEFITS

PART FOUR
BUSINESS AND ECONOMY

INTRODUCTION

Coronavirus disease 2019 (COVID-19) is caused by severe acute respiratory syndrome coronavirus 2 (SARS-CoV-2), a novel human coronavirus. The virus was detected when multiple severe pneumonia cases of unknown etiology emerged in December 2019 in Wuhan City, China. The earliest date of symptom onset was December 1, 2019, with patients displaying symptoms of fever, malaise, dry cough, and dyspnea and given the diagnosis of viral pneumonia (Liu et al., 2020). Initially, the disease was known as Wuhan pneumonia, as reporters termed it in early media reports (Liu et al., 2020) and the 2019-novel coronavirus (2019-nCoV; Ruiz-Medina et al., 2021). Colloquially, it has been termed COVID, corona, and the coronavirus.

By March 11, 2020, the number of cases of COVID-19 had increased to over 118,000 cases, spread to 114 countries, and caused 4,291 deaths, according to the World Health Organization (WHO, 2020). At that time, the WHO officially declared the health crisis a pandemic. To date, COVID-19 is responsible for millions of deaths worldwide (Ruiz-Medina et al., 2021).

Crises are defined as undesirable and unexpected situations that possess latent harm to people, organizations or society (Canyon, 2020). The pandemic can be regarded as one of the most impactful crises in history for its far-reaching aftershocks at the micro, meso, and macro levels. This book attempts to evaluate the crisis responses, the decisions made by leaders as they attempted to react to the pandemic expediently. Making consequential decisions where risk and uncertainty abounded was no small feat and it is apparent that mistakes were made along the way.

These mistakes made throughout the pandemic decision processes led to interpersonal, intragroup, intergroup, and interorganizational conflicts. You will read about some of them within this collection. A vital step in conflict mitigation and management is to listen to all sides. While this was not always possible due to the urgency of crisis decision making, at some point, it is important to gain alternative perspectives. Often during the pandemic, individuals and groups tuned the "other side" out, disregarding the root causes of various conflicts associated with pandemic-related issues, while intensifying distrust and polarization. Thus, when we were planning what we had in mind for this collection as co-editors, we shared a goal that the collection would offer accounts from various perspectives, while remaining scholarly in nature. Week after week, as we both collaborated when coediting this collection, we discovered that we disagreed on quite a few aspects of the COVID-19 pandemic responses. Despite that fact, we respected each other and in some instances, moved closer to common ground. That is our hope for the readers of this collection. We would like our readers to seek a greater understanding of the "other," the person with the opposing stance on the issues of this polarizing pandemic. It is our wish that a more civil response to alternate views may be considered.

Our book consists of four sections. Section A of this book highlights the multiple disruptions that individuals, families, and communities faced as their customary lives were turned upside down. Remote work, online schooling, and social isolation became the new normal and individuals were left grieving the loss of what was left behind and trying to grasp the reality of their current situation. Section B tackles the difficult subject of social inequities. Unequal distribution of resources led to disparities in suffering and death. The pandemic provided the reminder that the time to fight for social justice is now. Section C offers the readers a chance to determine if suppression measures such as lockdowns, school closures, and public temperature testing were necessary and effective, excessive and ineffective, or somewhere in between. The final section, Section D, focuses on business and the economy. As government and business leaders made decisions to help those affected, they found that their actions came with a tradeoff. Was it worth it? Readers can be the judge.

We wish to thank our chapter authors, experts in various fields, for their eclectic contributions. Without them, this collection would not be possible. We also thank you, our readers. We sincerely hope that you enjoy reading this collection and, once completed, you are able to broaden your perspective on this most difficult crisis, the COVID-19 pandemic.

In order to retain our authors' authentic voice, we preserved their use of American and British English spelling and styling.

References

Canyon, D. (2020). Definitions in crisis management and crisis leadership. *Security Nexus, 21.* https://apcss.org/nexus_articles/definitions-in-crisis-management-and-crisis-leadership/

Liu, Y-C., Kuo, R-L., & Shih, S-R. (2020). COVID-19: The first documented coronavirus pandemic in history. *Biomedical Journal, 43*(4), 328-333. https://doi.org/10.1016/j.bj.2020.04.007

Ruiz-Medina, B. E., Varela-Ramirez, A., Kirken, R. A., & Robles- Escajeda, E. (2022). The SARS-CoV-2 origin dilemma: Zoonotic transfer or laboratory leak? *BioEssays, 44,* e2100189. https://doi.org/10.1002/bies.202100189

WHO (2020b). Virtual press conference on COVID-19. *World Health Organization.* https://www.who.int/docs/default-source/coronaviruse/transcripts/who-audio-emergencies-coronavirus-press-conference-full-and-final-11mar2020.pdf?sfvrsn=cb432bb3_2

ABOUT THE EDITORS

Dr Cheryl Patton serves as a Ph.D. Dissertation Advisor and Adjunct Professor in the Ph.D. in Organizational Leadership program at Eastern University, St. Davids, Pennsylvania. Her previous career was in the healthcare sector, where she spent two decades as a medical imaging technologist in a tertiary care center. Her research interests include healthcare leadership, workplace conflict, workplace ethics, and phenomenology.

Dr Eleftheria Egel is a scholar, business mentor for female entrepreneurs and startup founder. Her scholarly research focuses on female leadership & entrepreneurship, sustainability and spiritual leadership. Her vision is to inspire and support positive transformative change in the way we interact by breaking down conventional barriers (assumptions); promoting new ways of thinking (holistic attributes such as compassion); and expanding the boundaries (sense-giving) of what is possible (sense-making) in our personal understanding and socio-organizational setting.

PART ONE
Disruption is the New Normal

ETHICAL MANAGEMENT IN THESE UNPRECEDENTED TIMES: COVID-19, GENDER, REMOTE WORK, AND THE SEARCH FOR EMPLOYEE WORK-LIFE BALANCE

Bethany Huxford Davis[1]

Abstract: For many engaged in the workforce, the onset of the COVID-19 pandemic led to a reevaluation of the intersection of work and life. Employees—especially women for whom the pandemic impact has been felt more sharply—are pondering the sustainability of experiencing an imbalance between work and life. The temporary shift to remote work for employees forced both organizational and individual assessment as the world reopened and many began to push for a return to "normal." Employees are not always willing to return to a fully in-office job and are demanding more flexibility to attend to life, to shorten commutes, and to alter schedules. This wide-ranging change in workplace norms demands a sharp attention to ethical managerial practices. Questions surrounding logistics and feasibility remain and are vital for employers to address. Critically, the equitable decision making needed around who *can* work remotely, and who *should* do so must be considered. Solutions for the future must be made in partnership with employees rather than in managerial silo. This chapter explores the impact of the sudden shift to workplace flexibility created by COVID-19, offering practical solutions for individuals and organizations seeking to address the future with a priority on ethical approaches.

Facing a once-a-century pandemic tests every facet of work and life, and not insignificantly, the collision of the two spheres. Management during such unprecedented times presents major challenges and demands an acute attention to ethics (Allen et al., 2021). Almost overnight, employees who might not otherwise have been approved for working from home were being remotely managed. Managers were unexpectedly overseeing teams scattered across living rooms and kitchen islands, frequently needing to

---

[1] Dean of Academic Operations, Point University, West Point, Georgia, USA

make schedule exceptions for parents supervising virtual learning and adapting to employees being unable to work due to quarantine or illness. Employers tending towards sharper managerial oversight found themselves considering just how invasively to supervise suddenly remote employees. Ethical challenges abound in the "how to" of managing a remote employee *without* a pandemic. This is only complicated further by adding in pandemic factors such as extreme stress, concern for health, and for many employees the complication of additional caring responsibilities (Allen et al., 2021).

The push for returning to "normal" as soon as possible has been prevalent throughout the pandemic, and increased with the dawn of vaccines, reduced hospital counts, and expired patience. In writing on this phenomenon, Chang (2022) notes, "We still want to get back to normal, and we can't acknowledge the realities of our current world" (para. 19). The process of determining who should return to the physical office remains at the forefront for many professionals and their employers. Whose job *can* be done at home? Whose job *should be allowed* to be done at home? Are workplace leaders and managers equipped to make these decisions as we collectively move towards a "new normal"? In a not-quite-post-pandemic reality, employers find themselves faced with the challenge of determining how to move forward equitably and ethically.

In the months immediately preceding the pandemic the International Labour Organization (2020) brought the complicated reality of family needs to the forefront, noting most of the "family work" is handled by women. The ILO also notes "the issues of work-life balance are relevant to all workers and have become a priority in both urban centres and rural areas across the globe" (p. 1). The ILO maintains a goal to ensure that "workers with family responsibilities – women as well as men – are not disadvantaged in relation to other workers and, in particular, that women with family responsibilities are not disadvantaged in comparison to men with family responsibilities" (p. 2). These are not new issues, but rather issues that were amplified by the dawn of a pandemic and the struggle to "make it all work" when the sustainability of such a concept was already shaky at best.

COVID-19's Immediate Workplace Impact

Nearly as soon as we could get our collective minds around what was happening to us in the wake of COVID-19, news outlets began reporting on the uneven impact on women attempting to balance career and family responsibilities during a global pandemic (Cain Miller, 2021a, 2021b; Cohen & Hsu, 2020; Robertson & Gebeloff, 2021). Writing for NBC news in 2021, Jessica Denson said this of the balancing act:

Don't misunderstand me. My husband has helped out a lot by doing laundry and assisting with the mopping and sweeping. But, honestly, the messy kitchen, the dirty bathroom and the cluttered dining room table just don't bother him like they do me. So I have felt personally responsible for taking care of them much more often and have generally done so. (para. 4)

Again, this tendency for women to hold more of the household burden is not new. Thoreau (n.d.) reporting on the She-Cession, includes this summation, "the pandemic did not create new gender inequalities in the workforce, but it is noteworthy that it did substantially worsen existing inequalities" (section 2, para. 1). Of course, the "second shift" of household work after one's job present in many women's lives morphed into what seems to be more a third shift when making considerations for the challenges of caregiving, managing remote learning, and navigating pandemic health concerns. This pressure to "do all the things" is only amplified for single mothers as Cohen and Hsu shared in a 2020 article for *The New York Times.* Also in *The New York Times,* in 2021, a series of images and profiles of women and how they were navigating this tightrope were portrayed. Chapman et al. (2021) share, women seem to have more options and yet, "that also means that whether they work for pay or stay at home with children is considered a personal choice, and one they're often judged for. It's different for men, because society expects them to work. Women's identities feel hard-earned" (para. 5).

For women who left outside employment during the pandemic, and those who did not, considerations for the future are important for employers. Many women will mull their options for returning, staying, finding something new, or some other solution. A part of the equation must be employers reconsidering the equitable and ethical priorities they set. The impact of COVID-19 did not create a new focus on how to treat employees equitably and ethically. Indeed, in their 2011 report, *Equality at Work*, the International Labour Organization outlined many areas of concern, including several that largely impact women, such as gender inequality, maternity and paternity protection, and sexual harassment. These inequalities must be addressed at both the national and workplace level (ILO, 2011). This ILO report was written on the heels of the global economic crisis of 2008 and emphasizes that economic uncertainty can increase discrimination (p. 5). In the recovery from the financial crisis, the ILO warned, "whatever has been the social impact of the financial crisis, post-crisis recovery strategies and measures must not ignore the principles of non-discrimination and equality" (p. 5). This warning holds true now, in the earliest days of recovery from the COVID-19 pandemic—days when hospital rates and case counts and booster shots are still a glaring part of an emerging new norm. As the world begins to move forward from COVID-19, employers must seek to impact employee work-life balance via flexible and remote schedules, helping employees to find a reasonable path toward work-life balance.

The Sudden Shift to Flexibility

To determine next steps for employers, it is necessary to understand the context of the past and the present. Long before the impact of a global pandemic, there was a sense of frustration or confusion in trying to find a healthy balance at the intersection of work and life (Akanji et al., 2015; Huxford Davis, 2017) that seems to feel more immediate and frustrating for many in the current reality (Sun et al., 2020, Veal, 2020). Various factors entangle the struggle towards balance, such as parenting responsibilities (Orel, 2019); the sense of a breakdown of the psychological contract between employer and employee (Kaya & Kartepe, 2020); being single and childless (Akanji et al., 2019); and being a female professional (Chung & van der Lippe, 2018; Høg Utoft, 2020).

A part of the complication around understanding the push to remote work during COVID-19 is the idea that the shift was not voluntary (Allen et al., 2021; de Klerk et al., 2021; McGloin et al., 2022; Zhang et al., 2021). This was true for employees who previously were not given the opportunity to remotely work or did not desire the shift (Zhang et al., 2021). The loss of the physical separation between work and home for many was a challenge to boundary management (Allen et al., 2021; Awada et al., 2021; de Klerk et al., 2021; Mirchandani, 2008). Indeed, the shift to widespread remote work during the beginning of the pandemic might best be described as abrupt or jarring, forcing organizations, "even those with a reluctance to change—to modify practices and processes that influenced the employee experience far faster than would have occurred without the crisis" (Nyberg et al., 2021, p. 1968; see also Zhang et al, 2021).

Organizations were forced into quick decisions and the vital nature of "clear, authentic communication" became more critical as employer and employee struggled with health concerns, capabilities of remote work technologies, and the unrelenting anxieties of pandemic uncertainty (Nyberg et al., 2021, p. 1968; see also McGloin et al., 2022). Even when attempting to communicate clearly and deliberately, many organizations discovered that confusion often remained prevalent, leading them to focus on "continuous messaging, consistent messaging, and the power of listening" (Nyberg et al., 2021, p. 1968). The sudden shift to widely dispersed and unsettled remote work, must be understood according to Awada et al. (2021) in three ways: "the work (the what), the workspace (the where), and the worker (the who)" (p. 1172). The intersection of the "what, where, and who" Awada et al. refer to, created a work-life collision for many.

Feelings about work-life boundaries, of course, vary from person to person, but these "preferences are important to the extent that individuals are able to act in ways consistent with their needs and preferences" (Allen et al., 2021, p. 63). The sense of organizational-individual fit and the collective sense of role conflict was rather complicated already pre-pandemic (Awada et al., 2021). Divisions between work and life have "become more permeable," leading to people switching roles more frequently (Leroy et al., 2021). The loss of separation and privacy for remote workers is not a new concept, but it quickly became a prevalent one in early 2020. Mirchandani (2008) describes it as "the spheres of work and nonwork" being "under perpetual threat from one another" (p. 92). The boundary violation involved "reinforces the publicness of work and the privateness of nonwork" (p. 92). Suddenly work was encroaching on one's home life in new ways, and life was simultaneously pushing back on the boundary of work.

The ability to maintain these boundaries in terms of physical space and working schedules is a key aspect of successful remote work (Mirchandani, 2008). As de Klerk et al. (2021) note, "The absence of natural daily structures made it complicated to distinguish between work and personal life and to create distance between home and work, making it challenging to maintain a healthy work-life balance" (p. 7). No doubt this is challenging enough for those who participated in working from home pre-pandemic, but in a time when many of us stayed home for weeks and months without so much as going to a grocery store, the loss of distinguishing moments between "who I am as a human" and "who I am as a worker" began to fade quickly.

An important caveat to all of this is the privilege of being able to work from home in relative safety rather than being an essential worker serving the public with little protection, as seen frequently in the earliest days of the pandemic. The challenge for nonessential workers was figuring out the adaptation of working remotely and doing so quickly (Zhang et al., 2021). As Jacks (2021) argues, this shift is not all positive, but indeed has highlighted digital inequities, wherein "white-collar knowledge workers" could shift to remote work while blue collar workers did not see the same benefit (p. 94). This is complicated further when moving outside the United States' context, as "the digital disparity between 'haves' and 'have nots' increases further in countries that lack IT infrastructure and stable/cheap Internet access" (p. 94).

For those able to work from home, some of the known benefits of more flexibility were immediately seen. Of course, there are some obvious benefits to working from home for many professionals, including a more flexible management of one's life, saving time and money without a commute, and saving the expense of more formal work attire (de Klerk et al., 2021; Jacks, 2021). Interestingly, the lack of commute seems to be primarily a benefit but for many it also serves as "a tangible boundary between work and home" (de Klerk et al., 2021, p. 8). This leads some teleworkers to "develop rituals of going to work which replace the traditional commute to the workplace"

(Mirchandani, 2008, p. 91). Notably among the benefits, one particularly vital during the pandemic, is flexibility around childcare options (Jacks, 2021). There is also a benefit for employees with disabilities (Goldfarb et al., 2022) in terms of accessibility, comfort, and opportunity for specific kinds of work that had previously been more limited.

In addition, flexible work arrangements lead to fewer physical health issues for some, positively impact "psychological well-being" and lead to fewer illness-related absences (Senthanar et al., 2021, pp. 295-296). Not all work from home (WFH) experiences are positive, of course. The "initial excitement" of the early-pandemic arrangement was often tempered by the reality of the need to find space, quiet, and focus in one's home for one's job (de Klerk et al., 2021). While those participating in remote work have long appreciated "having a 'flexibility' to meet nonwork demands" throughout the day, this is tempered with the process of dividing and labeling household and childcare as "not work" (Mirchandani, 2008, pp. 94-95). Challenges in finding the oft-recommended "dedicated workspace" or a moment of quiet to focus away from the people one lives with were immediately apparent for many (Allen et al., 2021; Awada et al., 2021). Workers trying to make do in a new reality were frequently forced to shuffle—physically and mentally—around the complications of life. These included such factors as children doing remote learning and finding time for care responsibilities, which included enhanced cleaning in many cases (Awada et al., 2021). Challenges with a lack of privacy when housemates are a part of the equation, including sound from video meetings were also quickly apparent (Natomi et al., 2022). Other challenges include the technology used for remote working, as software such as Zoom, Microsoft Teams, and others used for team connectivity could increase worker anxiety. If an employee was already nervous about some of these tools, they may have become more so when suddenly required to use them with increased frequency and urgent need (Prodanova & Kocareve, 2021).

Natomi et al. (2022) illuminate one of the greatest challenges of this time in striking language, saying, "…while the way that we work has changed dramatically, the residences of many employees have remained the same. It is conceivable that employees are being forced to bear the brunt of both changes" (p. 12). For those who shifted to remotely working from home during the pandemic, the sudden experiment led to work and life encroaching on each other in significant ways.

Work–family boundary stressors capture the blurriness or dysfunctional permeation of work–family boundary during the COVID-19 outbreak. Although existing research has shown that increased family needs and demands can promote employee adoption of telework (Shockley & Allen, 2010), working from home may also make it easier for family activities to encroach upon work time, blurring the work–family boundary (Golden et al., 2006; Hill et al., 1996). This is especially true as COVID-19 outbreak engenders an abrupt increase in family demands (e.g., taking care of children due to school closure) that may interfere with working at home (Kanfer et al., 2020). Not surprisingly, these stressors are more likely to occur and interfere with work activities in the home setting, as it involves more frequent interactions between the employee and his/her family members. (Shao et al., 2021, p. 827)

Tangled into the family demands outlined by Shao et al. (2021) above, are the ways in which we now must learn to live with COVID-19. As we move from the immediate crisis into living with the virus, employees find themselves at times making daily choices or "just-in-time decisions" about where to work (Shao et al., 2021, p. 825). Shao et al. note this is part of a "coping strategy to manage stress-eliciting demands and events from the previous day" which is "particularly relevant and informative to daily work location choices" based on pandemic uncertainty and related demands (Shao et al., 2021, p. 826). It is critical that organizations seek to understand the ways in which employees are *permanently* changed by the pandemic and experience daily decisions about remote work, family care dynamics, and quarantine choices that most could not have reasonably imagined before 2020.

Organizational Issues

There is pressure now on organizations to be more flexible and allow more permanent remote work arrangements and schedule options for employees. The arguments of "your job cannot be done from home" or "your job must be done between these set hours" are harder to make when the pandemic forced us to see that many jobs *can* be done from home *and* at varied times. Sensibly, there are more considerations than "can X be done at home," when we are aware of technological challenges (Messenger & Gschwind, 2016) and benefits of being in group settings for some tasks. As Shao et al. (2021) note, "many necessary (or even specialized) infrastructures, equipment, and software remain more accessible or operate more efficiently at the work sites" (p. 828). Workers at home tend to be more productive but do lose out on collaboration and can feel isolated (de Klerk et al., 2021). While one might communicate less with coworkers, there are potentially more interruptions, including those "emanating from the nonwork domain" (Leroy et al., 2021, p. 1448). Employers and employees alike must grapple with new concepts like the "fatigue that can be associated with a heavy reliance on videoconferences" (Bennett et al., 2021 as cited in Nyberg et al., 2021, p. 1971). Beyond technical challenges, building on the work of Jett and George (2003), Leroy et al. (2020) note employees working from home might experience many types of other interruptions, labeled as: intrusions, distractions, breaks, multitasking, and surprises. People you live with, people who are making deliveries, laundry buzzers, and the noises of one's neighborhood are all contenders for distraction.

It is, of course, not just the individual that varies in preferences and fit for remote work, but also the organizational approach taken by each workplace (de Klerk et al., 2021). As Allen et al. (2021) point out, "workplaces vary with regard to the extent that they supply conditions that facilitate integration [and] segmentation" (p. 65). Not all organizations were prepared in practice or policy to support a major transition to WFH for employees, especially so suddenly (Awada et al., 2021). Challenges for organizations include communication, training for roles and the required skill set, and adaptation to organizational culture (Nyberg et al., 2021). These challenges, combined with personal preference and organizational needs contribute to a "fit" equation for each job and its capability for being done remotely. The challenge for organizations to determine "fit" must also include doing so equitably across the organization.

As the International Labour Organization points out, within flexibility there is a greater chance to increase inequality (ILO, 2022). McGloin et al. (2022) describe that the shift to remote work may have caused on-site employees to experience disruptions in managerial rapport, which is a critical piece of the supervisor and employee relationship with impacts on "job satisfaction, employee retention, and reduced stress" (Swarnalatha & Prassanna, 2013 as cited in McGloin et al., 2022, p. 45). A key aspect of this idea of remote work functioning well includes trust. The "the tone at the top" matters in determining how to move forward, including how leaders communicate, behave, prioritize, and manage (Lašáková & Remišová, 2019). As Hungerford and Cleary (2021) define it, "high-trust work environments are those where the workplace culture supports and engenders trust between colleagues: leaders and team members alike" (p. 506). Employees generally start with a "willingness to trust" and hold expectations for that to "develop over time" (p. 507). For example, the inherent lack of employer trust seen in excessive monitoring is, understandably, not taken well by employees and can lead to turnover (Nyberg et al., 2020).

Organizations have been forced to trust *more*. This includes trusting new employees to work remotely, often hired without ever meeting in person, for jobs that will later be expected to be largely on site. The loss of opportunity for training, settling into in-person team dynamics, and developing communication routines is a significant challenge for organizations and their employees (Waizenegger et al., 2020 as cited in McGloin et al., 2022). Video substitution for in- person interactions leads to losing out on things like spontaneity as well as "shared identity, shared context, and reduce[d] conflict" (Hinds & Mortensen, 2005 as cited in McGloin et al., 2022, p. 50). This trust is a part of the organizational climate and this matters for flexible work arrangements. Organizational climate has a "negative and significant effect on work stress" meaning a "conducive organizational climate will reduce the level of work stress and vice versa" (Pradoto et al., 2022, p. 352). Senthanar et al. (2021) concur, noting:

> Flexible work arrangements are in large part dictated by organizational climate. Organizations that have a supportive organizational climate value nonwork aspects of people's lives and seek to accommodate the multiple needs of employees to create a positive work environment and enhance organizational productivity. Conversely, a hindering organizational climate requires that employees prioritize work over nonwork activities which can mean putting in extra time to get the work done or the embedded

understanding within the organization's practices that nonwork activities may negatively impact career progression. (p. 296)

Both job stress and organizational climate have an impact on overall employee performance (Pradoto et al, 2022). Organizations must consider how they focus on goals, foster communication, create an environment of respect, and reward performance as part of the move to more flexibility (p. 352).

It is critical that leaders are involved in the process of building *and* supporting these structures, processes, policies, and practices related to trust-building *with* employees (Hungerford & Cleary, 2021). A lack of trust leads to higher stress, which impacts mental health and feelings of safety. This is resolved, in part, via improved work and life balance which should include "respect and kindness" as a key focus in the work environment (p. 512). It's not just paperwork to create a policy, rather "leaders need to understand how their decisions are intertwined with the company culture and climate" (Lašáková & Remišová, 2019, p. 26).

Beyond the availability of specific technology to make remote work a reality, organizations need to focus on business continuity planning and the infrastructure that supports remote work (Jacks, 2021). An important part of this is the need to pay attention to those who may not be able to take advantage of remote work in an industry where it is more prevalent (Kawaguchi & Motegi, 2021). The question *who can work from home?* is a key starting point for the conversation organizations need to have internally for moving forward.

Dingle and Neiman (2020) estimate that 37% of jobs can be done at home when allowing for characteristics that make it impossible (i.e., a grocery store cannot likely accommodate remote work for cashiers). They note "jobs in finance, corporate management, and professional and scientific services" are more easily done at home (p. 3). The Pew Research Center estimates that 60% of workers "*don't* have jobs that can be done from home, and others who do have these types of jobs are going into their workplace at least sometimes. For a large majority of these workers, their jobs continue to involve at least some in-person interaction with others at their workplace" and we cannot ignore that about half of those who ever interact with other people at their workplace say they're very (19%) or somewhat (32%) concerned about being exposed to the coronavirus" (Parker et al., 2022, para. 6). As Kawaguchi and Motegi (2021) see it, it makes sense that jobs focused in telecommunication and information can shift to a remote setting, but "workers in transportation, the postal industry and the public sector, who are considered essential workers are less likely to engage in remote work" (p. 6). Those with higher incomes tend to have more availability for remote work as well (Kwakguchi & Motegi, 2021). All of this has been at play for many years in various contexts and industries, but the COVID-19 pandemic has clarified a need to be more intentional and consistent in making calls about flexible and remote work for employees where possible.

Considerations for a Flexible Future

An abrupt shift in the separation of work and life unfolded rapidly with COVID-19. The increased shift to more employees working from home is likely here to stay on at least some level (Awada et al., 2021). Many who began working from home in early 2020 find themselves uncertain that a return to 40 hours a week in an office building is a sustainable future. With this shift, employers must address the new tensions in the ever-elusive search for work-life balance. As employers reopen buildings, are employees truly needed in a shared workspace five days a week or are we longing to justify a shift back to "the before times"? Of course, remote work is not practical for some industries, but where it can be, there is a louder push for it than perhaps ever before. For companies continuing to use a mostly hybrid or remote approach, are employees able to find rest and balance away from the job now being done at their dining room table? Who is allowed to work at home? How can employees function best when childcare is shut down or quarantine is required by a school? How do we set procedures during the ever-changing dynamic of COVID variants *and* a mandate from employees that we do better when it comes to balance?

Lopez-Leon et al. (2020) note we can learn from this experience – and must – that "we need to systematize the lessons learned in times of crisis to be able to implement them efficiently and successfully if and when the need arises to do so again" (p. 374). The push of the pandemic has "forced people to rethink their traditional ways of working, but [infection epidemics] have also provided an opportunity to change their conventional work practices" (Natomi et al., 2022, p. 2). Data from the Pew Research Center, notes that about 60% of U.S. workers can and are doing their work from home (Parker et al., 2022). Those who could be physically in their workplace but continue to choose to work from home, have shifted in their reasoning for doing so. The Pew data shows less concern about exposure to coronavirus and more preference for working from home, including due to relocation away from the office. Of those "currently work[ing] from home all or most of the time, 78% say they'd like to continue to do so after the pandemic" which is up 14% from 2020 (section 1, para. 5). Other factors are at play in understanding the population of employees who can work from home. Those with college degrees are more likely to be able to work from home, as are those with higher incomes (Parker et al., 2022). Simply put, organizations cannot assume employees will accept a return to the before times.

While COVID-19 concerns continue to be a part of the deciding factor for about half of those surveyed, the Pew data showcases that the reasons for wishing to work from home when it is not essential to do so, have shifted since the fall of 2020. The *preference* to do so is far more a part of the equation now, with 76% of those surveyed indicating they prefer to work from home even if their workplace is available to them, which is up from a 60% response rate in 2020. Childcare remains a significant part of a desire to work from home with 64% of those surveyed and working from home noting the shift to WFH "has made it easier to balance work and their personal life" (Parker et al., 2022, section 4, para. 1). Interestingly, those who are fully vaccinated and boosted report more concern about virus exposure if returning to the office. Most workers are "at least somewhat satisfied with the measures their workplace has put in place to protect them from coronavirus exposure" though only 36% are "very satisfied" (Parker et al., 2022, section 1, para. 10). Of note, "these assessments vary considerably by race and ethnicity, income and age" (Parker et al., 2022, section 7, para. 1). Organizations must pay attention to this early data to better understand a direction forward. Critically, this must also include a focus on understanding the pandemic-related gender dynamics.

Gender Dynamics

Understanding the gendered workplace is vital to moving forward ethically, if for no other reason than interest by employees. Forbes reported that only 7% of men are in favor of not returning to the office compared to 19% of women (Beheshti, 2022). More critically, however, as the International Labour Organization (2011) describes it, "women continue to suffer discrimination in almost all aspects of employment, including the jobs they can obtain, their renumeration, benefits and working conditions, and their access to decision-making positions" (p. 19). The pandemic has had the worst impact on young women, already impacted by gender inequality in pay (ILO, 2022). Of note, "the flexibility of remote work offers the opportunity to better balance domestic responsibilities with income generation, which has important ramifications when women carry a disproportionate burden of household work" (ILO, 2022, p. 31).

Awada et al. (2021) argue that "Overall, female workers, older workers, and those at higher income levels were found to be significantly more productive than their counterparts while WFH during the pandemic," allowing for creation of a "much-needed balance between work-family-home responsibilities" (p. 1183). As illuminated in news media and academic research women have "borne the brunt of the impact" of COVID-19 related job losses, including a "disproportionate number" of minorities (Jacks, 2021, p. 94). There are gender imbalances with childcare, scheduling, and other aspects of the "life" part of work-life balance (Leroy et al., 2021) even with a male and female set of partners both working from home during the pandemic (see also ILO, 2022).

This outcome is interesting, when well before the pandemic Mirchandani (2008) supposed that "teleworking women and men, it would seem, are appropriately placed to actualize the feminist vision of challenging the organization of social life into public and private spheres" (p. 89). Importantly, the teleworkers Mirchandani referenced were working from home voluntarily – or even fought for the option to do so. Most noted that it "allows them to gain greater control over the environment within which they work while managing responsibilities with less stress" and increasing productivity while saving on commute times (p. 89). However, some form of separation is key:

Both male and female teleworkers felt that without a separation between work and non-work, their work productivity would fall. The language which they use to refer to their reasons for separating their work and family domains differs qualitatively. For men, the family is a 'temptation,' for women, a 'responsibility'; the distinction between a temptation and a responsibility lies in the location of control. Men have to exercise self-control in managing their option to do family-related activities. Women, on the other hand, also have to negotiate their responsibility in the home with their paid work obligations. (Mirchandani, 2008, p. 12)

Employer concerns come back into play as well, as "when a clear separation between work and nonwork is not made, the legitimacy and value of work is called into question" (Mirchandani, 2008, p. 103). While women are often required to defend the "legitimacy" of their work, "men face an alternative pressure; that of being perceived as doing women's work" (Mirchandani, 2008, p. 104). Understanding these dynamics is an important piece of employers structuring the future of post-pandemic work.

The willingness to view employees as people who desire to balance work and life – or at least manage both – demands attention to the functionality of flexibility for employee and employer. Employees are not just their lives and not just their work, but rather are complete beings, or what the literature often describes as "whole people" desiring to be effective and engaged both in work and life responsibilities (Dehler & Welsh, 2010; Duchon & Plowman, 2005; Lips-Wiersma & Mills, 2013; Lund Dean et al., 2008; Miller, 2007; Zinnbauer & Pargament, 2005). What does it look like to ethically address concerns for employees as *whole people* as the pandemic continues to shape our view of both work and life?

Moving Forward Ethically

The pandemic has necessarily impacted every aspect of life across the globe. For workers and their employees, these "lessons and changes in the workforce are likely to have long-lasting ramifications" (Nyberg et al., 2021,

p. 1968). The dynamic has shifted from one of "few if any employees can possibly work from home" to "who needs to be physically in the office and how frequently." Considerations for employers must include onboarding and productivity, but also considerations for physical space needs. Further, there are complications of agreements for employees to remain fully remote and out-of-state in some cases (Nyberg et al., 2021). As the ILO (2022) notes, those "with access to technology and higher skills, who tend to work in larger businesses, will have options to participate in remote work while those who do not, will not be able to do so. This is widening the chasm between the haves and have-nots" (ILO, 2022, p. 31). Employers who are concerned with avoiding deepening these existing concerns and challenges, should endeavor to approach flexible working arrangements ethically.

To get to this point, it is necessary to understand some basics of organizational ethics. Lowery and Duesing (2014) summarize the ethical framework neatly, "Ethics in organizations is determined by the individuals in the organization, so while contextual variables can have an impact, it is the individual employee's personal ethical framework that likely has the largest influence on individual ethical behavior" (p. 411). Some professionals, like accountants, might have a formal code of ethics, though training and instruction are also important across industries (Lowery & Duesing, 2014). Organizations that provide this training either internally or through contracting with an outside organization find a positive relationship to "perceptions of workplace ethics; thus it appears employers might be able to take proactive steps to influence their employees' views toward acceptable behavior in the workplace" (p. 416). Interestingly, spirituality also is important here as those identifying with a "a higher degree of spirituality might have more of a tendency to view ethically questionable behaviors as wrong," and thus, "may be less likely to engage in manipulative behavior at work, to conceal errors at work, to falsify reports, and to engage in other such unethical behaviors" (p. 416). Lowrey and Duesing also found that older employees tend to "become more ethical in their view of questionable workplace behaviors" which may serve as a useful mentorship tool for younger employees (p. 417).

Regardless of the organizational structure and focus on ethics, leader behavior matters here and "is believed to influence the ethical climate in the company substantially" (Lašáková & Remišová, 2019, p. 27). Employees are watching for an "adherence to a common set of comprehensibly articulated group norms" in order to see how omit "to model, regulate, motivate and control human ethical conduct" in an organization (Lašáková & Remišová, 2019, p. 27). As we collectively have observed with scandals like those seen at Enron and AIG, employees need to feel safe in order to speak up about ethical problems. Employers endeavoring to set the correct "ethical tone" create an impact for employees' feelings of safety and to them behaving more ethically themselves (Mayer et al., 2013 as cited in Lašáková & Remišová, 2019, p. 27). Perhaps most critically in this conversation is a need to acknowledge the reality of a pandemic and coming post-pandemic world. The dynamic has already shifted – a return to "the way things were" is unlikely to be fully realized. Employees want more flexibility, and the ethical employer must make considerations – and likely concessions – to retain a satisfied workforce.

Practical Solutions for a Flexible Framework

What then should employers who choose to move forward mindfully towards more flexible arrangements for employees consider? Chang (2022) notes that some advice from Gerderman (2021) and the Harvard Business School is helpful here. Practical steps might include: (1) setting specific priorities for times when employees are in the office physically, (2) being direct and honest with employees, including about company needs (3) considering the risks of loneliness for remote employees, (4) maintaining a flexibility and willingness to look at a hybrid approach for future work arrangements, finding ways to talk about caregiving needs, and (5) showing compassion. Through the pandemic we have learned that in many ways we are all stressed out together. Employers and those tasked with leading teams must maintain sensitivity around the trauma and burnout we are collectively experiencing. This must include the emotional intelligence to lead empathetically, as well as the need to prove to employees it is safe for them to be on site in employer facilities. Organizations must strive to be fair and consistent when deciding who can work remotely and who cannot. These steps are both helpful and necessary for a United States' culture where Chang (2022) notes, "no matter how good a back-to-office plan is, they're all a reminder that we're insistent on building a post-pandemic world that mirrors the pre-pandemic one" (para. 21). Organizations and employers must work together in considering what changes they can make for a flexible and remote arrangement to be sustainable.

Additionally, employees must be willing to consider changes at home to make flexibility feasible. This might include things like setting up a dedicated workspace to cut down on distractions and interruptions (Awada et al., 2021; Leroy et al., 2021). While employers should strive to create a culture of trust, employers and employees need to work together to figure out the balance between concerns of management that all workers are "slacking off" and the reality that some will (Kawaguchi & Motegi, 2021). Clear training around ethical working from home behaviors for managers and employees alike should be a priority (Lašáková & Remišová, 2019).

Employers and employees can work together to develop strategies for success for employees utilizing a remote work option. Lopez-Leon et al. (2020) write specifically to remote educators, but include several recommendations for working from home that are applicable to any professional, including: (1) create routines, (2) be organized, (3) have an adequate home office, (4) enhance your productivity, (5) be responsible, (6) avoid extreme multitasking, (7) facilitate communication and networking, (8) be balanced, (9) use available computer programs and platforms, and (10) learn from the challenges (pp. 372-374). The admonition to "learn from the challenges" is of vital import. Indeed Lopez et al. (2021) indicate that working to systemize what we learned during the peak of the pandemic serves to better support a need to be flexible in the future.

Managers can be trained to help employees structure their days just as they would if present on site, but in cases of remote work with a special focus on maintaining boundaries. For example, Zhang et al. (2021) argue for attention on several factors like, improved work-life boundaries, physical space, technology, training, taking regular breaks, and finding ways to make personal connections (Zhang et al., 2021, p. 805). Research from Ohio State University indicates a need to also be specific in preparing for complications in the workforce for women. The researchers note "the pandemic did not create new gender inequalities, but it is noteworthy that it did substantially worsen existing inequalities" (Thoreau, n.d., section 2, para. 1). The report from Ohio State indicates a need for "businesses and institutions to start taking a hard look at changes they can make now to help women stay employed and to welcome them back into the workforce" (section 3, para 1). This includes a focus on policy and for organizations to "rethink how to configure their work environment to equitably accommodate and support women" (section 3, para 1). Practical changes employers can make include (1) allowing flexibility, (2) simplifying communication channels and technologies, (3) predictably scheduling meetings, (4) reconsidering the hours required for a full workday or week, including how employee productivity is measured, (5) moving away from the pressures of billable hours, (6) focusing more on hybrid/remote models for work, (7) designing work more around human behavior and less around specific locations and timeframes, (8) focusing on equitable changes, (9) ceasing caregiver bias, including in performance evaluations, and (10) focusing on retention programs (section 5). Employers need to move forward with an acceptance that "'in-person meetings' are important, but 'virtual facetime' is effective, efficient, and expanding use and value" (section 6, para. 3). Special care must be given to avoid employees with responsibilities for caregiving, including acknowledging that "the childcare system is broken, and employers must be part of the solution" (section 6, para. 4-5). Forcing employees—most often women—to ultimately choose between family and career is a broken part of our culture and one that reared its biased head again during the pandemic when mostly women took on the remote learning role for families with children learning at home (section 3). Those forced to leave the workforce should not be penalized as they return (section 6, para. 6).

Conclusion

The pandemic provided a pivotal impetus for change in remote and flexible work arrangements. Employees are demanding change, and the employers seeking to find and retain talent will need to listen to the shift in our collective acceptance of work arrangements as a culture. The impact of COVID-19 on workplace behaviors is far from fully understood, but the visibility into push back from employees on a "return to normal," is clear. Employees desire more flexibility, increased opportunities to work from home, and a better balance from work's encroachment on life. Employers who find ways to meaningfully and thoroughly address these concerns — not just through policy, but through action — will likely find a more satisfied and engaged workforce moving forward.

References

Akanji, B., Mordi, C., & Ojo, S. (2015). Reviewing gaps in work-life research and prospecting conceptual advancement. *Economic Insights, IV* (3), 21-30.

Akanji, B., Mordi, C., Simpson, R., Adisa, T. A., & Smart Orush, E. (2019). Time biases: Exploring the work-life balance of single Nigerian managers and professionals. *Journal of Managerial Psychology, 35*(2), 57-70. doi:10.1108/JMP-12-2018-0537

Allen, T. D., Merlo, K., Lawrence, R. C., Slutsky, J., & Gray, C. E. (2021). Boundary management and work-nonwork balance while working from home. *Applied Psychology, 70*(1), 60–84. https://doi.org/10.1111/apps.12300

Awada, M., Lucas, G., Becerik-Gerber, B., & Roll, S. (2021). Working from home during the COVID-19 pandemic: Impact on office worker productivity and work experience. *Work, 69*(4), 1171–1189. https://doi.org/10.3233/WOR-210301

Cain Miller, C. (2021a, May 17). The pandemic created a child-care crisis: Mothers bore the burden. *The New York Times.* https://www.nytimes.com/interactive/2021/05/17/upshot/women-workforce-employment-covid.html

Cain Miller, C. (2021b, October 30). Working moms are struggling: Here's what would help. *The New York Times.* https://www.nytimes.com/2021/02/04/parenting/government-employer-support-moms.html

Chang, A. (2022, March 21). Workplaces are in denial over how much Americans have changed. *The Guardian.* https://www.theguardian.com/lifeandstyle/2022/mar/21/workplaces-are-in-denial-over-how-much-americans-have-changed?mc_cid=2b35b58ba8&mc_eid=090a4132f6

Chung, H., & van der Lippe, T. (2020). Flexible working, work-life balance, and gender equality: Introduction. *Social Indicators Research, 151,* 365-381. doi:10.1007/s11205-018-2025-x.

Cohen, P., & Hsu, T. (2020, June 30). Pandemic could scar a generation of working mothers. *The New York Times*. https://www.nytimes.com/2020/06/03/business/economy/coronavirus-working-women.html

de Klerk, J. J., Joubert, M., & Mosca, H. F. (2021). Is working from home the new workplace panacea? Lessons from the COVID-19 pandemic for the future world of work. *SA Journal of Industrial Psychology, 47*, 2071-0763. https://doi.org/10.4102/sajip.v47i0.1883

Dehler, G. E., & Welsh, M. A. (2010). The experience of work: Spirituality and the new workplace. In R. A. Giacalone & C. L. Jurkiewicz (Eds.), *Handbook of Workplace Spirituality and Organizational Performance* (2nd ed., pp. 108-122). M. E. Sharpe.

Denson, J. (2021, March 18). The Covid shift to remote work is placing another burden on women: Housecleaning. *NBC News*. https://www.nbcnews.com/think/opinion/covid-shift-remote-work-placing-another-burden-women-housecleaning-ncna1261251

Golden, T. D., Veiga, J. F., & Simsek, Z. (2006). Telecommuting's differential impact on work-family conflict: Is there no place like home? *Journal of Applied Psychology, 91*(6), pp. 1340–1350. https://doi.org/10.1037/00219010.91.6.1340

Goldfarb, Y., Gal, E., & Golan, O. (2022). Implications of employment changes caused by COVID-19 on mental health and work-related psychological need satisfaction of autistic employees: A mixed-methods longitudinal study. *Journal of Autism and Developmental Disorders, 52*(1), 89–102. https://doi.org/10.1007/s10803-021-04902-3

Hill, E. J., Ferris, M., & Märtinson, V. (2003). Does it matter where you work? A comparison of how three work venues (traditional office, virtual office, and home office) influence aspects of work and personal/family life. *Journal of Vocational Behavior, 63*(2), 220–241. https://doi.org/10.1016/S0001-8791(03)00042-3

Hinds, P. J., & Mortensen, M. (2005). Understanding conflict in geographically distributed teams: The moderating effects of shared identity, shared context, and spontaneous communication. *Organization Science, 16*(3), 290–307. doi:10.1287/orsc.1050.0122

Høg Utoft, E. (2020). 'All the single ladies' as the ideal academic during times of COVID-19? *Gender, Work, and Organization, 27*(7), 778-787. doi:10.1111/gwao.12478

Hungerford, C., & Cleary, M. (2021). 'High trust' and 'low trust' workplace settings: Implications for our mental health and wellbeing. *Issues in Mental Health Nursing, 42*(5), 506–514. https://doi.org/10.1080/01612840.2020.1822480

Huxford Davis, B. (2017). *Workplace faith integration in nonprofit Christian camp and retreat center organizations: A grounded theory* (Unpublished doctoral dissertation). Eastern University, St. Davids, PA.

Jacks, T. (2021). Research on remote work in the era of COVID-19. *Journal of Global Information Technology Management, 24*(2), 93–97. https://doi.org/10.1080/1097198X.2021.1914500

International Labour Organization. (2011). *Equality at work: The continuing challenge*. https://www.ilo.org/wcmsp5/groups/public/---ed_norm/---relconf/documents/meetingdocument/wcms_154779.pdf

International Labour Organization. (2020). *Workers with family responsibilities convention, 1981 (No. 156)*. https://www.ilo.org/wcmsp5/groups/public/---ed_norm/---normes/documents/publication/wcms_752428.pdf

International Labour Organization. (2022). *World employment and social outlook: Trends 2022*. https://www.ilo.org/wcmsp5/groups/public/---dgreports/---dcomm/---publ/documents/publication/wcms_834081.pdf

Jett, Q. R., & George, J. M. (2003). Work interrupted: A closer look at the role of interruptions in organizational life. *Academy of Management Review, 28*(3), 494–507. https://doi.org/10.5465/amr.2003.10196791

Kawaguchi, D., & Motegi, H. (2021). Who can work from home? The roles of job tasks and HRM practices. *Journal of the Japanese and International Economies, 62*, 101162. https://doi.org/10.1016/j.jjie.2021.101162

Kaya, B., & Karatepe, O. M. (2020). Attitudinal and behavioral outcomes of work-life balance among hotel employees: The mediating role of psychological contract breach. *Journal of Hospitality and Tourism Management, 42*, 199-209.

Lašáková, A., & Remišová, A. (2019). The relationship between demographic factors and managers' perception of unethical tone at the top. *Journal of Management Development, 38*(1), 25–45. https://doi.org/10.1108/JMD-07-2018-0213

Leroy, S., Schmidt, A. M., & Madjar, N. (2021). Working from home during COVID-19: A study of the interruption landscape. *Journal of Applied Psychology, 106*(10), 1448–1465. https://doi.org/10.1037/apl0000972

Lips-Wiersma, M., & Mills, A. J. (2013). Understanding the basic assumptions about human nature in workplace spirituality: Beyond the critical versus positive divide. *Journal of Management Inquiry, 23*(2), 148-161. doi:10.1177/1056492613501227

Lopez-Leon, S., Forero, D. A., & Ruiz-Díaz, P. (2020). Recommendations for working from home during the COVID-19 pandemic (and beyond). *Work, 66*(2), 371–375. https://doi.org/10.3233/WOR-203187

Lowery, C. M., & Duesing, R. J. (2014). A research note on the relationships among spirituality, contextual variables, and perceptions of ethics in the workplace. *Journal of Managerial Issues, XXVI* (4), 408-423.

Lund Dean, K., Fornaciari, C. J., & Safranski, S. R. (2008). The ethics of spiritual inclusion. In J. Biberman & L. Tischler (Eds.), *Spirituality in business: Theory, practice, and future directions* (pp. 188-202). Palgrave Macmillan.

McGloin, R., Coletti, A., Hamlin, E., & Denes, A. (2022). Required to work from home: Examining transitions to digital communication channels during the COVID-19 pandemic. *Communication Research Reports, 39*(1), 44–55. https://doi.org/10.1080/08824096.2021.2012757

Miller, D. (2007). *God at work.* Oxford University Press.

Mirchandani, K. (2008). Legitimizing work: Telework and the gendered reification of the work-nonwork dichotomy. *Canadian Review of Sociology/Revue Canadienne de Sociologie, 36*(1), 87–107. https://doi.org/10.1111/j.1755-618X.1999.tb01271.x

Natomi, K., Kato, H., & Matsushita, D. (2022). Work-related stress of work from home with housemates based on residential types. *International Journal of Environmental Research and Public Health, 19*(5), 3060. https://doi.org/10.3390/ijerph19053060

Nyberg, A. J., Shaw, J. D., & Zhu, J. (2021). The people still make the (remote work) place: Lessons from a pandemic. *Journal of Management, 47*(8), 1967–1976. https://doi.org/10.1177/01492063211023563

Parker, K., Menasce Horowitz, J., & Minkin, R. (2022, February 16). COVID-19 pandemic continues to reshape work in America. *Pew Research Center.* https://www.pewresearch.org/social-trends/2022/02/16/covid-19-pandemic-continues-to-reshape-work-in-america/

Pradoto, H., Haryono, S., & Wahyuningsih, S. H. (2022). The role of work stress, organizational climate, and improving employee performance in the implementation of work from home. *Work, 71*(2), 345–355. https://doi.org/10.3233/WOR-210678

Prodanova, J., & Kocarev, L. (2021). Is job performance conditioned by work-from-home demands and resources? *Technology in Society, 66,* 101672. https://doi.org/10.1016/j.techsoc.2021.101672

Robertson, C., & Gebeloff, R. (2021, September 22). How millions of women became the most essential workers in America. *The New York Times.* https://www.nytimes.com/2020/04/18/us/coronavirus-women-essential-workers.html

Orel, M. (2019). Supporting work-life balance with the use of coworking spaces. *Equality, Diversity and Inclusion, 39*(5), 549-556. doi:10.1108/EDI-01-2019-0038

Senthanar, S., Varatharajan, S., & Bigelow, P. (2021). Flexible work arrangements and health in white-collar urban professionals. *NEW SOLUTIONS: A Journal of Environmental and Occupational Health Policy, 30*(4), 294–304. https://doi.org/10.1177/1048291120976642

Shao, Y., Fang, Y., Wang, M., Chang, C.-H. (Daisy), & Wang, L. (2021). Making daily decisions to work from home or to work in the office: The impacts of daily work- and COVID-related stressors on next-day work location. *Journal of Applied Psychology, 106*(6), 825–838. https://doi.org/10.1037/apl0000929

Shockley, K. M., & Allen, T. D. (2010). Investigating the missing link in flexible work arrangement utilization: An individual difference perspective. *Journal of Vocational Behavior, 76*(1), 131-142. https://doi.org/10.1016/j.jvb.2009.07.002

Swarnalatha, C., & Prasanna, T. S. (2013). Leveraging employee engagement for competitive advantage: Strategic role of HR. *Review of HRM, 2,* 139–148.

Sun, X., Xu, H., Köseoglu, M. A., & Okumus, F. (2020). How do lifestyle hospitality and tourism entrepreneurs manage their work-life balance? *International Journal of Hospitality Management, 85.*

Thoreau, M. (n.d.). The She-cession: How the pandemic forced women from the workplace and how employers can respond. *Ohioline – Ohio State University Extension.* https://ohioline.osu.edu/factsheet/cdfs-4110

Veal, A. J. (2020). Is there enough leisure time? Leisure studies, work-life balance, the realm of necessity and the realm of freedom. *World Leisure Journal, 62*(2), 89-113.

Waizenegger, L., McKenna, B., Cai, W., & Bendz, T. (2020). An affordance perspective of team collaboration and enforced working from home during COVID-19. *European Journal of Information Systems, 29*(4), 1–14. doi:10.1080/0960085X.2020.1800417

Zhang, C., Yu, M. C., & Marin, S. (2021). Exploring public sentiment on enforced remote work during COVID-19. *Journal of Applied Psychology, 106*(6), 797–810. https://doi.org/10.1037/apl0000933

Zinnbauer, B. J., & Pargament, K. I. (2005). Religiousness and spirituality. In R. F. Paloutzian & C. L. Park (Eds.), *Handbook of the Psychology of Religion and Spirituality* (pp. 21-42). The Guilford Press.

COVID-19 SCHOOL CLOSURES AND THE FLOURISHING OF OUR CHILDREN

Steve Jeantet[1]

Abstract: One of the first responses to the outbreak of the COVID-19 pandemic was to close schools around the world. With limited information on the severity of the virus to children and of how contagious it would be to children, school closures were thought a necessary step to mitigate the spread of COVID-19. Further research has since revealed the limited extent to which the virus spread through children and the mild cases that were typical of children who contracted the virus. While closing schools may have mitigated some of the spread of the virus, it did so at the cost of the flourishing, both in the near term and potentially long-term, of children. This chapter explores five ways that closing schools negatively affected the flourishing of children: 1) delays in learning and loss of learning, 2) food insecurity, 3) loss of physical health contributing to childhood obesity, 4) undiagnosed abuse and neglect, and 5) loss of important milestones in social development of children.

Every society has a moral responsibility to protect its children and seek the flourishing of its children. Thus, children, both as those who are potentially vulnerable and as a means of transmission, were among the most important of the upended arenas of life to consider as COVID-19 went from small phenomenon outbreak in China covered in passing on the news to global pandemic. "Children are thought to be vectors for transmission of many respiratory diseases including influenza. It was assumed that this would be true for COVID-19 also" (Heavey et al., 2020, p. 1). Any experienced educator would have intuitively understood the risk of spread within schools, having certainly witnessed hundreds of absences within a few days as a virus such as influenza ran through the school.

Even as COVID-19 was rapidly spreading, so little else, including the contagiousness and severity to children, was known. Educators and school

---

[1] Principal, Radical Greatness Leadership Consulting, Sarasota, Florida, USA

administrators immediately went into emergency response mode responding to government mandated lockdowns and rapidly shifting advice from health officials. Moreover, the research on the efficacy of closing schools as a mitigation intervention during a pandemic is mixed. For example, Hoffman and Miller (2020) state, "Few would argue that school closures are an important a necessary policy action in fighting COVID-19. Indeed, evidence from past pandemics suggests that closing schools can have a significant effect on reducing infection rates and flattening the curve (p. 2). And yet, Ferguson et al. (2006), whom Hoffman and Miller (2020) directly reference, found that "school closure during the peak of a pandemic can reduce peak attack rates by up to 40%, but has little impact on overall attack rates" (p. 448). That is, school closures can be an effective measure on the dual conditions of 1) being combined with other measures and 2) schools being a place of meaningful transmission.

School officials were thrust into the unenviable (and, at least in many parts of the world, unprecedented) position of closing schools with limited information and mixed messages from past research in an attempt to mitigate the spread and protect the health of students and educators alike. A one-week spring break was extended to a second week before declaring there would be no more in-person school that year, leaving teachers to experiment on the fly with how to teach online, parents scrambling to gather the technology required for remote-learning, and everyone rearranging schedules given the need to be home with their kids (all while simultaneously trying to learn how to work remotely themselves).

If those school interventions and alternative approaches to learning had only lasted the remainder of that school year, it would be cause for sadness, but the effects likely could have been overcome or, at least, minimized. Alas, that has not been the case. During the week of January 10, 2022, 7462 K-12 schools across the United States were disrupted, defined as not offering in-person learning as a result of the pandemic (K-12 School Opening Tracker, n.d.).

Compounding the devastation to children, not all of the closures have been directly a result of public health concerns or understaffing that led to an inability to provide in-person learning (such as when too many teachers are out sick). Labor disputes and national policy debates over COVID-19 protocols also directly led to school closures, as evidenced by the Mayor of Chicago closing schools in the nation's third largest school district in January 2022 as part of a lockout following a confrontation regarding pandemic response with the teacher's union (Tareen, 2022).

Globally, the situation is much the same. Many schools in France were closed in January, including nearly 200 schools in Paris, due to a teacher strike over pandemic policies (Lumetta, 2022). One estimate states that the education of more than 120 million children around the world effectively ended when all learning was moved online because the children did not have access to (or, at least, reliable access to) the internet (Schmall & Yasir, 2022). A UNICEF report states that over 102 million students are from 14 countries "which either fully or partially closed their classrooms for at least half of the COVID-19 pandemic" (United Nations, 2021a, para. 1).

So as not to lose the effect on individual stories in the midst of these large numbers, consider one 14-year-old boy in India, who, having begun to work to help provide for his family, states, "If schools open, I'm not sure I will go back. Only if there is no work" (Schmall & Yasir, 2022, para. 19). Or consider the single mom from Maryland who works in health care and concludes, "But in talking with other parents, we all feel like we're witnessing the death of public education up close and personal" (Kamenetz, 2021). These anecdotes – just two among millions of similar stories from around the globe – highlight the ways in which children and families have been alienated from the critical services, nurturing, and compassion that have previously been provided by their local schools.

Now in the third school year since those inauspicious beginnings, enough time has passed, and enough research has been conducted to consider the efficacy of these interventions and their effect on an entire generation of school-aged children. "It's worth remembering that the point of those measures is to maximize people's health and well-being. And maximizing health and well-being is not the same thing as minimizing Covid" (Leonhardt, 2021, para. 19). Leonhardt identifies a key moral dilemma present throughout all COVID-19 related discussions: How do we think about that intersection of minimizing COVID-19 (which may call for more drastic and, hopefully, short-term steps) and maximizing overall well-being (which certainly accounts for matters of public health but also considers matters such as economic factors and long-term flourishing)? The present discussion is focused specifically on the decision to prioritize COVID-19 containment through school closures over and against the overall well-being of the children affected by that decision.

"You're risking too much," declared one parent concerned for his child's health with regards to efforts to keep his child's school open (Shapiro et al., 2022, para. 17). And yet, what is being risked when kids are not in school? "Closing schools, for example, almost certainly harms children more than it protects them, given the minuscule rate of severe childhood Covid, even lower than that of severe childhood flu" (Leonhardt, 2021, para. 16). The risk to both the short- and long-term flourishing of an entire generation of children caused by COVID-19 related school closings may be far greater.

The duration and extent of the interruption in the normal learning of kids in their most formative years has had at least five profound moral effects. First, there is the loss of learning and the possibility that kids never recover from the delays in their reading experienced because schools were closed. Second, food insecurity is a major moral issue as schools are the place where many children eat their only healthy, and sometimes only, meals. Third, kids' long-term physical health has been compromised as physical fitness deteriorates and childhood obesity escalates. Fourth, kids have potentially been in physical danger as educators are often the first to recognize signs of potential abuse of children. Fifth, early childhood is important for social development and yet kids have been forced to stay at a distance when they need to be learning important skills such as listening, following routines, and sharing. These are moral issues because of the responsibility of one generation to the next generation and because the decisions made on behalf of this generation of children may have long-term implications upon the flourishing and thriving of an entire generation (van der Dussen, 2016).

Loss of Learning

The first, and maybe most obvious, question to ask when considering the effect of COVID-19 related school closures is this: What effect has closing schools had on the learning of children? A primary responsibility of any generation is to seek the flourishing of the generation that comes after it.

The outcomes of education for the individual have been well-documented in research. Lifetime earnings, probability of being employed, reduction in incarceration rates, happiness, and even life expectancy are all positively correlated to levels of education (Cuñado & de Gracia, 2011; Education and Lifetime Earnings, 2015; Lochner & Moretti, 2004). To the extent this research is accurate, loss of learning now, especially if not recovered, projects a future for this generation of children where they will earn less, be less happy, have higher incarceration rates, and, potentially, have a decrease in life expectancy.

In addition to the individual outcomes, education predicts desirable societal outcomes as well. In the enduring words of Nelson Mandela, "Education is the most powerful weapon which we can use to change the world" (Mandela, 1990, 9:19). Increased education typically leads not only to higher individual earnings, but also acts as an accelerant for the economy. One analysis concludes that, unless the pandemic-related deficit in learning is overcome, individuals will earn $49,000 to $61,000 less over the course of their lifetimes. Their analysis continues, "The impact on the US economy could amount to $128 billion to $188 billion every year as this cohort enters the workforce" (Dorn et al., 2021, para. 3). Societal thriving is certainly not limited to individual or even collective earning potential, but it is reflective of the tremendous cost of the lost learning. This is best captured by understanding the correlation between education and poverty. According to UNESCO, "Nearly 60 million people could escape poverty if all adults had just two more years of schooling, and 420 million people could be lifted out of poverty if all adults completed secondary education" (Rodriguez, 2020, para. 16).

So, given the importance – both for the individual and society – to educate young people well, what has been the impact? Are they thriving academically? Or has learning been hindered such that there are both meaningful near term and long-term implications?

The short answer is that the impact has been "dramatic" (Mervosh, 2021, para. 5). Anecdotally, one high school math teacher who teaches the same subject but at three different levels (honors, general and intermediate) reports, "They don't know how to be students anymore. Their motivation to study and do homework and achieve on their own is non-existent. They are not understanding anymore that in order to pass, they need to pay attention." Here is a case where rudimentary skills, significant not only for flourishing in education but also in life and future career, are lacking as a direct result of the interruptions in the normal learning patterns these students have encountered.

More than just that one anecdotal story, the emerging research is compelling. Longitudinal research studies have asked the question: Do students struggling to read ever catch up? The findings clearly suggest that – statistically speaking – they never catch up and the gap is even wider than one might presume. "There is nearly a 90 percent chance that a poor reader in first grade will remain a poor reader" (American Federation of Teachers, 2017, para. 4). One seminal study found that if a child was a poor reader at the end of first grade, there was only a 13% probability of that student being an average reader at the end of fourth grade. But if the student was already an average reader in first grade, there was an 88% probability of being an average reader in fourth grade (Juel, 1998).

As research emerges from the pandemic, the results are staggering. In Virginia, 25% of kindergarten and first grade students were behind in early literacy skills, a 10% increase from before the pandemic (McGintey et al., 2021, p. 3). Another report found that 40% of first graders and 35% of second graders were well below grade level in reading in 2020, up from 27% and 29% in the year prior (Amplify, 2020). Capturing the deficit in learning in time lost, one report concludes that children are five months behind in math and four months behind in reading when compared against the same grade levels prior to the pandemic (McKinsey report). And one first grade teacher describes starting the 2021-22 school year by teaching kids how to form their letters, rather than by starting to write simple words like she did previously (Mader, 2021). One report from the UN concludes that it could take upwards of a decade to return to pre-pandemic learning levels for kids (United Nations, 2021b). The data is clear, unmistakable and dramatic: the attempts to mitigate the spread of COVID-19 by closing schools has left our kids struggling academically.

And, unfortunately, that is not the worst of it. Most disheartening about the data that is coming forth is the inequity of it all. Report after report shows that lower income students and racial minority students have disproportionately fallen behind, increasing already existing gaps in test scores. Even as all students have seen drops in test scores, the results are even more noticeable among these population groups. Consider this summation: "Achievement was lower for all student groups in 2020-21; however American Indian and Alaska Native (AIAN), Black, and Latinx students, as well as students in high-poverty schools were disproportionately impacted, particularly in the elementary grades we studied" (Lewis et al., 2021).

Or consider this report that states, "the increase in students considerably behind in early literacy skills from 2019 to 2020 was most pronounced among students who identify as Black, Hispanic, economically disadvantaged, and English learner" (McGintey et al., 2021, p. 3). Or consider the analysis that found that in math, students in majority Black schools were six months behind and students in low-income schools were seven months behind, compared with five months for their overall peer group (McKinsey report). It's also likely that some of the income gap in particular is actually *under*stated because those students were the least likely to take assessment tests during the course of the pandemic (Barshay, 2021). Education already had gaps in performance related to socio-economics and racial inequalities. Multiply that by the pace of reopening schools where, in the Spring of 2021, only 2% of majority White school districts stayed closed, but 18% of majority Black schools and nearly 25% of majority Hispanic schools stayed closed (Allen, 2021). The reasonable conclusion is simple: the closing of schools due to the pandemic most hurt the most disadvantaged students.

One analysis of education during the pandemic has coined the phrase "unfinished learning" (Dorn et al., 2021, para. 4) to describe the sense that students had not completed the amount of learning they would have during a typical year. And yet, inherent in that phrase is a sense of hopefulness and, maybe even a call to action to help students finish the learning and regain that which was lost. If we are unable to finish that *unfinished learning*, the end result will simply be that the loss of learning that occurred as a result of COVID-19 related school closures will follow an entire generation for the rest of their lives. For those students who are able to finish their learning, they may enter into their adulthood with the fortitude of character that allowed them to persevere in learning and the life experiences to be kind.

Food Insecurity

While the effect of COVID-19 related school closures upon the learning of students and the long-term implications thereof are dramatic and required special consideration, it is not the only moral issue highlighted by the closing of schools. Food insecurity is defined as "a household-level economic and social condition wherein, at times, one or more household members are unable to acquire adequate food because of insufficient money or other resources" (Kinsey et al., 2020, p. 1635). School closures exacerbated food insecurity for many children all around the world because school is the place where they receive their only healthy, and sometimes only, meals. For these students, to not attend school is to not eat at all or to eat extremely unhealthily, risking their future physical well-being.

The role of schools in providing nutrition for students is well established. The National School Lunch Program (NSLP) is the second largest anti-hunger initiative in the United States behind Supplemental Nutrition Assistance Program (SNAP). Even before the pandemic, there were conversations about food and nutrition surrounding low-income families whenever school was out for a holiday or summer break or for weather-related reasons (such as a hurricane or snow). It was well established that students suffered a lack of nutrition when school was not in session, including nearly half of families that benefit from school meal programs stating that they experience significant financial struggles during the summer when school is out (Borkowski et al., 2020).

In 2018-2019, the last full school year before the pandemic, over 26 million children across the United States, or 52.3% of public school students in the United States, were eligible for free or reduced-price lunch. Those numbers, both as total numbers and percentages, have been steadily on the rise from 38.3% in the 2000-2001 school year to 48.1% in the 2010-2011 school year to over 52% the last few years (National Center for Education Statistics, 2020). In that last full school year before the pandemic began, the National School Lunch Program served 21.8 million free or reduced-price lunches per day and its companion program, the School Breakfast Program, served free or reduced price breakfast to over 12.5 million students each day (School Nutrition Association, 2021).

"For some children, school meals may be the only ones they get in a day" (Turner, 2020). So, what happened when schools were closed? While school nutrition directors across the country sought to find creative ways to distribute meals, they saw a rapid and dramatic decrease in meals being served. One researcher estimated that only about 15% of children who qualified for free or reduced-price school meals were receiving them. In Charlotte, North Carolina, school meals were down 89%. Fulton County Schools in Georgia went from serving between 50,000 and 60,000 meals per day to distributing approximately 70,000 per week. And, in Arizona, the Tucson Unified School District went from serving 35,000 meals per day to 3,500 meals per day (Turner, 2020).

COVID-19 had a double effect on the most vulnerable populations of kids that resulted in a dramatic increase in food insecurity. First, their schools closed resulting in missed meals. Kinsey et al. (2020) continue, "We estimate that among students who receive free and reduced-price meals, more than 1.15 billion meals were not served as a result of school closures during the 9-week period between March 9 and May 1" (p. 1636). For these students, the effect of not eating their otherwise normally provided meals at school (and receive the associated nutritional value) was compounded by job losses from COVID-19. The result was a dramatic increase from about 14% to about 33% of children living in food-insecure households (Kinsey et al., 2020). The compounding effect is that the families who need the school meals the most saw a significant increase in food cost even as income evaporated due to job losses. Closing schools increased the number of students in need of food assistance even while it decreased opportunities to receive the nutrition they so desperately needed.

The situation around the globe was much the same. By the middle of April 2020, 192 countries, representing 1.6 billion students (90% of the world's students), closed schools (Donohue & Miller, 2020). UNICEF estimates that 370 million children missed more than 39 billion meals they would have otherwise received as a result of COVID-19 school closures (Buechner, 2021). Given that report estimate was from February 2021, it can safely be assumed the total count of meals missed is closer to 80 billion since the start of the pandemic. As the director of the World Food Programme, David Beasley, summarized, "For millions of children around the world, the meal they get at school is the only meal they get in a day. Without it, they go hungry, they risk falling sick, dropping out of school, and losing their best chance of escaping poverty (UNICEF, 2020).

Much could be said about the effect of proper nutrition for children's physical development, cognitive development, academic performance, lifetime earnings, escape from poverty, and more. But let's keep this simple: one study found that, for students from low-income families, school meals accounted for 47% of their daily caloric intake and represented 41% of their consumption of vegetables (Cullen & Chen, 2017). Schools play an instrumental part in the nourishment of kids. And yet, by closing schools, these kids were kept away from a place where they are provided meals and we more than doubled the number of kids in the food-insecure risk category.

Just as it was the most vulnerable of students who experienced the worst of the learning delays from closing schools, so also it was the vulnerable students who were most at risk nutritionally as a result of closing schools. As Florida's Agriculture Commissioner so helpfully summarizes, "Healthy nutrition is so critical to our children, because without food in our schools, they can't succeed in school, which means they can't succeed in life" (Florida Department of Agriculture, 2021, para. 3).

Child Health and Physical Fitness

Compounding the challenge of food scarcity for many students is the effect on the physical health and safety of these students introduced by closing schools. Not attending school in-person had two significant and important negative effects on kids: deteriorated levels of physical fitness and decreased opportunity to recognize at-risk students experiencing harm or abuse at home.

Regarding physical fitness, closing schools allowed for two things to happen simultaneously: first, even when kids had access to food, they were eating more empty calories devoid of any nutritional value and, second, the level of physical activity decreased. School meals must meet certain nutritional standards. "As households stock up on shelf-stable foods they appear to be purchasing ultra-processed, calorie-dense comfort foods.... We anticipate that many children experience higher calorie diets during the pandemic response" (Rundle et al., 2020, p. 1008). At home, especially in a period of financial hardship, kids were eating more junk food and less fruits, vegetables, and healthy snacks.

Poor eating habits were amplified by a reduction in physical activity. Now, certainly not all the sedentary behavior of students during the pandemic is a result of closing schools. Parks and playgrounds were closed, youth sports leagues were canceled, and people were told to stay home. School closures certainly did, though, contribute to the lack of physical activity among students. With no in-person school, there were no physical education classes, no recess, and not even the ancillary times of physical movement such as walking to the lunch room or to get to the next class.

Research has shown that students experience unhealthy weight gain when they are not in school (Rundle et al., 2020). What is often experienced over summer breaks and holidays happened nonstop for months with kids out of school. One mom saw her 9-year-old gain 40 pounds during the time schools were closed, before eventually enrolling the child in private school to get her son back into a classroom (Goldberg, 2021). Unfortunately, her son's experience was not isolated as the "the number of children diagnosed with obesity rose five times faster during the pandemic than before" (Dunn,

2021). On average, during the time schools were closed due to COVID-19, students gained anywhere from two to six pounds more than expected against historical patterns (Dyer, 2021). Closing schools as a mitigation intervention against one health risk escalated another health risk among children: obesity, and its long-term risks such as diabetes and cardiovascular disease.

Child Safety

It was not only the nutritional health of kids that was risked during the COVID-19 response of closing schools, but also their physical safety and well-being. Every year, over half a million children and students are subjected to maltreatment. The various types of maltreatment include neglect, physical abuse, sexual abuse, and medical neglect (Child Welfare Information Gateway, 2021).

The physical and emotional harm experienced by kids is diametrically opposed to their flourishing as the path of thriving is replaced with a path of survival. While tragic under any circumstance, the present question is simple: how was the safety and security of children affected by closing schools?

Awareness of the mistreatment of kids typically surfaces either via medical intervention (such as emergency department visits) or by reporting of potential abuse. In most of the United States, school employees, including teachers, nurses, and other school personnel, are mandatory reporters meaning they are required to make a report when they become aware of abuse or have reasonable suspicion of abuse. Teachers, school counselors, school nurses, and school administrators are, then, among the most qualified to identify signs of potential harm in children because they are 1) mandated to report, 2) trained to recognize the signs of maltreatment and 3) interact with the same kids on a daily basis and have opportunity to observe changes in physical appearance or behavior that may be indicators of abuse or neglect.

Given the prominence and reliable presence of teachers in the lives of children, it is not a surprise that educators are the common source of maltreatment reports and are responsible for over 20% of all child welfare reports (Child Welfare Information Gateway, 2021; Rapoport et al., 2021). Other research has shown that "time spent in school increases the likelihood that abuse will be noticed and documented" (Mahnken, 2021, para. 8). Reports of maltreatment drop when school is out for the summer or over holidays. As such, unsurprisingly, there was a steep decline in reports to child welfare services while schools were closed. One study found that in New York City, during just the first three months of the pandemic and schools being closed, there were nearly 8,000 fewer reports of child maltreatment than expected when comparing against the same period in prior years. When they extrapolated across the country, they estimated "that approximately 276,293 allegations of child maltreatment which would have otherwise been reported nationally in March to May 2020 were not reported" (Rapoport et al., 2021, p. 4).

The precipitous drop in reports of maltreatment of kids leaves two possible conclusions: either there was less maltreatment occurring or those cases of maltreatment were not being identified and being reported. Given that the rates of medical evaluations or hospitalization attributed to child abuse remained constant or increased, the former conclusion of less maltreatment seems highly unreasonable and unlikely (Mahnken, 2021). Quite to the contrary, research has shown that factors present throughout the pandemic such as financial instability, unemployment, isolation, and substance use typically result in higher levels of child mistreatment (Rapaport et al., 2021). This leaves as the most plausible explanation that children have been endangered and/or mistreated and yet those cases have not been identified and reported. In other words, school closures have compromised the safety, security, and flourishing of many children and students.

Social Development

A final theme to explore concerning the effect of school closures upon the flourishing of our children concerns their social development. The value of schooling is certainly, but not exclusively, the academic enterprise of reading and writing and mathematics and social studies and science. School is also a formative place of social and interpersonal development.

As Robert Fulghum captured so wonderfully in the credo turned title of his collection of essays, "*Everything I need to know I learned in kindergarten.*" He goes on to describe a variety of important skills that are learned at the youngest ages and yet shape adult life on a daily basis such as how to play fair, share toys, apologize when you make a mistake, wash your hands, and much more (Fulghum, 2004). It is in school that these important skills are learned and practiced. Play fair is training for the ethics of business. Sharing toys prepares children to share office equipment. Apologizing when you make a mistake as a kid raises people of integrity that know how to accept blame when they say or do something they regret as adults. Washing your hands, well, we should all do this before we eat, right?

So, what happens when you remove that environment by closing schools or schools are open, but distancing and masks are enforced? Kids don't learn those important interpersonal skills. They don't learn how to read facial expressions. They don't learn how to tell by a smile that someone is joking or by the frown which, unaccompanied by words, tells the story of sadness. They don't do group projects where they learn how to work together toward a goal for an assignment that anticipates those moments to come where they have to work together as part of a team on the rollout of a new product or even as a team to parent well their children. They don't get to be the line leader on the way to recess where they rotate the role each week and learn the importance and opportunity of being both leader and follower in different environments. They don't learn to raise their hands to ask a question or how to even ask questions out of curiosity to further learning. They don't learn how to resolve conflict over playing with a specific toy that will prepare them to resolve conflict when the stakes are much higher as adults.

Part of social development is also the milestones involved in growing up. My son's 5th grade graduation was not walking across a stage, but a drive-by selfie with the principal. For high school seniors, it all just stopped. Proms were canceled. Graduations were canceled. So many of those moments that could never be replicated or repeated were gone forever.

School is a place of personal social development where students learn how to work with and alongside one another. It is also the context for many parts of the journey of growing up where students experience those moments that shape their lives. We have an entire generation of students who missed those moments that could have served as milestones in the journey of their personal growth and development. School closures hindered the social development of our children.

Conclusion

As is readily admitted at the opening of this chapter, educators and school administrators were thrust into an unforeseen and unprecedented situation both out of concern for students and staff and out of government-mandated shutdowns. With little to no information about severity or contagiousness for kids (and staff), decisions were made to close schools.

And yet, the undesired nature of the events does not remove the accountability of asking how the decisions made and the paths walked have affected kids, both in the short- and the long-term. If a primary responsibility of any generation is to seek the flourishing – most simply defined as the peak of well-being – of its children, then school closures accomplished the opposite. Given the significant moral issues that closing schools presented, doing so "almost certainly harms children more than it protects them" (Leonhardt, 2021, para. 16).

Through setbacks in learning, food insecurity and poor nutrition, degraded physical fitness, increased opportunity for abuse along with decreased opportunity to recognize it, and delayed social development, our children are not thriving and flourishing.

They are languishing. "Languishing is a sense of stagnation and emptiness…. Languishing is the neglected middle child of mental health. It's the void between depression and flourishing – the absence of well-being" (Grant, 2021, para. 3, 7). They have forgotten how to study. They take longer to do homework. They stare at screens without moving for hours on end and put on unhealthy weight as a result. They are experiencing the absence of well-being. Our kids are languishing.

"We are meant to flourish – not just to survive, but to thrive; not just to exist, but to explore and expand" (Crouch, 2016, p. 10). School closures hindered the flourishing of an entire generation of children. The choice now is if, into a still unknown future, we will leave them languishing or guide them back to the path of flourishing.

References

Allen, J. G. (2021, December 20). We learned our lesson last year: Do not close schools. *The New York Times*. https://www.nytimes.com/2021/12/20/opinion/omicron-schools-do-not-close.html

American Federation of Teachers. (2017, December 18). *Waiting rarely works: Late bloomers usually just wilt*. Reading Rockets. https://www.readingrockets.org/article/waiting-rarely-works-late-bloomers-usually-just-wilt

Amplify. (2020, December). Instructional loss due to COVID-19 disruptions. https://amplify.com/wp-content/uploads/2020/12/mCLASS_Flyer_CovidBrief-LearningLoss_v10.pdf

Barshay, J. (2021, August 9). Proof points: Three reports on student achievement during the pandemic. *The Hechinger Report*. https://hechingerreport.org/proof-points-three-reports-on-student-achievement-during-the-pandemic/

Buechner, M. (2021, February 1). *UNICEF reports: Over 39 billion meals missed since schools shut down*. UNICEF USA. https://www.unicefusa.org/stories/unicef-reports-over-39-billion-meals-missed-schools-shut-down/38134

Borkowski, A., Hares, S., Minardi, A. L. (2020, March 24). *With schools closed, hundreds of millions of children are not receiving school meals*. Center For Global Development. https://www.cgdev.org/blog/schools-closed-hundreds-millions-children-are-not-receiving-school-meals

Child Welfare Information Gateway. (2021). *Child maltreatment 2019: Summary of key findings*. U.S. Department of Health and Human Services, Administration for Children and Families, Children's Bureau. https://www.childwelfare.gov/pubs/factsheets/canstats/

Cullen, K. W., & Chen, T. (2017). The contribution of the USDA school breakfast and lunch program meals to student daily dietary intake. *Preventive Medicine Reports 5*. 82-85. https://doi.org/10.1016/j.pmedr.2016.11.016

Crouch, A. (2016). *Strong and weak*. InterVarsity Press.

Cuñado, J., & de Gracia, F.P. (2012). Does education affect happiness? Evidence for Spain. *Social Indicators Research 108*, 185-196. https://doi.org/10.1007/s11205-011-9874-x

Donohue JM, Miller E. (2020). COVID-19 and School Closures. *JAMA, 324*(9):845–847. https://doi:10.1001/jama.2020.13092

Dorn, E., Hancock, B., Sarakatsannis, J., & Viruleg, E. (2021, July 27). *Covid-19 and education: The lingering effects of unfinished learning*. McKinsey & Company. https://www.mckinsey.com/industries/education/our-insights/covid-19-and-education-the-lingering-effects-of-unfinished-learning

Dyer, O. (2021). Obesity in US children increased at an unprecedented rate during the pandemic. *BMJ, 374(2332)*. https://doi.org/10.1136/bmj.n2332

Dunn, L. (2021, November 17). *Post-pandemic, PE teachers warn of lost skills*. WORLD. https://wng.org/roundups/post-pandemic-p-e-1637179902

Education and Lifetime Earnings. Research summary: Education and lifetime earnings. (2015, November). https://www.ssa.gov/policy/docs/research-summaries/education-earnings.html

Ferguson, N. M., Cummings, D. A., Fraser, C., Cajka, J. C., Cooley, P. C., & Burke, D. S. (2006). Strategies for mitigating an influenza pandemic. *Nature, 442*(7101), 448–452. https://doi.org/10.1038/nature04795

Florida Department of Agriculture. (2021, July 6). *Commissioner Nikki Fried announces $93 million in school nutrition emergency relief funding* [Press release]. https://www.fdacs.gov/News-Events/Press-Releases/2021-Press-Releases/Commissioner-Nikki-Fried-Announces-93-Million-in-School-Nutrition-Emergency-Relief-Funding

Fulghum, R. (2004). *All I really need to know I learned in kindergarten*. Ballantine Books.

Goldberg, M. (2021, December 17). We desperately need schools to get back to normal. *The New York Times*. https://www.nytimes.com/2021/12/17/opinion/randi-weingarten-schools.html

Grant, A. (2021, April 19). There's a name for the blah you're feeling: It's called languishing. *The New York Times*. https://www.nytimes.com/2021/04/19/well/mind/covid-mental-health-languishing.html

Heavey, L., Casey, G., Kelly, C., Kelly, D., & McDarby, G. (2020). No evidence of secondary transmission of COVID-19 from children attending school in Ireland. *Euro Surveillance, 25*(21), 1-4. https://doi.org/10.2807/1560-7917.ES.2020.25.21. 2000903

Hoffman, J. A., & Miller, E. A. (2020). Addressing the consequences of school closure due to COVID-19 on children's physical and mental well-being. *World Medical & Health Policy,* 10.1002/wmh3.365. Advance online publication. https://doi.org/10.1002/wmh3.365

Juel, C. (1988). Learning to read and write: A longitudinal study of 54 children from first through fourth grades. *Journal of Educational Psychology, 80*(4), 437–447. https://doi.org/10.1037/0022-0663.80.4.437

K-12 school opening tracker. (n.d.). K-12 School Opening Tracker. https://cai.burbio.com/school-opening-tracker/

Kamenetz, A. (2021, November 23). Parents are scrambling after schools suddenly cancel class over staffing and Burnout. *NPR.* https://www.npr.org/2021/11/23/ 1057979170/school-closures-mental-health-days-families-childcare-thanksgiving-break

Kinsey, E. W., Hecht, A. A., Dunn, C. G., Levi, R., Read, M. A., Smith, C., Niesen, P., Seligman, H. K., & Hager, E. R. (2020). School closures during COVID-19: Opportunities for innovation in meal service. *American Journal of Public Health, 110*(11), 1635–1643. https://doi.org/10.2105/AJPH.2020.305875

Leonhardt, D. (2021, December 10). Covid malaise. *The New York Times.* https://www.nytimes.com/2021/12/10/briefing/us-economy-covid-malaise.html

Lewis, K., Kuhfield, M., Ruzek, E., & McEachin, A. (2021, July). *Learning during COVID-19: Reading and math achievement in the 2020-21 school year.* Center for School and Student Progress. https://www.nwea.org/content/uploads/2021/07/ Learning-during-COVID-19-Reading-and-math-achievement-in-the-2020-2021-school-year.research-brief-1.pdf

Lochner, L., & Moretti, E. (2004). The effect of education on crime: Evidence from prison inmates, arrests, and self-reports. *American Economic Review, 94*(1), 155-189.

Lumetta, C. (2022, January 13). French teachers strike over pandemic policies. *WORLD.* https://wng.org/sift/french-teachers-strike-over-pandemic-policies-1642100596

Mader, J. (2021, November 15). The reading year: First grade is critical for reading skills, but kids coming from disrupted kindergarten experiences are way behind. *The Hechinger Report*. https://hechingerreport.org/the-reading-year-first-grade-is-critical-for-reading-skills-but-kids-coming-from-disrupted-kindergarten-experiences-are-way-behind/

Mahnken, K. (2021, July 21). *Stuck at home, separated from teachers, children may have faced more severe abuse during pandemic, research suggests*. The 74. https://www.the74million.org/stuck-at-home-separated-from-teachers-children-may-have-faced-more-severe-abuse-during-pandemic-research-suggests/

Mandela, N. (1990, June 23). *The words that change the world* [Speech audio record]. YouTube. https://www.youtube.com/watch?v=b66c6OkMZGw

McGinty, A., Gray, A., Partee, A., Herring, W., & Soland, J. (2021). (rep.). *Examining early literacy skills in the wake of COVID-19 spring 2020 school disruptions*. Phonological Awareness Literacy Screener. https://pals.virginia.edu/public/pdfs/login/PALS_Fall_2020_Data_Report_5_18_final.pdf

Mervosh, S. (2021, July 28). The pandemic hurt these students the most. *The New York Times*. https://www.nytimes.com/2021/07/28/us/covid-schools-at-home-learning-study.html

National Center for Education Statistics. (2020). *Number and percentage of public school students eligible for free or reduced-price lunch, by state: Selected years, 2000-01 through 2018-19*. Digest of Education Statistics, 2020. https://nces.ed.gov/programs/digest/d20/tables/dt20_204.10.asp

Rapoport, E., Reisert, H., Schoeman, E., & Adesman, A. (2021). Reporting of child maltreatment during the SARS-COV-2 pandemic in New York City from March to May 2020. *Child Abuse & Neglect, 116*, 104719. https://doi.org/10.1016/j.chiabu.2020.104719

Rodriguez, L. (2020, February 6). *Understanding how poverty is the main barrier to education*. Global Citizen. https://www.globalcitizen.org/en/content/poverty-education-satistics-facts/

Rundle, A. G., Park, Y., Herbstman, J. B., Kinsey, E. W., & Wang, Y. C. (2020). COVID-19-related school closings and risk of weight gain among children. *Obesity (Silver Spring, Md.), 28*(6), 1008–1009. https://doi.org/10.1002/oby.22813

Schmall, E., & Yasir, S. (2022, January 27). India schools stay closed, and hopes fade for a lost generation. *The New York Times*. https://www.nytimes.com/2022/01/27/world/asia/india-schools.html

School meal trends and stats. (2021). School Nutrition Association. https://schoolnutrition.org/aboutschoolmeals/schoolmealtrendsstats/

Shapiro, E., Wong, A., & Zraick, K. (2022, January 7). New Yorkers reflect on a stressful week back at school amid omicron wave. *The New York Times*. https://www.nytimes.com/2022/01/07/nyregion/nyc-schools-omicron.html

Tareen, S. (2022, January 7). As Chicago Teachers Union negotiations continue, school closures enter third day. *PBS*. https://www.pbs.org/newshour/nation/as-chicago-teachers-union-negotiations-continue-school-closures-enter-third-day

Turner, C. (2020, September 8). Children are going hungry: Why schools are struggling to feed students. *NPR*. https://www.npr.org/2020/09/08/908442609/children-are-going-hungry-why-schools-are-struggling-to-feed-students

UNICEF. (2020, April 29). *Futures of 370 million children in jeopardy as school closures deprive them of school meals – UNICEF and WFP*. [Press release]. https://www.unicef.org/eap/press-releases/futures-370-million-children-jeopardy-school-closures-deprive-them-school-meals

United Nations. (2021a, October 28). Millions missing out on remote learning during emergencies: UNICEF. *UN News*. https://news.un.org/en/story/2021/10/1104362

United Nations. (2021b, March 26). 100 million more children fail basic reading skills because of COVID-19. *UN News*. https://news.un.org/en/story/2021/03/1088392

van der Dussen, J. (2016). Responsibility for Future Generations. In: *Studies on Collingwood, History and Civilization*. Springer, Cham. https://doi.org/10.1007/978-3-319-20672-1_13

FINDING GOOD WORK IN COVID-19: LEGAL AND ETHICAL CHALLENGES FOR SUSTAINABILITY

Janis Balda[1] and Joanna Stanberry[2]

Abstract: This chapter explores, through a case study, the legal and ethical responses by individuals in the business context to the reality of limited resources in the time of COVID-19. It looks at how an individual seeking to do "good work" can be supported or hindered by workplace and societal expectations, and advances possibilities for using the case study to help us think more ethically about future demands on limited resources. It raises questions about how we prepare students, co-workers, and others within our sphere of influence to exercise personal and corporate responsibility for making tough calls about how to distribute limited resources and how to make ethical decisions. We connect this effort to the principles of Good Work and Sustainability, seeing in COVID-19 and this case a microcosm of the even more far-reaching demands placed on the planet and humanity. As we increasingly encounter resource limitations in all its forms, natural and manufactured, we will be forced as individuals and as communities to negotiate the complex limbo of "the new normal." In this murkiness, we need narratives to help navigate short-term and long-term demands, complex decision-making, and to find innovative solutions - all of which demand our most creative and moral selves.

Marcia Bastion got what she considered her dream job right out of college and at just the right time. Scratch Exports (SE)[3], was in the import business, sourcing suppliers and handling the sale, distribution, and delivery of personal protective equipment (PPE), with disposable vinyl gloves its primary product. The job

---

[1] Senior Lecturer, University of Texas Rio Grande Valley, USA

[2] Doctoral Student and Postgraduate Researcher, University of Cumbria, UK

[3] Except for Eagle Protect, all names and titles used in the case scenario are pseudonyms. Eagle Protect PBC is an actual company and graciously agreed to its use in this case study. The firm identifies itself as a certified B Corporation® since 2012 and the world's only disposable glove and clothing specialist to be B Corp™ certified.

challenged Marcia who was responsible for her own accounts and included overseeing the supply chain of some of its importers.

Located in a temporary office in East Los Angeles Marcia's new company had entered the PPE market about four years earlier and Marcia joined in 2019, the year the U.S. had used 228,000 disposable gloves every minute, 328 million gloves a day and 120 billion gloves every year, or about 40-50% of the world's production. She had been sent out to visit a few of the manufacturing sites in Asia as part of her orientation and came back thinking about whether greater oversight of the production might be necessary to improve glove quality as well as the working conditions in the factories.

Then the COVID-19 pandemic hit and as Marcia struggled to deliver the large and profitable orders she had negotiated; her concern grew to include SE's entire PPE supply chain. While her only real connection was by Zoom, she could imagine what was taking place in the factories located in far-flung places that were primitive, employing exhausted workers run by questionable supervisors, and with poor quality control. The deal-making required included watching factories change hands frequently with some unsavory characters who seemed intent on maintaining a low profile while meeting demand.

Marcia knew the job had the potential to be lucrative but also addressed an important need, so she was willing to work hard. Six months in, however, Marcia read an article in an industry magazine that noted the increased demand for PPE had made it even more difficult to ensure safe workplaces and ethical labor practices globally. Then a little later she saw a piece by the World Health Organization saying that there were places in the world where the shortage of PPE meant that choices would need to be made of who to treat based upon the seriousness of the need for protection. They recommended that health providers take steps such as extended use of PPE, prioritizing patients, and limiting the use of supplies. She tried to let go of thinking about it, rationalizing that after all, she was doing her best to get orders filled as fast as possible.

No one else at Scratch Exports seemed to share her concerns and Marcia's main worry became the quality of the gloves. On more than one sale's call she pulled out samples that were mangled together and completely useless or stuck to the box and in shreds. Marcia's boss Beryl insisted that she only had to get orders, get them filled in time, and deliver the profits. But her disquiet grew.

One Monday morning Beryl announced that Scratch Exports staff were required to attend a meeting at the office that Friday. When Marcia walked into the conference room federal agents were there and notified the staff that they were investigating the importation of disposable gloves and other PPE.

The agents provided more information than Marcia wanted to know. Not only was there the issue of forced labor at factories operated by one of the largest producers in Malaysia, (which had resulted in banning imports of that particular glove), but there was also involvement in counterfeit and substandard medical equipment, including PPE. Incredible to her, it appeared that organized criminal groups used the opportunities arising from the pandemic to exploit the vulnerabilities and gaps existing in health and criminal justice systems, and quickly adapted by providing substandard and falsified medical products. Some had sold non-existent supplies of products to defraud individuals and procurement agencies. One case in Europe involved EUR 15 million worth of face masks.

Deeply shocked, Marcia texted her resignation to Beryl by the end of the day. She had a few months of salary saved, wanted to stay in the industry, but emphatically wanted to work at a place where her conscience could be clear.

That evening online she found Eagle Protect PBC (EP), a firm founded in New Zealand with a branch in California. EP supplied approximately 80% of the primary food processing Industry in New Zealand with responsibly sourced disposable gloves and protective clothing. They seemed to have thought of most of these issues - and others, such as what to do about the disposal of gloves. EP seemed to have devised a business model that addressed many of them proactively - something Marcia was keen to experience. Anxious to send off an application, Marcia sat down to write out ideas for her cover letter. She wanted to frame her knowledge of the industry's abuses while connecting to EP's strengths.

The Good Work Project was conceived in the 1990s by three psychologists - Csikszentmihalyi, Damon, and Gardner - when they were "inspired and troubled by the hegemony of market–oriented thinking." They were asking: "Is it possible to have individuals, institutions, and societies that are at once creative and innovative, yet at the same time are also humane, providing for those who cannot fend for themselves?" (Gardner, 2008, p. 204). Good work can also be identified as "quality for the end user, meaningfulness to the worker, and social responsibility to the wider society" (Gardner et al., 2008, as cited in Moran, 2010, p. 128). This social responsibility to the wider society encompasses sustainability - a boundary term linking shared understandings of, and common commitments to environmental and economic development concerns (Scoones, 2007, p. 589) and recognizes that constructing pathways to a sustainable world is inevitably a normative struggle, rooted in political and moral choices. (Scoones, 2016). This is what the domain of sustainability is asking from us, we consider those who do not have a voice - future generations as well as the natural world.

It is within this nexus that we examine the complexities of legal and ethical challenges post COVID-19, examining the connections between professional roles and personal ethics. "Good Work" is defined as work that is simultaneously excellent in quality (excellence), responsive to the needs of the broader community (engagement), and personally meaningful (ethical) (Gardner et al., 2001). Good work is most likely to emerge when four factors are in alignment: when the individual beliefs, the values of the domain, the forces of the field, and the reward system of the society all point in the same direction (Gardner, 2010). Contrary actions are referenced as "compromised work" (Nakamura, 2010, p. 118, Figure 2). In practice it presumes a preliminary step of assessing our own work before advancing toward ethical theories for decision making, acknowledges the role of personal responsibility and accountability, yet recognizes that positive change requires concerted action by many (Mucinskas & Gardner, 2013, p. 462). Sustainability connects the ideas of good work – individually and corporately – offering a source from which to consider one's practices and activities. It involves assessing the four areas of the Good Work Project as portrayed in Figure 1.

Good Work is most likely to emerge when all of the four factors are in alignment – when the individual beliefs (C), the values of the domain (A), the forces of the field (C), and the reward system (D), of the society all point in the same direction (Gardner, 2010). As Gardner (2009) summarized, "All four of these forces are always present. The ways in which they operate and interact determine the likelihood of good work" (p. 210).

This arena is not static. In any field or domain, and particularly with sustainability, there is a need to be aware of and attentive to the need to align the worker and their domain to achieve the purposes of Good Work. Fields and professions have ethical values in them and, when well-aligned, enable workers to feel empowered that they can do Good Work, since the field points them in the direction of their purpose. What COVID-19 did was misalign many fields. First, it became less clear what the practitioner had to do to accomplish Good Work - work that is simultaneously excellent in quality, responsive to the needs of the broader community, and personally meaningful. Thus COVID-19 made it even more difficult to figure out what Good Work looks like in the domain, and resulted in the individual being less able to connect to their values and purpose. Secondly, the growing gap between resources and consumption evident around the globe became secondary to meeting the immediate demands of the pandemic. The result is that the domain of sustainability, being relatively new and thrown into some of the most pressing global issues and complexities of our day, has never really had its field defined.

Reflecting these processes, the model shown in Figure 1 recognizes the interactions of all four dimensions.

Figure 1. *Good Work Model*

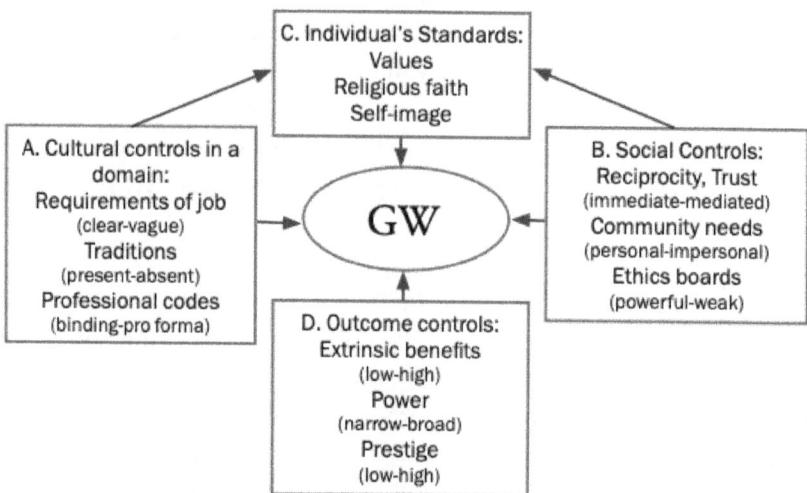

Source: Gardner, 2008, p. 209

A. The domain, discipline, or profession under study.

In the Marcia case we examine the domain of business in which the individual has had training, received orientation, visited sites, and interacted with suppliers and customers. Outside of that it is unlikely that she has received any training in the nature of professional ethics or responsibility in the business in which she operates.

The way that work is grouped into domains is a societal construct and consists of practices and knowledge with their accompanying beliefs and values, that are encoded in a symbol system and passed down generationally among workers (Gardner, 2009, Csikszentmihályi, 1990, p. 200). "Cultural controls" in this description has broad meaning. It includes the requirements of the job - whether well-defined or vaguely sketched, traditions that have arisen and either been kept or discarded, and rules and codes that prescribe behavior.

B. The Field or social ambit within which the domain is situated.

In this case we find Marcia's field of business having few controls by accrediting or other bodies or regulations directly affecting operations she is engaged in. In addition, since her business is addressing a crisis, many of the standard forms of regulation do not apply or are being superseded due to the urgency of the pandemic. There are intersecting fields such as global health, international logistics, and import-export frameworks that have some bearing but do not provide clear guidance.

The forces that operate on the domain regulate its operation. It includes a loosely organized orchestration of gatekeepers, training schools, and awards, as well as punitive agencies, that together act on a domain to create a "social ambit" that encompasses the work of individuals and organizations. These are devised by those having an interest in the domain to regulate its operation. These social controls are diverse and vary in strength as they include layers of relationships (Gardner, 2009, p. 10). A field can be exceedingly varied in scope and scale, including an organization, or a profession provided it develops its own organizing logic around what matters with its own, implicit and explicit rules of behavior.

C. The individual worker

Marcia, as the protagonist in the case, is caught in a web of issues over which she has little control. However, she sees herself as a professional with a sense of agency in the situation and is seeking to not only advance her career (a utilitarian view) but to do so in a way that puts her on a solid foundation for principled decision-making and the expression of her own values, fashioned through her family, community and education.

The person is situated in relationship to the standards of the field and is the origin of work. As such, the focal point of Good Work is the individual who positions herself with regard to her beliefs, values and goals, but also her motivations, personality, temperament, and how the field rewards or penalizes such work.

D. The control mechanisms of society.

Within the business sector in the U.S. and in the academic preparation for it, there is significant lip-service to observing legal and ethical parameters with most businesses recognizing that in their need to find professional talent, they have to acknowledge social and environmental responsibilities. However, these are also frequently in conflict with the profit motive and require the ability of business to negotiate adaptive or grand challenges such as the tensions presented here with the need to ensure profitability although some would argue that the focus must be on prosperity for all rather than the financial bottom line of the business.

The larger reward system of the ambient society is part of the control mechanisms from the broader societal system that interact with the field, the domain, and the individual. Economic incentives (or disincentives), how productivity is determined, drivers for equity (or inequity), and other pushes and pulls duly act on the other factors, resulting in responses at various levels (Gardner, 2009, p. 10). Individuals in their specific domain are impacted by broader forces within society - "the opportunities available, the prevalent rewarding and punishing mechanisms, the messages prevalent on the street and in the media" (Gardner, 2009, p. 10). It involves macro-social conditions as well, such as the labor market.

Legal issues and ethical conundrums from COVID-19

The conflux of the dimensions described above and expressed in Marcia's case raise particular legal and ethical issues that directly bear on the situational challenges. Examples (identified below in Figure 2) connect the good work dimensions to the domain, discipline, or profession under study ("A"), for example in situations that arise from considerations of counterfeit goods that become common in the supply chain and how businesses as a whole address the challenges while attempting to remain competitive in the market. Similarly, considerations arising from the field or social ambit within which the business is situated ("B") influences how the broader context aligns itself when businesses take advantage of less structure or regulation in a crisis. Do they ignore the situation, seek to find immediate remedies through legal challenges, or gather support for post-crisis regulatory solutions? These inputs can of course influence the control mechanisms of society ("D") and the type of restrictions that can meet the challenges, sometimes recognizing that less formal mechanisms (such as allegations of greenwashing or establishing the impact of unethical actions on vulnerable workers) can lead to the requisite changes. And of course, there is always the principal - the protagonist - who positions herself with regard to her beliefs, values and goals ("C") in light of the external factors to which she is exposed.

Drawing from the ethical and legal issues arising from the supply of personal protective equipment (PPE) during COVID-19, we examine in Figure 2 the legal and ethical factors enacted – some directly and some indirectly - in individual, corporate, and industry dynamics at a global level. Issues of allocating limited resources are key drivers to the challenges of sustainability as well. To understand this connection, we provide a brief background on sustainability and corporate social responsibility, and the manner in which PPE became a central issue to business during the pandemic.

Sustainability from a business perspective rests on three pillars: environmental, socially responsible, and economic /governance practices. Social responsibility requires a broad view of stakeholders and seeks to benefit the company's employees, consumers, and the wider community.

Identifying and addressing the firm's stakeholders, includes both those at the community or local level as well as those in its global network. The economic includes governance (rules, practices, and processes by which a firm is directed and controlled), and is frequently referenced as ESG. It includes compliance, using managerial practices such as internal controls, regulatory compliance and disclosure, and requires honest and transparent financial practices. It also involves ethical behavior, corporate strategy, compensation and workplace practices, and risk management. Corporate Social Responsibility (CSR), among many other functions, seeks to hold the corporation and the industry accountable for proactive innovations to create value-added sustainable solutions and solutions to mitigate less desirable outputs such as reducing carbon or replacing water usage.

Some of the traditional efforts globally to address supply chains and sustainable development include the Organisation for Economic Co-operation and Development (OECD) Guidelines for Multinational Enterprises and relate to due diligence guidance. Their intent is to "lay out the expectation that businesses contribute to sustainable development while avoiding and addressing adverse impacts of their activities, including throughout their supply chains." (OECD, 2020, p. 1).

Companies in vital sectors such as health care or food production during COVID-19 were particularly concerned with protecting the health and safety of workers and clients or customers, and creating as safe an environment as possible, given the conditions of the pandemic. The World Health Organization specifically mandated that management of PPE should be coordinated through essential national and international supply mechanisms that included monitoring and controlling waste management streams and appropriate processes for discarding used PPE (WHO, 2020). For a number of reasons, often overlapping, this directive was not seen to be effective.

Interpol and the World Customs Organization (WCO) reported that seizures of substandard and falsified medical products, including PPE, increased for the first time in March 2020. The United Nations Office on Drugs and Crime (UNODC) considered the emergence of trafficking in PPE to be a significant shift in organized criminal group behavior "that is directly attributable to the COVID-19 pandemic," which created a huge demand for PPE over a relatively short period of time (UNODC, 2020, p. 7).

The UNODC (2020) further identified challenges in pandemic preparedness as including weak regulatory and legal frameworks as well as the prevention of the manufacturing and trafficking of substandard and falsified products. Though these were evident before COVID-19, the pandemic exacerbated them. Challenges like these cannot be improved over the short term, during the crisis itself, while law enforcement, customs agencies, and international health and human rights institutions are overwhelmed in addressing the upfront issues of health and safety. "Public pressure on health systems to acquire sufficient PPE for a country's needs created an opportunity for criminals to take advantage of the situation and supply substandard and falsified PPE with lower good governance checks" (p. 9).

Below we consider some of the significant legal challenges that impacted the business of PPE, both directly and indirectly, and that offer a platform from which to consider the principles of Good Work. Each of the challenges is identified as having some impact on one or more of the elements in the model - (A) the domain, (B) the field, (C) the individual or (D) the control mechanisms of society. Each legal category on the following list includes documented evidence of pandemic effects applied across the global landscape.

Figure 2. *Legal and ethical issues*

Legal Issues pertaining to PPE during the COVID-19 Pandemic		Example of issues with ethical dimensions & Good Work Principal Element: A, B, C, D
Counterfeit and Substandard Goods:	The sale of counterfeit healthcare, sanitary/pharmaceutical products and personal healthcare equipment has become one of the main areas of criminal activity (EU); allegations of forced labor in the supply chain (Brew, et al., 2021; Butler, 2022).	How do businesses manage competition in the supply chain where counterfeit goods are common? How do they promote transparency? - A
Inadequate Regulatory and Legal Frameworks:	Among the vulnerabilities that have been exposed are the weaknesses in supply chains and the dependence on third party providers, often operating without traditional accountability channels (McClean, et al., 2022). New hindrances to investigation, the collection of evidence and the possibility of a consequent prosecution (UNODC, 2020).	In thinking of the corporate social responsibility of business and particularly ESG Reporting what duty is there? - A Is it different for small businesses without shareholders? - A Has Marcia inadvertently contributed to this? – C What is "decent work" for the individual and does Marcia in her procurement role needs to establish new avenues of accountability? - A, B, C
Unfair Market Practices:	Price gouging and sales of substandard medical supplies and devices (Gibson Dunn, 2020). The U.K. government's Department of Health and Social Care Annual report and accounts 2020-21, writes off almost £10bn of spending on PPE that was either unusable, above market price, or was not delivered (Iacobucci, 2022).	What can be done and by whom to promote consumer protections while addressing unnecessary barriers to doing business? What is the impact on global South inequities in terms of economic development? - C
Competition Law:	In most "free market" economies there is a commitment to furthering competition - an underlying presupposition that competition produces lower	What happens when businesses take advantage of less structure or regulation in a crisis in order to reap a profit? - B

	prices, better service, and higher quality for the consumer. As a result, governments prohibit agreements and arrangements between businesses that restrict competition, however these restrictions were loosened during the pandemic (CMA, 2020).	
International Trade and Import/Export Controls:	Issues include restricting exports to support the "national defense" (George Washington Univ., n. d.)	Is it right to withhold needed goods (PPE, vaccines, equipment) to reserve their use for a county's own population? - D
Personal Attacks:	More than two-thirds of scientists who have commented about COVID-19 reported negative experiences as a result of their media appearances or their social media comments, and 22% had received threats of physical or sexual violence. Some have been sued (Nature, 2022).	While not related to Marcia directly does this type of fear and intimidation affect her? - C
Criminal Activity and Law Enforcement Capacity:	Substandard and falsified medical product investigation requires a high level of collaboration among agencies nationally and internationally to trace traffickers over borders using all available resources. This cooperation is hampered by resource deficiencies, challenges in investigation, and prosecution (UNODC, ND; Europol, 2020). Enforcement mechanisms in response to the issues include new national regulatory initiatives, expanded investigative authority, alliances among law enforcement agencies to share data, addressing crimes carried out across borders, and tracking international crime trends (Forman & Mossialos, 2021).	Does this threaten Marcia and//or her firm directly? - C What is the nature of working in a business that law enforcement is cracking down on? - A

Organized Crime:	Criminals exploit corruption, the relaxation of due diligence checks and systemic weaknesses exacerbated by COVID-19. Shortages of medical products create opportunities for medical product traffickers. Organized criminal groups in the Western Balkans involved in possible money laundering and illicit gains in the production and trafficking of falsified medical products and PPE (UNODC, n. d,). Organized criminal groups exploited gaps and discrepancies in national legislation and criminal justice systems. Weak and/or inconsistent regulatory and legal frameworks for preventing, deterring and punishing offenders who manufacture or traffic in falsified medical products became more evident in the rapidly evolving circumstances of the pandemic (UNODC, n. d.).	Does Marcia need to do her own investigation and determine whether she or her firm has potential risk? - C What is the nature of working in a business that is complicit? - A
Financial Services Sector:	FinCEN, the unit of the US Department of the Treasury that collects, analyzes, and disseminates intelligence on financial crimes, advises financial institutions by alerting them to the rising number of scams relating to PPE and other medical products (Cavanaugh, et al., 2020).	What is the role of regulation across sectors to reinforce the equitable ends we seek? - D
Privacy and Cybersecurity Issues:	The Cyberspace Administration of China (CAC) released a formal notice regarding privacy and cybersecurity principles in connection with the collection, use, and disclosure of personal information for purposes of containing COVID-19 (Luo, 2020).	Are restrictions on personal freedoms and invasion of what some consider the right to privacy legitimate in a pandemic? - D

| Fraud: | Pandemic disrupted global shipping supply chains. With increased demand there was an opportunity for criminals to defraud purchasers through non-delivery of merchandise. Various instances of fake companies advertising test kits, masks, drugs, and other goods. Victims include companies, hospitals, governments, and consumers (Cavanaugh, et al., 2020; Interpol, 2020). | What are the impacts on the industry as a whole and how can reputable companies thrive? - A, B, D |
| Securities Law: | Insider trading on material nonpublic information on the Coronavirus in the United States (Gibson Dunn, 2020). | Is it important to enforce prohibitions on insider trading to ensure fairer and more equitable expenditures and reduce corruption? - D |

The impact of these significant institutional factors caused by COVID-19 created more pressure on the already overstretched national and international bodies and across sectors – public, plural, and private. Those results enable us to extrapolate for social and environmental sustainability learning where resource limitations that have been around for some time are becoming more apparent. Additionally, COVID-19 brought the public's attention to the notion of scarce resources as being newsworthy. In an article explaining the broken supply chain and scarcity of goods that dominated the news during many months, *The New York Times* noted that it did not even have a way for reporters to write about supply chains and logistics prior to the pandemic - but it does now (Goodman, 2021).

What is now more clearly recognized is the political dimension of decision-making in complex social ecological systems (Clark et al., 2016). With COVID-19 we saw certain nations and groups were privileged to receive protective equipment and exports were restricted. In sustainability we see the same in relation to the resource of water, for example. Scarcity of the resource is not only natural but is embedded in a dynamic of social relations and power where the naturalization of the resource scarcity can abet the powerful (Mehta, 2005). We can be challenged to consider the allocation of scarce resources as an ethic that goes beyond mere facts of quantities. As with COVID-19, the challenge is not mathematical – but emotional and stems from trust and relationships. Creating sustainability partnerships is one way to address the political process. "True community is defined by these kinds of bonds of trust and shared purpose, collectively sharing resources where our mutual interests lie (instead of competition)" (Brothers, 2021, para. 9).

While businesses wrestled with decision-making over constraints and resource limits before the pandemic, the challenge has only increased. The decisions individuals made, and are making, about the work they will and will not do, sparked the "great resignation" in the United States. The ethical challenge for business sustainability after COVID-19 is also a challenge of workers facing "time poverty" that exacerbates inequities, especially for unpaid laborers (BBC, 2021).

The Individual and "Good Work"

We know that in times of crisis, little attention is paid to the ideal as day-to-day exigencies can seem to defeat the best intentions. To address what is important and respond, despite the obstacles identified among the legal factors, we can focus as individuals on exercising "practical moral guidance" in the midst of the complex dynamic, approaching "gray area issues as managers and resolv[ing] them as human beings" (Badaracco, 2016). By interweaving ethical, social, emotional, and cognitive perspectives, we can find tools to parse the legal and ethical challenges ahead.

As a former Good Work researcher explains it for herself: "[Good Work ideas] allow me to perceive and understand the social events and trends with more complexity. It informs my critical eye and provides a way to consider action that could lead to healthier, more ethical professional and social circumstances" (Barendsen, 2010, p. 283). It is this understanding of the work world and our role in it that needs to inform our view of the future and our response to it.

One of the key concepts to emerge from the Good Work Project encompasses the idea of responsibility and resulted in a publication built out of just one of their 60-plus questions: "To whom or what do you feel responsible?" In evaluating the responses, Gardner posits that the ethical worker "takes the challenges of responsibility seriously and seeks to behave in as responsible a way as possible" (Gardner, 2010, p. 13). It introduces CSR through some of its originators including Anita Roddick, founder of The Body Shop (Gardner, 2010, p. 166).

Advancing the model of Good Work can assist individuals, business, and societies toward potential solutions. It has the potential to redirect business (the "field") toward ethical decision-making that results in positive change. It can also prepare us for better responses to the forces acting on that field, including climate change and global inequality (Schmidt, 2021) which are on our doorstep. Allocating limited resources - and the actual potential found in constraints - in a globally interdependent world is essential to taking personal responsibility and determining accountability particularly where structural injustice exists.

In practice, considering Good Work presumes a step back toward assessing our own work within the system before advancing toward particular ethical theories for decision resolution. In the management literature it acknowledges the role of personal responsibility and accountability, through thinkers such as Peter Drucker (Malcolm & Hartley, 2009) and the ethicist, Joseph Badaracco (2016).

From this vantage point, sustainability in a post-COVID-19 world enables individuals to confront the major questions before them. Sustainability acknowledges the complex interdependence of social and environmental systems (SES) and relies on tested processes for making progress on seemingly intractable challenges (Matson et al., 2016). What are the questions we can ask to navigate the turbulence? Sustainability can reframe good work for all professions, proposing a way to envision the situation, and enabling integration. As a field Sustainability invokes all of the Sustainable Development Goals (SDGs) interwoven through Goal 17 for partnerships, toward the flourishing of society now and in the future (Goransson, 2021). The marching orders from every nation's sign-on of the SDGs are clear – "all hands-on deck" through collaboration, formal partnership, and collective engagement (UN DESA, n.d., para. 1).

How does this move us toward better understanding the urgency of sustainability and addressing post-COVID-19? It can provide a personal framework that can be brought to the workplace, the corporation, the organization, or to society in identifying areas where Good Work matters and that helps us identify the actions required within organizations to move positively toward a flourishing world (Dutton et al., 2002). It applies, for example, in addressing the "great resignation." It also enables a connection to SDG 8 – "decent work for all" (UN DESA, 2022). In addition, it enables an attainable response to the multiple layers of complexity within CSR (Metcalf & Benn, 2013), for clarifying values (Benkert, 2020), and for adopting a worldview that embeds the natural environment into our understanding of society and economy (Hoffman & Jennings, 2015; Landrum, 2018). Finally, it provides a context for deciding to exit a given job, profession, or organization (Hirschmann, 1970).

We recognize that what is offered in the Good Work model is "not enough" in the sense of providing the framework from which to view all sustainability issues. As noted by those involved in the Good Work research, global, seismic issues, such as the financial collapse of 2008 and its corresponding irresponsible work, "require lenses and approaches from both psychology and sociology, among other disciplines," and in fact requires a "robust, interdisciplinary research agenda capable of understanding the workings of such complex domains, whose failures and successes affect us all" (Nakamura, 2010, p. 171) - which describes the very nature of sustainability. But we find this encouraging; the acknowledgement of the limitations of Good Work and the ideal of interdisciplinary research are mutually reinforcing. We would agree with Clark et al. (2016) that crafting usable knowledge for sustainable development requires humility in engaging multiple knowledges to build into sustainability the tools and processes to address its responsibilities and possibilities. Organizational cultures and authority structures demand attention, particularly given the inequality of proposed solutions when examined independently of historical and cultural inequities and injustices.

Conclusion

Can this model be applied to the situations we find ourselves in now and post-COVID-19? We believe so. The reality includes unsavory stories of fraud, dishonesty, slave labor, organized crime, and of powerful people taking advantage of position and influence in dehumanizing ways. But individuals are also on the front lines addressing the difficulties, providing oversight, offering direction, pursuing honest governance, and seeking fair and equitable solutions. Yet they too are facing individual challenges that can result in burnout and fatigue, at all levels.

Using the potential of finding good work offers a first step toward reducing this demoralization and frustration. Thinking back to the earlier analysis of the legal factors affecting the supply of PPE during COVID-19 we see that personal and corporate interventions can be applied strategically. Taken together, they offer the possibility of seeding thinking and reflection at both the personal and organizational level (Lippitt, 2021) which in turn, transmits the new learning to the next generation within the domain. This offers us a framework for considering our responses in a resource-limited but sustainable future.

References

Badaracco, J. L., Jr. (2016). Managing in the gray: Five timeless questions for resolving your toughest problems at work. *Harvard Business Review Press*.

Balda, J. & Cox, C. (2009, December) Conceptualizing palliative care for the developing world as "good work" [Conference session]. *International Conference of the International Development Ethics Association*, Valencia, Spain.

Barendsen, L. (2010). Do you see what I see: or, what has the GoodWork Project done to us! In H. Gardner (Ed.), *GoodWork: Theory and Practice* (pp. 273-291). GoodWork Project.

Benkert, J. (2020) Reframing business sustainability decision-making with value-focused thinking. *Journal of Business Ethics*, 174, 441-456. doi.org/10.1007/ s10551-020-04611-4.

Brew, J., Hadfield, F. P., Yerovi, M., Stepp, D., & Snyder, J. L. (2021, December 22). Withhold release orders (WRO)/findings archives. International Trade Law. https://www.cmtradelaw.com/category/withhold-release-orders-wro-findings/

Butler, B. (1 February, 2022). US bans imports of disposable gloves from Ansell supplier in Malaysia over allegations of forced labour. *The Guardian*. https://www.theguardian.com/global-development/2022/feb/01/us-bans-imports-of-disposable-gloves-from-ansell-supplier-in-malaysia-over-allegations-of-forced-labour

Brothers, J. (2021). Sharing sugar. *Stanford Social Innovation Review*. https://doi.org/10.48558/YJJ2-WS70

Cavanaugh, J. M., Oleynik, R. A., Werner, M. J., & Zhang, H. (30 July 2020). *FinCEN warns of scams*. Holland & Knight. https://www.hklaw.com/en/insights/publications/2020/07/fincen-warns-of-scams-relating-to-ppe-and-other-medical-goods

Competition and Markets Authority (CMA). (25 March, 2020). CMA approach to business cooperation in response to coronavirus (COVID-19). https://www.gov.uk/government/publications/cma-approach-to-business-cooperation-in-response-to-covid-19

Clark, W. C., van Kerkhoff, L., Lebel, L., & Gallopin, G. C. (2016). Crafting usable knowledge for sustainable development. *Proceedings of the National Academy of Sciences of the United States of America, 113*(17), 4570–4578.

Csikszentmihály, M. (2014). *The systems model of creativity*. Springer.

Csikszentmihályi, M. (1990). The domain of creativity. In M. A. Runco & R. S. Albert (Eds.), *Theories of creativity* (pp. 190–212). Sage Publications.

Csikszentmihályi, M. (1999). Implications of a systems perspective for the study of J. Sternberg (Ed.), *Handbook of creativity* (pp. 313–338). Cambridge University Press.

Desierto, D. (2021, February 1). Equitable COVID vaccine distribution and access: Enforcing international legal obligations under economic, social, and cultural rights and the right to development. EJIL. https://www.ejiltalk.org/equitable-covid-vaccine-distribution-and-access-enforcing-international-legal-obligations-under-economic-social-and-cultural-rights-and-the-right-to-development/

Dutton, J. E., Frost, P. J., Worline, M. C., Lilius, J. M., & Kanov, J. M. (January, 2002), Leading in times of trauma. *Harvard Business Review, 80*(1), 54-61.

European Anti-Fraud Office (20 March 2020). OLAF launches enquiry into fake COVID-19 related products. *European Commission,* Press Release No 07/2020. https://ec.europa.eu/anti-fraud/media-corner/news/olaf-launches-enquiry-fake-COVID-19-19-related-products-2020-03-20_en

Europol. (24 March 2020). Rise of fake 'corona cures' revealed in global counterfeit medicine operation. https://www.europol.europa.eu/media-press/newsroom/news/rise-of-fake-%E2%80%98corona-cures%E2%80%99-revealed-in-global-counterfeit-medicine-operation

Europol. (Update 06 Dec. 2021). Pandemic profiteering: How criminals exploit the COVID-19 crisis. https://www.europol.europa.eu/publications-events/publications/pandemic-profiteering-how-criminals-exploit-COVID-19-19-crisis

Forman, R. & Mossialos, E. (September 2021). The EU response to COVID-19-19: From reactive policies to strategic decision-making. *Journal of Common Market Studies, 59*(S1), 56-68. https://onlinelibrary.wiley.com/doi/full/10.1111/ jcms.13259

Gardner, H. (2010). *Responsibility at work: How leading professionals act (or don't act) responsibly.* John Wiley & Sons.

Gardner, H. (2009). I. What is good work? II. Achieving good work in turbulent times (G.B. Petersen, Ed.). *The Tanner Lectures on Human Values, 28,* 199-233.

Gardner, H., Csikszentmihály, M. & Damon, W. (2001). *Good work: How excellence and ethics meet.* Basic Books.

George Washington University, (n. d.). *Temporary FEMA export restrictions on certain PPE products.* https://researchintegrity.gwu.edu/ COVID-19-19-and-export-controls

Gibson Dunn Law Firm, (8 April 2020). *Fraud in the COVID-19 age: Examining and anticipating changing enforcement activity.* https://www.gibsondunn.com/wp-content/uploads/2020/04/fraud-in-the-COVID-19-19-age-examining-and-anticipating-changing-enforcement-activity.pdf

Goodman, P. S. (31 October, 2021). How the supply chain broke, and why it won't be fixed anytime soon. *The New York Times.* https://www.nytimes.com/2021/10/22/business/shortages-supply-chain.html

Goransson, O. (2021, April 30). *UN/DESA Policy brief #103: Transformational partnerships and partnership platforms*. Department of Economic and Social Affairs. United Nations. https://www.un.org/development/desa/dpad/publication/un-desa-policy-brief-103-transformational-partnerships-and-partnership-platforms/

Hirschman, A. O. (1970), *Exit, voice, and loyalty: responses to decline in firms, organizations, and states*. Harvard University Press.

Iacobucci, G. (03 February 2022), Covid-19: Government writes off £10bn on unusable, overpriced, or undelivered PPE. *The BMJ, 376*. https://doi.org/10.1136/bmj.o296

Interpol. (14 April 2020). Unmasked: International COVID-19 fraud exposed. https://www.interpol.int/en/News-and-Events/News/2020/Unmasked-International-COVID-19-19-fraud-exposed

James, C. (2010). Reflections on The GoodWork Project: A sociologist's perspective. In H. Gardner (Ed.), *GoodWork: Theory and practice*. GoodWork Project.

Landrum, N. L. (2018). Identifying worldviews on corporate sustainability: A content analysis of corporate sustainability reports. *Business Strategy and the Environment, 27*, 128–151.

Lippitt, M. (2021). Situational mindsets: A context-based leadership framework. *Journal of Leadership Studies, 15*(2).

Luo, Y. (11 February 2020). Cyberspace Administration of China releases notice on the protection of personal information in the fight against coronavirus. https://www.insideprivacy.com/international/china/cyberspace-administration-of-china-releases-notice-on-the-protection-of-personal-information-in-the-fight-against-coronavirus/

Malcolm, S. B. & Hartley, N. T. (2009). Peter F. Drucker: Ethics scholar par excellence. *Journal of Management History, 15*(4), 375-387. doi: 10.1108/17511340910987301

Matson, P., Clark, W. C., & Andersson, K. (2016). *Pursuing sustainability: A guide to the science and practice*. Princeton University Press.

McLean, S., Davey-Attlee, F., Olarn, K. & Lister, T. (24 October 2021). Investigation: Tens of millions of filthy, used medical gloves imported into the US. *CNN*.

https://www.cnn.com/2021/10/24/health/medical-gloves-us-thailand-investigation-cmd-intl/index.html

Mehta, L. (2005). *The politics and poetics of water: The naturalisation of scarcity in Western India*. Orient Blackswan.

Metcalf, L. & Benn, S. (2013) Leadership for sustainability: An evolution of leadership ability. *Journal of Business Ethics, 112*, 369–384.

Moran, S. (2010). Returning to the GoodWork Project's roots: Can creative work be humane? In H. Gardner (Ed.), *GoodWork: Theory and practice*. GoodWork Project.

Mucinskas, D. & Gardner, H. (December 2013). Educating for Good Work: From research to practice. *British Journal of Educational Studies, 61*(4), 453-470.

Nakamura, J. (2010). Defining and modeling good work. In H. Gardner (Ed.) *GoodWork: Theory and practice* (pp. 107-126). GoodWork Project.

Nogrady, B. (13 October, 2022). "I hope you die": How the COVID-19 pandemic unleashed attacks on scientists. *Nature*.

Organisation for Economic Co-operation and Development (OECD). (2021). COVID-19 and responsible business conduct. https://www.oecd.org/coronavirus/policy-responses/covid-19-and-responsible-business-conduct-02150b06/

Romar, E. J. (2004). Managerial harmony: The Confucian ethics of Peter F. Drucker. *Journal of Business Ethics, 51*(2), 199-212.

Schwartz, M. (2002). Peter Drucker's Weimar experience: Moral management as a perception of the past. *Journal of Business Ethics, 41*(1/2), 51-68.

Schwartz, M. S., & Carroll, A. B. (2003). Corporate social responsibility: A three-domain approach. *Business Ethics Quarterly: The Journal of the Society for Business Ethics, 13*(4), 503– 530.

Scoones, I. (2007). Sustainability. *Development in Practice, 17*(4/5), 589–596. http://www.jstor.org/stable/25548257

Scoones, I. (2016). The politics of sustainability and development. *Annual Review of Environment and Resources, 41*(1), 293–319.

Sim, M. (2007). *Remastering morals with Aristotle and Confucius*. Cambridge University Press.

United Nations Office on Drugs and Crime (UNODC) (2020). COVID-19-related trafficking of medical products as a threat to public health. https://www.unodc.org/documents/data-and-analysis/covid/COVID-19_research_brief_trafficking_medical_products.pdf

United Nations Department of Economic and Social Affairs (UN DESA). (ND). Multi-stakeholder partnerships and voluntary commitments.

World Health Organization (WHO). (23 December 2020). Rational use of personal protective equipment for COVID-19 and considerations during severe shortages. *Interim guidance*. https://www.who.int/ teams/health-product-policy-and-standards/assistive-and-medical-technology/medical-devices/ppe/ppe-COVID-19

THE IMPACT OF THE COVID-19 PANDEMIC ON INDIVIDUALS AND THEIR INTRA- AND INTERGROUP RELATIONS

Islam Borinca[1], Mariuche Gomides[1], and Sevim Mustafa[2]

Abstract: In this chapter, we address how the COVID-19 pandemic has impacted people on an individual level as well as affected their intra- and intergroup relationships. At the individual level, many people have suffered from anxiety, depression, and inadequate sleep during the pandemic, the prolonged nature of which has also made them feel lonely and isolated. However, simultaneously feeling connected to their in-group members during the pandemic has made them feel as if their well-being has improved. Added to that, their (dis)trust of national institutions has influenced their willingness to comply with measures to mitigate COVID-19. Furthermore, in-group normativity (e.g., information about in-group members' compliance with health advice) brought people together and encouraged them to believe fewer conspiracy theories about COVID-19. However, in relation to out-group members, the pandemic has resulted in individuals' heightened prejudice, dehumanization, distrust, and negative affect.

Keywords: COVID-19 pandemic, health, social relations, groups, misinformation, social norms

Introduction

The COVID-19 pandemic, a global crisis caused by a new coronavirus-induced disease (World Health Organization, 2020), has presented considerable challenges for people's lives, in particular jeopardizing their health and economic livelihood, as well as their freedom of movement and social relationships (Krahé, 2020). Among other things, many people have had to work from home, either alone or alongside their spouses and/or loved ones, while children have had to attend school virtually. Such

---

[1] School of Psychology, University College Dublin, Ireland

[2] Department of Psychology, Kolegji AAB, Kosovo

transitions have brought about an entirely new set of problems, including isolation and loneliness, feelings of stagnation, tension due to working in close quarters with family, frustration with trying to secure the appropriate equipment, and fatigue from Zoom and Microsoft Teams meetings, among many others (Accenture, 2021). In their magnitude, the crisis and its consequences have spawned widespread fear, uncertainty, and anxiety that, when coupled with social isolation, altered work and family routines, cabin fever, and economic insecurity, have caused suffering for public mental health. Moreover, because the trajectory of the pandemic has been impossible to predict and because people's circumstances have changed rapidly, many have come to feel powerless, almost as if they no longer have control over their lives (Jacinta, 2021).

In view of those challenges, in this chapter we address how the COVID-19 pandemic has impacted people on an individual (personal) level as well as affected their relationships at the intragroup (i.e., including family, friends, other citizens, intragroup norms, and national institutions) and intergroup levels (i.e., including relations with people in other social and/or ethnic groups known as *out-groups*; see Borinca et al., 2020, 2021a).

The COVID-19 pandemic and its consequences at the individual level

The COVID-19 pandemic has exerted numerous detrimental effects on various aspects of individuals' personal lives. On that topic, Vindegaard and Benros (2020) found that anxiety and depression have increased in the general public as well as among health care professionals, the latter of which have also experienced psychological distress and poor sleep quality. They also discovered high levels of depression and symptoms of post-traumatic stress among patients who had contracted COVID-19 (see also Al-Omiri et al., 2021; Tsamakis et al., 2021). Along similar lines, other research has revealed a relatively high prevalence of symptoms of post-traumatic stress disorder (PTSD) related to the COVID-19 pandemic among health care workers, a potential predictor of which has been a lack of social support (d'Ettorre et al., 2021). Epidemiological research has also shown that 17% of adults in the general population experienced symptoms of PTSD during the early stages of the pandemic (Karatzias et al., 2020).

Although traumatic events can indeed cause symptoms of PTSD, they can also be catalysts for positive change. In fact, studies have shown that up to 50% of individuals who have faced traumatic events experience some form of post-traumatic growth. That post-traumatic growth was characterized by less depression and a greater sense of well-being (i.e., positive affect, self-esteem, and life satisfaction; Vicki et al., 2006). Thus, increasing evidence suggests that post-traumatic growth results from an adaptive response to and ability to cope with trauma (Schubert et al., 2016; Wu et al., 2019). Similarly, research has begun documenting the positive psychological effects of the COVID-19 pandemic even despite the unprecedented challenges that it has created (Matos et al., 2021). For example, carers of children in Portugal and the United Kingdom have reported increased post-traumatic growth that researchers have associated with higher levels of well-being (e.g., experiencing positive feelings, such as being able to stop worrying and hoping that COVID-19 will end soon, satisfying interpersonal relationships, and positive functioning; Stallard et al., 2021). Added to that, moderate levels of post-traumatic growth observed among frontline nurses were found to positively relate to social support (Peng et al., 2021).

The COVID-19 pandemic and intragroup relations

As a result of the pandemic, relationships among group members in society have also been affected. In that context, the term *group members* refers to one's family members, friends, relatives, other nationals and their national institutions and local media.

The negative effect of COVID-19 pandemic on intra-group relations

In the first year of the pandemic, an analysis of messages that had been forwarded on the messaging app WhatsApp in Singapore found that 35% of those messages were based on falsehoods, while another 20% combined true as well as false information. This resulted in confusion among nationals and a rift in their understanding of the governmental recommendations regarding COVID-19 health advice (Tandoc & Mak, 2020). Also, fake news spread via social media (i.e., WhatsApp and Facebook) during the first year of COVID-19 in Brazil was characterized by political content, misinformation about the number of cases and deaths, and a dispute among the population regarding COVID-19 health advice (de Barcelos et al., 2021). In addition, Roozenbeek and colleagues (2020) found a negative association between believing in misinformation about COVID-19 and self-reported compliance with health guidelines.

Accordingly, a polarization has emerged among group members (i.e., nationals) relating to the COVID-19 vaccine (Bolsen & Plam, 2022; Henkel et al., 2022) and thus threatening social cohesion within nations (McCoy et al., 2018). During preparations for the release of the vaccines, social media posts presented a wide range of alarming claims. Such claims included that the government would alter individuals' DNA and negatively affect their fertility. Another spurious claim stated the government was injecting microchips into people in order to monitor their behavior (Romer & Jamieson, 2020). Therefore, many nationals (i.e., anti-vax nationals) started to maintain that vaccinations are a personal decision and should not be mandated by the government. These nationals were less likely to follow COVID-19 governmental health recommendations and felt less empathy for other nationals who were trying to adhere to these recommendations. As an example, anti-vax protesters clashed with police in multiple locations across Western Europe due to their attempts to gather at malls when they were not advised to do so or to disrupt public transportation as a means of expressing their opposition (Hardinges, 2021).

The positive effect of COVID-19 pandemic on intra-group relations

Overall, however, feeling connected to group members during lockdowns predicted better well-being and a decrease in perceived stress (Landmann & Rohmann, 2022). In a similar vein, Matos and colleagues (2021) found that perceiving social connectedness plays a crucial role in coping with crises such as the COVID-19 pandemic. In fact, having social connections that are caring and supportive can significantly improve individuals' mental and physical health (Brown & Brown, 2015; Ditzen & Heinrichs, 2014) as well as reduce symptoms of depression, anxiety, and post-traumatic stress (Maheux & Price, 2016).

Another factor in encouraging people's compliance with the governmental health advice during the COVID-19 pandemic has been the way the majority of in-group members act or *in-group normative compliance*—that is, perceptions of whether other in-groups such as family, friends and other nationals are engaging in preventive behaviors or normative influence—which can influence an individual's personal compliance with policy (Goldberg et al., 2020; Martínez et al., 2021). Policymakers, for example, have increasingly used normative influence to prompt individuals in diverse contexts to pursue goals such as improving their health behaviors, including by changing their diet, exercising, and quitting smoking (Mollen et al., 2013; Okun et al., 2002; Reid et al., 2010), as well as decreasing their dependence upon medical prescriptions, increasing their tax compliance, and reducing their energy and water consumption (Allcott, 2011; Bhanot, 2021; Coleman, 2007; Ferraro et al., 2011; Hallsworth et al., 2016). Normative influence can also affect individuals' willingness to enforce and sanction violations (Acemoglu & Jackson, 2017; Traxler & Winter, 2012).

As such, in-group normative compliance is also relevant to explaining behaviors during the COVID-19 pandemic because it has also influenced those same behaviors (Lunn et al., 2020a, 2020b). Past research has shown that health interventions may be more effective when they alter instead of maintaining the status quo of others' actions in one's group, which can indirectly influence their personal behaviors (Bond et al., 2012; Van Bavel et al., 2020). By extension, if a behavior becomes a social norm, then its normativity can influence personal behavior as a result of processes of conformity (e.g., Deutsch & Gerard, 1955; Neville et al., 2021), including injunctive norms—that is, what others approve of—and descriptive norms—that is, what others do (e.g., Borinca, 2021; Borinca et al., 2022b; Cialdini et al., 1991). For instance, Goldenberg and colleagues (2020) found that witnessing family and friends adhere to COVID-19 regulations had the potential to positively influence individuals' behavior in the same direction, while Smith and colleagues (2020) in the United Kingdom discovered that believing that other people of one's age were complying with restrictions was associated with relatively better compliance with lockdowns. Further evidence stems from experimental manipulations of "what others are doing" in response to vignettes depicting adherence to COVID-19 guidance, both in general behavior and in specific scenarios (e.g., attending a birthday party). In the latter context, when informed others did not (vs. did) attend such a party, individuals were more likely than not to comply with restrictions (Bicchieri et al., 2021; Martínez et al., 2021).

Research by Borinca and colleagues (2022c) has additionally shown that when in-group norms indicate that in-group members do in fact comply with COVID-19 measures (vs. in-group norms indicating that in-group members do not comply with those measures or a control condition with no information provided related to the measures), beliefs in conspiracy theories about COVID-19 decreased (e.g., that the pharmaceutical industry is involved in spreading COVID-19 and that the coronavirus was intentionally created in a laboratory), and national solidarity with other in-group members involved in the fight against COVID-19 pandemic improved.

In addition, participants were more willing to comply with measures to mitigate COVID-19 and to perceive others as doing the same when in-group norms indicated that in-group members were also complying with those measures (vs. in-group norms indicating that in-group members do not comply with those measures or a control condition with no information provided related to the measures). Their study also revealed that participants were less willing to participate in collective action against COVID-19 health advice when in-group norms indicated that in-group members were complying with the measures. Those dynamics were examined across two cultural groups in western Europe (i.e., Ireland) and southeastern Europe (i.e., Kosovo).

Institutional trust and compliance with COVID-19 health recommendations

Other research has additionally identified trust in national institutions (e.g., in governments and health care institutions) as an important factor in citizens' compliance with government policies and interventions. Several scholars have posited that the public's trust in the government encourages ordinary citizens to comply with such policies (Chanley et al., 2000; Levi & Stoker, 2000; Scholz, 1998; Shi, 2001) and/or be more likely to comply with laws when they perceive the government as being trustworthy (Levi & Stoker, 2000; Murphy, 2005; Tyler, 1990). Findings from empirical research also suggest that trust in government not only promotes compliance with policy but also facilitates its implementation (Cui et al., 2015; Güzel et al., 2019).

During pandemics, a high level of public trust in government tends to positively influence citizens' compliance with policy directives. For example, during the influenza A virus subtype H1N1 (i.e., "swine flu") pandemic, a high level of trust in government increased citizens' likelihood of adopting recommended countermeasures (Gilles et al., 2011; van der Weerd et al., 2011). In another example, despite not knowing much about the nature of severe acute respiratory syndrome (i.e., SARS), individuals adhered to control measures due to a high level of trust in the government, thereby signaling that the public was satisfied with the government's response (Deurenberg-Yap et al., 2005). Of particular relevance to this chapter, research conducted during the COVID-19 pandemic has shown that specific types of trust in national institutions (i.e., confidence in one's health care system) predicts longer-lasting adherence to social distancing (Chan et al., 2020; Woelfert & Kunst, 2020). On top of that, cross-sectional data demonstrate that trust in institutions (e.g., health care institutions and COVID-19 committees) predicted greater adherence to social distancing measures in Slovakia (Caplanova et al., 2021), and across 23 countries, trust in governments was associated with greater engagement in behaviors to mitigate COVID-19 (Pagliaro et al., 2021).

The COVID-19 pandemic and intergroup relations

Along with affecting people personally and in their relations with ingroup members, the COVID-19 pandemic has also shaped relationships between different groups. The term *between group members* refers to people's perception and reaction toward other groups perceived as different such as immigrants, refugees, or other ethnic minorities within one's nation (Borinca et al., 2021b, 2021c, 2022a).

The outbreak of COVID-19 dramatically changed the ways in which people were able to view, feel about, and interact with other people. First, diseases and pathogenic threats such as COVID-19 increase prejudice toward people perceived as being different or out-groups because they activate the behavioral immune system, a bodily network of psychological processes aimed at detecting and avoiding potential sources of pathogenic infection (Murray & Schaller, 2012). In addition, crises and other threatening times (e.g., the 1918 influenza pandemic and the Great Recession) tend to activate imagery of wartime such that citizens identify an enemy (i.e., the out-group) against which to defend the in-group (Fritsche et al., 2006; Sabucedo et al., 2020). Thus, individuals may attempt to direct their hostility toward out-groups in order to establish a sense of control and reduce their negative affect (Glick, 2002; Rothschild et al., 2012).

Research has begun identifying the repercussions of the COVID-19 pandemic on intergroup relations and attitudes. In the pandemic's early phases, xenophobic reactions toward Asian individuals, especially those of Chinese descent, increased in non-Asian countries, as did discrimination toward people from minority subgroups, including light-skinned people in some African countries and even citizens from Wuhan in China (Roberto et al., 2020). Other empirical evidence suggests that worrying about COVID-19 was positively associated with both xenophobia and less positive attitudes toward Asian American individuals in the United States (Reny & Barreto, 2022), while a study in Poland showed that people who frequently sought out and shared information about COVID-19 reported higher anxiety and negative affect toward Italian individuals—that is, the people most affected by COVID-19 in Europe at the time (Sorokowski et al., 2020).

Research examining the Italian context has additionally shown that perceptions of common belonging (i.e., belonging to a common group, sharing a common destiny, and perceiving the difficulties faced by other groups) with disadvantaged and national out-groups were associated with perceptions of COVID-19 as a threat and of prejudice against certain individual differences, namely a social dominance orientation, the need for cognitive closure, deprovincialization, and positive and negative face-to-face contact with immigrants before the pandemic (Fuochi et al., 2021). Meanwhile, research examining the Israeli context has shown that higher levels of exposure to COVID-19 predicted less willingness to aid out-groups and that out-group dehumanization mediated that association (Adler et al., 2021).

Recent work by Borinca and colleagues (2022d) examining post-conflict relations in Kosovo between Kosovars and Serbs has revealed that the COVID-19 crisis has impacted intergroup relations involving the former opponents. Their findings indicated that people with low levels of prejudice reacted negatively to prosocial actions of former opponents by showing more negative emotions when their former enemy had helped them with fighting COVID-19 than when they had not. Beyond that, individuals with high levels of prejudice reacted negatively regardless of whether their past rival had helped them or not. Those authors also reported similar findings regarding people's perceptions of social dominance and trust, such that ones with less prejudice perceived more negative intentions from the out-group (i.e., attempts to dominate them) and trusted them less when they, as their former enemy, had helped them with combating COVID-19 than when they had not. In addition, individuals with a high level of prejudice reacted negatively (i.e., trusted less and exhibited a more negative perception of dominance) regardless of whether their former enemy had helped them or not.

Their additional data suggest that individuals with low levels of prejudice tended to like their former enemy less when the latter had helped them with COVID-19 than when they had not. In addition, individuals with high levels of prejudice tended to dislike their former enemy regardless of whether the latter had helped them or not. Accordingly, COVID-19 has resulted in negative attitudes towards outgroups, a decrease in trust, and a higher level of negative affect in various intergroup settings.

Practical implications

This chapter has sought to illustrate how the COVID-19 pandemic has affected people on a personal level as well as in relation to others, including both in-group members (e.g., family, friends, and other nationals and national institutions) and out-group members. As mentioned, on a personal level many people experienced anxiety, depression, and poor sleep during the COVID-19 lockdowns, as well as feelings of loneliness and isolation. In spite of these difficulties, the more that people have reported post-traumatic growth, the more they have also reported improved well-being. That dynamic suggests that challenging circumstances can in fact change how people think about the world and themselves, which can result in deeply meaningful personal changes (Tedeschi & Calhoun, 2004).

At the intergroup level, the more people exchanged false information about COVID-19 with other in-group members, the less likely they were to follow COVID-19 guidelines. The same was true when such information was transmitted via social media. However, despite all of these challenges, the more that individuals have reported feeling connected with others close to them during the COVID-19 pandemic, the more that they have also reported improved well-being. Research has additionally shown that in-group normativity (e.g., information about the majority of in-group members' compliance with health advice) has brought group members together because they believe less in conspiracy theories, do not participate in actions against the government's measures to mitigate COVID-19, and respect public health advice (Borinca et al., 2022c). Indeed, the more that individuals have reported believing in their national institutions, the more that they have also reported following their countries' health advice and regulations. It therefore seems that, in times of crisis, governments and health institutions should always strive to use in-group norms as a means to increase unity within their countries and minimize misinformation and division among their citizens.

At the intergroup level, the COVID-19 pandemic has worsened perceptions of and reactions toward out-group members (Borinca et al., 2022d). A consequence of the initial threat of COVID-19 was an increase in reports of people's xenophobic reactions against members of out-groups and of their desires to distance themselves from out-groups living in areas most affected by the pandemic. The out-group has also been perceived as being less human during the pandemic, such that in-groups have been less willing to aid out-group members. Added to that, when out-group members offered to assist in-group members, the latter distrusted such help because they didn't trust the intentions of out-group members. As a result, it is reasonable to conclude that social crises such as the COVID-19 pandemic harm intergroup relations and that methods and interventions that bring people from different groups together need to be examined in order for all groups to be united in the future.

Conclusion

The considerations raised in this chapter shed light on people's experiences at the individual level and on intra- and intergroup processes during the COVID-19 pandemic. On the negative side, the COVID-19 pandemic has been challenging for people on a personal level because it has risked their psychological well-being. The pandemic has also intensified the circulation of misinformation and thus confused people about the ethical issues involved in the pandemic and measures to mitigate it, such that they have lost sight of human ethics when considering out-group members as a consequence of increased out-group prejudice and hostility. On the positive side, by contrast, maintaining healthy relationships with in-group members has allowed people to cope more effectively with the pandemic. In addition, inclusive in-group norms and unending institutional efforts appear to have brought people together to eventually defeat the pandemic. Even so, to construct and maintain a harmonious society, each group's identity needs to be recognized, especially during times of crisis, as a way of protecting humanity as a whole from division, hatred, and dehumanization both within and between groups.

References

Accenture. (2021). COVID-19's impact on people with disabilities. https://www.easterseals.com/shared-components/document-library/media-room/easterseals-study-on-the-impact-of-covid-full.pdf

Acemoglu, D., & Jackson, M. O. (2017). Social norms and the enforcement of laws. *Journal of the European Economic Association, 15*(2), 245-295. doi:org/10.1093/jeea/jvw006

Adler, E., Hebel-Sela, S., Leshem, O. A., Levy, J., & Halperin, E. (2022). A social virus: Intergroup dehumanization and unwillingness to aid amidst COVID-19– Who are the main targets? *International Journal of Intercultural Relations, 86*, 109-121. doi:org/10.1016/j.ijintrel.2021.11.006

Al-Omiri, M. K., Alzoubi, I. A., Al Nazeh, A. A., Alomiri, A. K., Maswady, M. N., & Lynch, E. (2021). COVID-19 and personality: A cross-sectional multicenter study of the relationship between personality factors and COVID-19-related impacts, concerns, and behaviors. *Frontiers in Psychiatry, 12*, 608730. doi:org/10.3389/fpsyt.2021.608730

Allcott, H. (2011). Social norms and energy conservation. *Journal of Public Economics, 95*(9-10), 1082-1095. doi:org/10.1016/j.jpubeco.2011.03.003

Bhanot, S. P. (2021). Isolating the effect of injunctive norms on conservation behavior: New evidence from a field experiment in California. *Organizational Behavior and Human Decision Processes, 163*, 30-42. doi:org/10.1016/j.obhdp. 2018.11.002

Bicchieri, C., Fatas, E., Aldama, A., Casas, A., Deshpande, I., Lauro, M., Parilli, C., Spohn, M., Pereira, P., & Wen, R. (2021). In science we (should) trust: Expectations and compliance across nine countries during the COVID-19 pandemic. *PloS One, 16*(6), e0252892. doi:org/10.1371/journal.pone.0252892

Bolsen, T., & Palm, R. (2022). Politicization and COVID-19 vaccine resistance in the US. *Progress In Molecular Biology and Translational Science, 188*(1), 81. doi.org/10.1016/bs.pmbts.2021.10.002.

Bond, R. M., Fariss, C. J., Jones, J. J., Kramer, A. D., Marlow, C., Settle, J. E., & Fowler, J. H. (2012). A 61-million-person experiment in social influence and political mobilization. *Nature, 489*(7415), 295-298. doi:org/10.1038/nature11421

Borinca, I. (2021). (Mis) understanding out-group pro-social behaviors (Doctoral dissertation, University of Geneva). doi:org/10.13097/archive-ouverte/unige: 148613

Borinca, I., Çelik, P., & Storme, M. (2022a). Can conservatives who (de) humanize immigrants the most be able to support them? The power of imagined positive contact. *Journal of Applied Social Psychology*. doi:org/10.1111/jasp.12864

Borinca, I., Andrighetto, L., Valsecchi, G., & Berent, J. (2022b). In-group norms shape understanding of out-group prosocial behaviors. *Group Processes & Intergroup Relations, 25*(4), 1084-1106. doi:org/10.1177/1368430220987604

Borinca, I., Falomir-Pichastor, J. M., & Andrighetto, L. (2020). "How can you help me if you are not from here?" Helper's familiarity with the context shapes interpretations of prosocial intergroup behaviors. *Journal of Experimental Social Psychology, 87*, 103944. doi:org/10.1016/j.jesp.2019.103944

Borinca, I., Griffin M, S., McMahon, G., Maher, P., & Muldoon, O. (2022c). Normative compliance attenuates conspiracy theories about COVID-19 among people who distrust science: Findings from Western and Southeastern Europe. *Manuscript Submitted for Publication.*

Borinca, I., Moreno-Bella, E., Sánchez-Rodríguez, Á., & Muldoon, O. (2022d). Crisis complicates peacebuilding in post-conflict societies: COVID-19 support triggers negative out-group emotions among individuals with low and high prejudice. *Peace and Conflict Journal of Peace Psychology.* Advanced Online Publication. doi:org/10.1037/pac0000631

Borinca, I., Tropp, L. R., & Ofosu, N. (2021a). Meta-humanization enhances positive reactions to prosocial cross-group interaction. *British Journal of Social Psychology, 60*(3), 1051-1074. doi:org/10.1111/bjso.12435

Borinca, I., Falomir-Pichastor, J. M., Andrighetto, L., & Durante, F. (2021b). Out-group prejudice and perceptions of prosocial intergroup behaviors. *European Journal of Social Psychology, 51*(1), 40-53 doi:org/10.1002/ejsp.2712.

Borinca, I., Falomir-Pichastor, J. M., Andrighetto, L., & Halabi, S. (2021c). Overcoming negative reactions to prosocial intergroup behaviors in post-conflict societies: The power of intergroup apology. *Journal of Experimental Social Psychology, 95*, 104140. doi:org/10.1016/j.jesp.2021.104140

Brown, S. L., & Brown, R. M. (2015). Connecting prosocial behavior to improved physical health: Contributions from the neurobiology of parenting. *Neuroscience & Biobehavioral Reviews, 55*, 1-17. doi:org/10.1016/j.neubiorev.2015.04.004

Caplanova, A., Sivak, R., & Szakadatova, E. (2021). Institutional trust and compliance with measures to fight COVID-19. *International Advances in Economic Research, 27*(1), 47-60. doi:org/10.1007/s11294-021-09818-3

Chan, H. F., Brumpton, M., Macintyre, A., Arapoc, J., Savage, D. A., Skali, A., Stadelmann, D., & Torgler, B. (2020). How confidence in health care systems affects mobility and compliance during the COVID-19 pandemic. *PloS One, 15*(10), e0240644. doi:org/10.1371/journal.pone.0240644

Chanley, V. A., Rudolph, T. J., & Rahn, W. M. (2000). The origins and consequences of public trust in government: A time series analysis. *Public Opinion Quarterly, 64*(3), 239-256. doi:org/10.1086/317987

Cialdini, R. B., Kallgren, C. A., & Reno, R. R. (1991). A focus theory of normative conduct: A theoretical refinement and reevaluation of the role of norms in human behavior. *Advances in Experimental Social Psychology, 24*, 201-234.

Coleman, S. (2007). The Minnesota income tax compliance experiment: replication of the social norms experiment. *Available at SSRN 1393292.* doi:org/10.2139/ssrn.1393292

Cui, E., Tao, R., Warner, T. J., & Yang, D. L. (2015). How do land takings affect political trust in rural China? *Political Studies, 63*, 91-109. doi:org/10.1111/1467-9248.12151

d'Ettorre, G., Ceccarelli, G., Santinelli, L., Vassalini, P., Innocenti, G. P., Alessandri, F., Koukopoulos, A. E., Russo, A., d'Ettorre, G., & Tarsitani, L. (2021). Post-traumatic stress symptoms in healthcare workers dealing with the COVID-19 pandemic: A systematic review. *International Journal of Environmental Research and Public Health, 18*(2), 601. https://doi.org/10.3390/ijerph18020601

de Barcelos, T. D. N., Muniz, L. N., Dantas, D. M., DF, C. J., Cavalcante, J. R., & Faerstein, E. (2021). Analysis of fake news disseminated during the COVID-19 pandemic in BrazilAnálisis de las noticias falsas divulgadas durante la pandemia de COVID-19 en Brasil. *Revista Panamericana de Salud Publica= Pan American Journal of Public Health, 45*, e65-e65.

Deurenberg-Yap, M., Foo, L., Low, Y., Chan, S., Vijaya, K., & Lee, M. (2005). The Singaporean response to the SARS outbreak: Knowledge sufficiency versus public trust. *Health Promotion International, 20*(4), 320-326. doi:org/10.1093/heapro/dai010

Deutsch, M., & Gerard, H. B. (1955). A study of normative and informational social influences upon individual judgment. *The Journal of Abnormal and Social Psychology, 51*(3), 629. doi:org/10.1037/h0046408

Ditzen, B., & Heinrichs, M. (2014). Psychobiology of social support: The social dimension of stress buffering. *Restorative Neurology and Neuroscience, 32*(1), 149-162.

Ferraro, P. J., Miranda, J. J., & Price, M. K. (2011). The persistence of treatment effects with norm-based policy instruments: Evidence from a randomized environmental policy experiment. *American Economic Review, 101*(3), 318-322. doi:org/10.1257/aer.101.3.318

Fritsche, I., Moya, M., Bukowski, M., Jugert, P., de Lemus, S., Decker, O., Valor-Segura, I., & Navarro-Carrillo, G. (2017). The great recession and group-based control: Converting personal helplessness into social class in-group trust and collective action. *Journal of Social Issues, 73*(1), 117-137. doi:org/10.1111/josi.12207

Fuochi, G., Boin, J., Voci, A., & Hewstone, M. (2021). COVID-19 threat and perceptions of common belonging with outgroups: The roles of prejudice-related individual differences and intergroup contact. *Personality and Individual Differences, 175,* 110700. doi:org/10.1016/j.paid.2021.110700

Gilles, I., Bangerter, A., Clémence, A., Green, E. G., Krings, F., Staerklé, C., & Wagner-Egger, P. (2011). Trust in medical organizations predicts pandemic (H1N1) 2009 vaccination behavior and perceived efficacy of protection measures in the Swiss public. *European Journal of Epidemiology, 26*(3), 203-210. doi:org/10.1007/s10654-011-9577-2

Glick, P. (2002). Sacrificial lambs dressed in wolves' clothing: Envious prejudice, ideology, and the scapegoating of Jews. In L. S. Newman & R. Erber (Eds.), *Understanding genocide: The social psychology of the Holocaust* (pp. 113–142). Oxford University Press. doi:org/10.1093/acprof:oso/9780195133622.003.0006

Goldberg, M. H., Gustafson, A., Maibach, E., van der Linden, S., Ballew, M. T., Bergquist, P., Marlon, J. R., Rosenthal, S.A., & Leiserowitz, A. (2020). Social norms motivate COVID-19 preventive behaviors. https://doi.org/10.31234/osf.io/9whp4

Güzel, S. A., Özer, G., & Özcan, M. (2019). The effect of the variables of tax justice perception and trust in government on tax compliance: The case of Turkey. *Journal of Behavioral and Experimental Economics, 78,* 80-86. doi:org/10.1016/j.socec.2018.12.006

Hallsworth, M., Chadborn, T., Sallis, A., Sanders, M., Berry, D., Greaves, F., Clements, L., & Davies, S. C. (2016). Provision of social norm feedback to high prescribers of antibiotics in general practice: a pragmatic national randomised controlled trial. *The Lancet, 387*(10029), 1743-1752. doi:org/10.1016/S0140-6736(16)00215-4

Hardinges, N. (2021). Anti-vaxx protesters clash with police while storming Westfield shopping centre. https://www.lbc.co.uk/news/anti-vacine-protesters-clash-police-storming-westfield-shopping-centre-london/

Helgeson, V. S., Reynolds, K. A., & Tomich, P. L. (2006). A meta-analytic review of benefit finding and growth. *Journal of Consulting and Clinical Psychology, 74*(5), 797. doi.org/10.1037/0022-006X.74.5.797

Henkel, L., Sprengholz, P., Korn, L., Betsch, C., & Böhm, R. (2022). Understanding the trouble spot: Does vaccination status identification fuel societal polarization? doi.org/10.31234/osf.io/mgqk5

Jacinta, J. (2021). The Challenges of Covid and how to deal with them. https://www.silvercloudhealth.com/us/blog/the-challenges-of-covid-19-and-how-to-deal-with-them#_ftn1

Karatzias, T., Shevlin, M., Murphy, J., McBride, O., Ben-Ezra, M., Bentall, R. P., Vallières, F., & Hyland, P. (2020). Posttraumatic stress symptoms and associated comorbidity during the COVID-19 pandemic in Ireland: A population-based study. *Journal of Traumatic Stress, 33*(4), 365-370. doi:org/10.1002/jts.22565

Krahé, B. (2020). Aggression in times of Covid-19: The social costs of the pandemic. https://www.routledge.com/blog/article/aggression-in-times-of-covid-19-the-social-costs-of-the-pandemic

Landmann, H., & Rohmann, A. (2022). Group-specific contact and sense of connectedness during the COVID-19 pandemic and its associations with psychological well-being, perceived stress, and work-life balance. *Journal of Community & Applied Social Psychology, 32*(3), 438-451. doi:org/10.1002/casp.2564

Levi, M., & Stoker, L. (2000). Political trust and trustworthiness. *Annual Review of Political Science, 3*(1), 475-507. doi:org/10.1146/annurev.polisci.3.1.475

Lunn, P., Belton, C., Lavin, C., McGowan, F., Timmons, S., & Robertson, D. (2020a). *Using behavioural science to help fight the coronavirus.* http://hdl.handle.net/10419/237928

Lunn, P. D., Timmons, S., Belton, C. A., Barjaková, M., Julienne, H., & Lavin, C. (2020b). Motivating social distancing during the Covid-19 pandemic: An online experiment. *Social Science & Medicine, 265,* 113478. doi:org/10.1016/j.socscimed.2020.113478

Maheux, A., & Price, M. (2016). The indirect effect of social support on post-trauma psychopathology via self-compassion. *Personality and Individual Differences, 88,* 102-107. doi:org/10.1016/j.paid.2015.08.051

Martínez, D., Parilli, C., Scartascini, C., & Simpser, A. (2021). Let's (not) get together! The role of social norms on social distancing during COVID-19. *PloS One, 16*(3), e0247454. doi:org/10.1371/journal.pone.0247454

Matos, M., McEwan, K., Kanovský, M., Halamová, J., Steindl, S. R., Ferreira, N., Linharelhos, M., Rijo, D., Asano, K., Vilas, S.P., & Márquez, M.G. (2021). The role of social connection on the experience of COVID-19 related post-traumatic growth and stress. *PloS One, 16*(12), e0261384. doi:org/10.1371/journal.pone. 0261384

McCoy, J., Rahman, T., & Somer, M. (2018). Polarization and the global crisis of democracy: Common patterns, dynamics, and pernicious consequences for democratic polities. *American Behavioral Scientist, 62*(1), 16-42. doi.org/10.1177/ 0002764218759576

Mollen, S., Rimal, R. N., Ruiter, R. A., & Kok, G. (2013). Healthy and unhealthy social norms and food selection. Findings from a field-experiment. *Appetite, 65*, 83-89. doi:org/10.1016/j.appet.2013.01.020

Murphy, K. (2005). Regulating more effectively: The relationship between procedural justice, legitimacy, and tax non-compliance. *Journal of Law and Society, 32*(4), 562-589. doi:org/10.1111/j.1467-6478.2005.00338.x

Murray, D. R., & Schaller, M. (2012). Threat (s) and conformity deconstructed: Perceived threat of infectious disease and its implications for conformist attitudes and behavior. *European Journal of Social Psychology, 42*(2), 180-188. doi:org/10.1002/ejsp.863

Neville, F. G., Templeton, A., Smith, J. R., & Louis, W. R. (2021). Social norms, social identities and the COVID-19 pandemic: Theory and recommendations. *Social and Personality Psychology Compass, 15*(5), e12596. doi:org/10.1111/spc3.12596

Okun, M. A., Karoly, P., & Lutz, R. (2002). Clarifying the contribution of subjective norm to predicting leisure-time exercise. *American Journal of Health Behavior, 26*(4), 296-305. doi:org/10.5993/AJHB.26.4.6

Pagliaro, S., Sacchi, S., Pacilli, M.G., Brambilla, M., Lionetti, F., Bettache, K., Bianchi, M., Biella, M., Bonnot, V., Boza, M., & Butera, F. (2021). Trust predicts COVID-19 prescribed and discretionary behavioral intentions in 23 countries. *PloS One, 16*(3), e0248334. doi:org/10.1371/journal.pone.0248334

Peng, X., Zhao, H.-z., Yang, Y., Rao, Z.-l., Hu, D.-y., & He, Q. (2021). Post-traumatic growth level and its influencing factors among frontline nurses during the

COVID-19 pandemic. *Frontiers in Psychiatry, 12,* 632360. doi:org/10.3389/fpsyt.2021. 632360

Reid, A. E., Cialdini, R. B., & Aiken, L. S. (2010). Social norms and health behavior. In A. Steptoe, K. Freedland, J. R. Jennings, M. M. Llabre, S. B. Manuck, & E. J. Susman (Eds.), *Handbook of behavioral medicine: Methods and applications* (pp. 263–274). Springer Science + Business Media.

Reny, T. T., & Barreto, M. A. (2022). Xenophobia in the time of pandemic: othering, anti-Asian attitudes, and COVID-19. *Politics, Groups, and Identities, 10*(2), 209-232. doi:org/10.1080/21565503.2020.1769693

Roberto, K. J., Johnson, A. F., & Rauhaus, B. M. (2020). Stigmatization and prejudice during the COVID-19 pandemic. *Administrative Theory & Praxis, 42*(3), 364-378. doi:org/10.1080/10841806.2020.1782128

Romer, D., & Jamieson, K. H. (2020). Conspiracy theories as barriers to controlling the spread of COVID-19 in the US. *Social Science & Medicine, 263,* 113356. doi:org/10.1016/j.socscimed.2020.113356

Roozenbeek, J., Schneider, C. R., Dryhurst, S., Kerr, J., Freeman, A. L., Recchia, G., Van Der Bles, A. M., & Van Der Linden, S. (2020). Susceptibility to misinformation about COVID-19 around the world. *Royal Society Open Science, 7*(10), 201199. doi:org/10.1098/rsos.201199

Rothschild, Z. K., Landau, M. J., Sullivan, D., & Keefer, L. A. (2012). A dual-motive model of scapegoating: displacing blame to reduce guilt or increase control. *Journal of Personality and Social Psychology, 102*(6), 1148. doi:org/10.1037/a0027413

Sabucedo, J.-M., Alzate, M., & Hur, D. (2020). COVID-19 and the metaphor of war (COVID-19 y la metáfora de la guerra). *International Journal of Social Psychology, 35*(3), 618-624. doi:org/10.1080/02134748.2020.1783840

Scholz, J. T. (1998). Trust, taxes, and compliance. *Trust and governance, 1,* 135.

Schubert, C. F., Schmidt, U., & Rosner, R. (2016). Posttraumatic growth in populations with posttraumatic stress disorder — A systematic review on growth-related psychological constructs and biological variables. *Clinical Psychology & Psychotherapy, 23*(6), 469-486. doi:org/10.1002/cpp.1985

Shi, T. (2001). Cultural values and political trust: A comparison of the People's Republic of China and Taiwan. *Comparative Politics,* 401-419. doi:org/10.2307/422441

Smith, L. E., Amlôt, R., Lambert, H., Oliver, I., Robin, C., Yardley, L., & Rubin, G. J. (2020). Factors associated with adherence to self-isolation and lockdown measures in the UK: A cross-sectional survey. *Public Health, 187*, 41-52. doi:org/10.1016/j.puhe.2020.07.024

Sorokowski, P., Groyecka, A., Kowal, M., Sorokowska, A., Białek, M., Lebuda, I., Dobrowolska, M., Zdybek, P., & Karwowski, M. (2020). Can information about pandemics increase negative attitudes toward foreign groups? A case of COVID-19 outbreak. *Sustainability, 12*(12), 4912. doi:org/10.3390/su12124912

Stallard, P., Pereira, A. I., & Barros, L. (2021). Post-traumatic growth during the COVID-19 pandemic in carers of children in Portugal and the UK: Cross-sectional online survey. *BJPsych Open, 7*(1). doi:org/10.1192/bjo.2021.1

Tandoc, E., & Mak, W. (2020). Forwarding a WhatsApp message on COVID-19 news? How to make sure you don't spread misinformation. *Channel News Asia*.

Tedeschi, R. G., & Calhoun, L. G. (2004). Target Article: "Posttraumatic Growth: Conceptual Foundations and Empirical Evidence". *Psychological Inquiry, 15*(1), 1–18. https://doi.org/10.1207/s15327965pli1501_01

Traxler, C., & Winter, J. (2012). Survey evidence on conditional norm enforcement. *European Journal of Political Economy, 28*(3), 390-398. doi:org/10.1016/j.ejpoleco.2012.03.001

Tsamakis, K., Tsiptsios, D., Ouranidis, A., Mueller, C., Schizas, D., Terniotis, C., Nikolakakis, N., Tyros, G., Kympouropoulos, S., Lazaris, A., & Spandidos, D. A. (2021). COVID-19 and its consequences on mental health. *Experimental and Therapeutic Medicine, 21*(3), 1-1. doi:org/10.3892/etm.2021.9675

Tyler, T. R. (1990). Why people obey the law: Procedural justice. *Legitimacy, and Compliance*.

Bavel, J. J. V., Baicker, K., Boggio, P. S., Capraro, V., Cichocka, A., Cikara, M., Crockett, M. J., Crum, A. J., Douglas, K. M., Druckman, J. N., & Drury, J. (2020). Using social and behavioural science to support COVID-19 pandemic response. *Nature Human Behaviour, 4*(5), 460-471. doi:org/10.1038/s41562-020-0884-z

Van der Weerd, W., Timmermans, D. R., Beaujean, D. J., Oudhoff, J., & Van Steenbergen, J. E. (2011). Monitoring the level of government trust, risk perception and intention of the general public to adopt protective measures during the influenza A (H1N1) pandemic in the Netherlands. *BMC Public Health, 11*(1), 1-12. doi:org/10.1186/1471-2458-11-575

Vindegaard, N., & Benros, M. E. (2020). COVID-19 pandemic and mental health consequences: Systematic review of the current evidence. *Brain, Behavior, and Immunity, 89,* 531-542. doi:org/10.1016/j.bbi.2020.05.048

WHO. (2020). Coronavirus. https://www.who.int/health-topics/coronavirus#tab=tab_1

Woelfert, F. S., & Kunst, J. R. (2020). How political and social trust can impact social distancing practices during COVID-19 in unexpected ways. *Frontiers in Psychology, 11,* 572966. doi:org/10.3389/fpsyg.2020.572966

Wu, X., Kaminga, A. C., Dai, W., Deng, J., Wang, Z., Pan, X., & Liu, A. (2019). The prevalence of moderate-to-high posttraumatic growth: A systematic review and meta-analysis. *Journal of Affective Disorders, 243,* 408-415. doi:org/10.1016/j.jad.2018.09.023

COVID-19 AND THE ETHICS OF GRIEF AND LOSS

Zachary C. Wooten[1] and Haley McDevitt[2]

Abstract: Pervasive throughout the ongoing COVID-19 pandemic is the experience of grief and loss. Losses of varying magnitudes challenged communities to endure sustained trauma, commit to personal and communal sacrifice, all while living with intensifying grief. Hospitalized individuals died alone, unable to hold the hands of loved ones in their final hours. Rites of passage never happened, leaving many with a lack of resolve and sense of closure. For many individuals, the grief was experienced without the coping mechanisms of gathering, embracing loved ones, or even rituals such as funerals. Eventually, recalling what was once "normal" felt like looking into a time capsule: decades from familiarity. Ethical issues continue to arise when considering the tension between public health and psychological, sociological, and spiritual needs for communities coping with loss and complicated grief. When considering how to work constructively with complicated grief, it is first important to make space for the naming of that which is lost. Then, one can identify the ethical dilemmas contributing to the strain of navigating such loss. Finally, it is essential to offer resources for a way forward with the ethics of grief and loss; in this case, a care ethics approach proves most useful.

The Choices of Grief

Early on during the COVID-19 pandemic, Amanda Gorman, the first United States' National Youth Poet Laureate, wrote a poem entitled, "The Miracle of Morning." Searching for hope and yearning for healing amidst grief and despair, she remarked, "Do not ignore the pain. Give it purpose. Use it" (Gorman, 2021, p. 174). She concluded another poem, "The Shallows," with the lines, "Watch us move above the fog / Like a promontory at dusk. / Shall this leave us bitter? / Or better? / Grieve. / Then

---

[1] Instructor, West Chester University, West Chester, Pennsylvania, USA

[2] Marketing Director, Marketing Insider Group, West Chester, Pennsylvania, USA

choose" (p. 24). Notably, Gorman did not invite her suffering and frayed country to ignore its pain, yet at the same time she did not give her fellow citizens permission to give way to the pull of apathy or despair. To choose between bitterness and betterment is one of many ethical dilemmas facing and awaiting individuals, organizations, and society at large. Those enacting leadership must hold the weight of their own decisions and the impact they have on others. Gorman's poetry called for a constructive approach to deal with the immense grief and immeasurable loss experienced due to a world ravaged by COVID-19. Scholarship and stories must reveal and explore the shadow the pandemic casted over life.

COVID-19's Shadow: Grief and Loss

Within a matter of months, COVID-19 spread to more than 189 countries and territories, and as a result, the World Health Organization declared COVID-19 as a pandemic (Sheposh, 2022). As of April 2022, there were "more than 495.49 million reported cases of COVID-19 around the world, [and m]ore than 6.16 million people ha[ve] died" (Sheposh, 2022). Furthermore, for all those who died there are even more who now must live without loved ones. Parents, siblings, children, friends, caregivers, teachers, and others cling to memories of the deceased; surely the choice between *bitter* and *better* is even more challenging for them. Though scholars and society at large will be dealing with the layered aftermath of the COVID-19 pandemic for decades to come, one area of inquiry is essential for consideration: grief, loss, and the ethical deliberations they require.

Pervasive throughout the ongoing pandemic is the experience of grief and loss. Synthesizing previous research looking at the impact of infectious disease outbreaks on experiences of grief and loss, Mayland et al. (2020) observed that previous pandemics included experiences of loss "both directly related to death itself and also in terms of disruption to social norms, rituals, and mourning practices" (p. 33). Thus, pandemics consistently lead to the increased likelihood of "complicated grief," an intense and layered grief that can limit one's day-to-day functioning, a grief that requires attention, intention, and genuine care (Burke & Neimeyer, 2013).

When considering how to work constructively with complicated grief, it is first important to make space for the naming of that which is lost. Then, one can identify the ethical dilemmas contributing to the strain of navigating such loss. Finally, it is essential to offer resources for a way forward with the ethics of grief and loss; in this case, a care ethics approach proves most useful. In the case of the complicated grief brought about by COVID-19, there is a true litany of loss that society and its leaders must acknowledge.

A Litany of Loss: Grief Upon Grief

Losses of varying magnitudes challenged communities to endure sustained trauma, commit to personal and communal sacrifice, all while living with intensifying grief. Though it may take years to unearth the layers of loss, several losses are front of mind for many. Such losses include the loss of self-concept, community, financial resources, autonomy and plans, life, grieving rituals, and still other losses whose full impact remains unknown.

Loss of Self Concept

Who am I? Loss itself can shake one's foundation and answers to this question. Who am I without my loved one? Who am I if I cannot do my work? Who am I apart from those I love? Who am I apart from the self I thought I would be? Who am I without my routines, rhythms, and rituals? Who am I now that everything has changed?

For those less close to suffering, the pandemic challenged narratives of predictability and invincibility. For those who knew the shadow of suffering as well as their own shadows, the new struggles compounded upon old scars and gaping wounds. For society at large, the pandemic in many ways serves as a historical marker of "before" and "after": a faultline of tragedy (Bowler, 2018). Will we ever be who we were before? What if *after* cannot be better than *before* (Bowler, 2018)? Such questions are disorienting, disheartening, and at times, dissatisfying. For better or worse, the self is a relational construct. We form our sense of self *because of* and *in spite of* our relationships, and thus the loss of self runs parallel to a loss of community.

Loss of Community

For many, life before the pandemic offered an unknown sense of stability in terms of support networks and social groups. COVID-19 was not the first struggle most humans faced, but it was a unique struggle due to the resources of relationship and community suddenly transformed to threats to wellbeing. To be human is to connect with others. How can we be human if we are not being human *together*? While some found ways to rally their communities virtually or through disease-mitigating efforts, others navigated solitude with resilience, taking up new hobbies or engaging in self-reflection. After all, often "the most lonely, frustrated people...[are] people who are addicted to social interaction" (Selby, 1998, p. 45). At the same time, there is a difference between chosen solitude and entrapped loneliness, and COVID-19 exacerbated an already existent public health crisis: the crisis of loneliness (Murthy, 2020). To be isolated and alone with one's thoughts can lead some to focus on their inability to escape themselves. At the most heightened states of the pandemic, many were met with staunch comparisons and contradicting ideas, especially since no one's experience of the pandemic was identical. People did not start on a level playing field, and like any crisis, some fared better than others. Additionally, according to the Center for Disease Control (2021), social isolation is not only "associated with about a 50% increased risk of dementia," but also "increases a person's risk of premature death from all causes." Loss of community and connection with others propelled many within our society into a desperate survival mode.

Such desperation and struggle captured the imagination of the public and artists. For instance, one story that made it to the public eye was told in the documentary "Life of Crime: 1984-2020" (Alpert, 2021), which follows the lives of three people caught in a toxic cycle of crime and drug abuse in New Jersey. One of the subjects of the film, Deliris, was a beacon of recovery in her community until COVID-19 derailed her life and her support center (and primary means of community) closed down. After thirteen years of sobriety and dedication to helping others, Deliris lost her battle to addiction during the lockdown period of the pandemic. Deliris' story requires society to reflect on the immense grief that comes with a lack of community. Such a community offers one a sense of belonging one finds in support networks and social groups, those who understand our experiences and struggles and empower us to choose better instead of bitter. Without those communities, the choice is not always so easy. While some were baking bread and downloading TikTok, not everyone found coping mechanisms that worked. Some could not find comfort in solitude, they only found loneliness.

Making matters worse, the loss of in-person interaction drove individuals online, a mode of interaction marked by comparison and heightened anxiety or depression (Turkle, 2015). The loss of community made some wonder if they were the only ones feeling as lonely, disconnected, and desperate as they were. The plight of comparison tempted individuals toward resentment, particularly if they were also facing financial struggles.

Loss of Financial Resources

Due to our efforts to halt the transmission of COVID-19, many individuals, organizations, and nations faced economic fallout (Han et al., 2021, p. 5). Inflation, layoffs, and closures marked many economic reports as the pandemic raged on. Some had sacrificed everything for years to open a new business, only to have to shut their doors in a matter of months. Others had just made their Broadway debut only to change industries altogether by necessity. Many retired earlier than anticipated and others resigned due to unsafe working conditions. It is worth mentioning that in the United States, many women disproportionately chose to exit the workforce to navigate the stressors of childcare and cyber schooling (Hsu, 2021). This occurrence is just one example of the complicated grief facing those who were no longer living a life they had imagined, constrained by circumstance and obligation.

Another financial result of the pandemic was the "Great Resignation," a mass exit from the workforce, argued to reach its peak in 2021 with record-high quit rates (Parker & Horowitz, 2022). During the early months of the pandemic, individuals clung to any source of income to survive. Once the dust settled a bit and workers adapted to this "new normal," 2021 brought about conversations surrounding workplace flexibility, benefits, treatment, and compensation. The economic fallout and shakeup across industries left many companies disoriented and struggling to plan.

Loss of Autonomy and Plans

In order to combat the virus, leaders took protective measures, many of which required personal and communal sacrifice. Some of that sacrifice involved the reduction of agency. As many individuals and families' worlds shrunk to the size of their home or "pod" (a small social group sharing similar levels of precautionary measures to combat COVID-19), the positive-thinking mantra of "Anything is possible" sounded silly, trite, and taunting.

Moreover, the loss of an imagined or plannable future made life challenging for many. What was rolled out as "fifteen days to slow the spread" (Trump White House, 2020) in the United States quickly became a seemingly unending "new normal" (Columbia Broadcasting Company, 2022). Weddings were canceled, postponed, or altered. Collegiate and Olympic athletes missed their "big shot" at their dreams. Maintenance and life-saving medical procedures were delayed due to the overflow of patients in hospitals. Mothers were delivering their babies without their partners by their sides. It will never be possible to lend a voice to each gut-wrenching circumstance; still, leaders must offer care, empathy, and a listening ear. The life that should have been– the life that was *supposed to be*– wasn't, and some are struggling to engage their capacity to dream.

For instance, Dustin Jones of *National Public Radio* (2021) reported a story of a young woman named Audrey Ellis. Along with her twin sister, Kelsey, Audrey was celebrating her twenty-ninth birthday when she was misdiagnosed with pneumonia. Five days later, she died of organ failure related to COVID-19. Audrey, like Amanda Gorman, wanted people to learn from their pain. Audrey often told her sister, "Life is a classroom…We are here to make a difference and to learn our lessons" (Jones, 2021). Yet, those lessons are not always readily apparent, and as Jones (2021) pointed out, not all the classes were chosen electives… "like how long a cremation takes, how to pick up an urn from a drive-through window at a funeral home or the procedure for checking in human remains at the airport." Many of the mantras and sentiments that may have brought us comfort in the past no longer worked.

While the loss of plans can seem trivial compared to the loss of life, traumatic events are marked by stress to our fragile nervous systems. Lack of resolve or sense of closure are enough to cause residual, compounding stress over time. During a period where we all lived and breathed helplessness and uncertainty, trauma took an innumerable number of shapes and sizes, and loss of plans often coincided with loss of life.

Loss of Life

As of July 2022, over 6.3 million people have died due to COVID-19. This amount of death exceeds the number of deaths statistical models offer for anticipated deaths; therefore COVID-19 is an event of excess mortality or "mass death" (Han et al., 2021, p. 5). If one counts the secondary deaths caused by COVID-19 (for instance, due to economic constraints or limited opportunities for hospitalization, the death count is likely much higher (Han et al., 2021, p. 5). Though far from the minds of those aiming to "move on" from the pandemic, history will remember the "images of struggling intensive care units, overflowing mortuaries, and the construction of mass graves" (Han et al., 2021, p. 5). Such horrific death, Han et al. (2021) argue, is reordering the world politically, socially, and psychologically.

If there was any bright spot for parents amidst COVID-19, it was that children were less likely to die; however, the high number of adult deaths meant that a high number of children lost parents and caregivers to COVID-19-associated deaths. From "April 1, 2020, through June 30, 2021, [more than] 140 000 children in the United States experienced the death of a parent or grandparent caregiver" (Hillis et al., 2021, para. 3). Some of these children lived in communities in which the predominant view was the politicized notion that COVID-19 was a hoax, further complicating their grief.

Perhaps some of the most haunting images of the pandemic were the scenes of those forced to say goodbye over video calls, unable to hold the hands of those who loved them. Such a death adds a sharpness to the broken hearts, shards of what should have been left lying on the ground for hospital workers to discard. Perhaps those who experienced such devastating loss may take comfort in the words of Nuland (1994): "The dignity that we seek in dying must be found in the dignity with which we have lived our lives...The art of dying is the art of living...Who has lived in dignity, dies in dignity" regardless of circumstance (p. 268). Such a sentiment may be comforting in retrospect, but at the time, no words could match the pain of being so disconnected from a loved one as they breathed their last breath.

Loss of Grieving Rituals

Many individuals experienced grief in response to the pandemic *without* the coping mechanisms of gathering, embracing loved ones, or even sacred rituals such as funerals. The precarity surrounding memorial services added to the already heavy and impossible feelings of grief. Amidst the standard yet tragic questions such as "What will we do without you?" and "Why did you have to go?" mourners faced an avalanche of new questions: "Are we allowed to have a service?", "Are we allowed to hug one another?", "Do we have to limit the number of attendees?" The questions were endless. The answers were unclear or dissatisfying.

Not to mention, for those left behind, life kept happening. COVID-19 was on the rise, but death loomed large over the living. It would be difficult to find someone untouched by COVID-19, indirectly or directly. In this upside-down universe, funerals were live-streamed on social media due to capacity limitations. Saying goodbye to one's grandmother over Facebook live was gut wrenching and deeply unsettling.

Some rituals were canceled altogether in fear of spreading the virus, and those who returned to such rituals during safer days may have felt removed from their grief and sense of time. Losing a loved one can be unbearable, and without the support offered by rites, rituals, and relationships, the loss is unfathomable. The withdrawal of coping methods impacted those experiencing first-hand loss, as in the loss of a loved one, but this loss also impacted hospital workers who had to fill in the emotional gaps while being overburdened with their own tasks and anxieties.

In May of 2020, Sam Foster, Chief Nurse at Oxford University Hospitals, wrote in the *British Journal of Nursing* about the challenges health leaders faced, particularly in the earliest months of the pandemic. For healthcare workers on the frontlines of the pandemic, their experience was marked with "little-to-no down time...and a steady stream of anxiety-provoking media" (p. 585). Furthermore, Foster (2020) revealed a number of concerns not only for healthcare providers enduring the worst of the health crisis, but also mentioned the toll the experience took on those who lived with or cared about such health professionals (p. 585). As evinced, the circles of complicated grief are ever-expanding.

Future Losses and Impact of Loss

While we have named a significant number of losses, tidily categorized yet disruptive and disorienting experiences, further discourse is necessary to unpack the losses, either unmentioned or still unknown. Perhaps the most dynamic loss, one of such magnitude that only time can reveal, is the loss of trust in our systems and one another, including but not limited to: media, politics, government, institutions, employers, and neighbors. In 2022, individuals are left to their own devices to piece together the truth, even now – in the aftermath of information overload and bias. How has our family or institution treated the media? Where do we stand politically on the matter, and should this even *be* a matter of politics? The politically fraught nature of leaders' response to the pandemic will take decades to parse out, if it is even possible for historians to eventually come to some kind uniform conclusion. Who do we trust to share unbiased, factual information?

For now, a vague picture exists. By March 2021, there had been "a deep decline (17 points) in trust for national health authorities such as the CDC [Center for Disease Control] and FDA [Food and Drug Administration] ..."

(Edelman, 2021). If trust in institutions and fellow humans continue to decline, it will take more than positive leaders to reshape and rebuild our societies. For now, it is worth exploring several ethical dilemmas facing leaders as a result of this litany of loss.

The Ethics of Grief and Loss Amidst COVID-19: Leadership Challenges

Ethical issues continued to arise when considering the tension between public health and psychological, sociological, and spiritual needs for communities coping with loss. Individuals at any level faced ethical dilemmas amidst grief and loss during the pandemic, but those engaged in roles and processes of leadership encountered ethical challenges in particularly pronounced ways. For instance, at many levels of political and corporate leadership, choices between economic health and public health competed in numerous ways. On one hand, if facing mass death, the economy would surely suffer, so apathy toward the public health crisis would be damaging economically in the long run anyway. On the other hand, mitigation efforts closed businesses that led to other public health concerns for those struggling to feed themselves or their loved ones. Individuals had to make decisions for themselves: "Is my job safe enough for me to go, but if I do not work, how will I pay my bills?" Those involved in leadership were responsible for themselves and their loved ones as well as the needs of their organizations, constituencies, and communities. This responsibility was a psychological burden not uncommon for leaders but magnified in the face of an extended crisis.

Evaluating the Past

Part of leaders' ethical deliberations need to evaluate the decisions of the past. Acknowledging that many decisions needed to be made before much scientific evidence existed, and recognizing that the virus was and is ever-evolving, leaders ought to consider the extent to which the emotional cost of the pandemic decision-making was weighed adequately. Moreover, leaders must evaluate if the decisions made were humane and whether or not they honored and supported the grief of those experiencing the worst of the pandemic's outcomes. Some individuals may have or currently be experiencing guilt– guilt for enjoying parts of COVID-19's impact, guilt for thriving during the pandemic, guilt for decisions made that hurt people, or survivor's guilt for somehow being less scathed by the virus than others. Leaders could very well be facing moral injury as an after-effect of COVID-19 decision-making– something that requires care and consideration in the years ahead (Griffin, 2019).

Looking Ahead: What Does it Mean to Value a Human Life?

During and after the pandemic, the value of health and our duty to one another took and will take center stage as competing values seemed to hover over every interaction, no matter how trivial. Han et al. (2021) asked the question, "How will, and should politics value human lives in the post-pandemic world" (p. 5)? One popular option for leaders, particularly political leaders, is to distance public narratives away from COVID-19 and instead shift from "mitigation" to "recovery" (Han et al., 2021, p. 6). To an extent, this response is unsurprising. Many individuals and communities cope with traumatic experiences through distancing from them in one way or another. Yet, as Gorman suggested, leaders cannot ignore pain, nor can they allow pain to crush them. Leaders must remember the loss of human life and the value of human life, especially the interconnectedness of human life. Amidst all these pressing ethical dilemmas, how should leaders respond?

Ethical discourse often begins with descriptive questions or claims, questions such as "What is going on?" Upon adequately describing an experience, prescriptive questions emerge: "What should be going on, and what should we do about it?" Now that we have described the gravity of grief and loss caused by the pandemic, we ought to pivot to prescriptive concerns of what should be done and what tools are available to leaders in the future.

Constructive Solutions: Employing an Ethic of Care

As individuals and communities struggle to find resources to assist them with navigating the ethical dilemmas related to grief, loss, and COVID-19, one ethical theory proves especially useful. Along with scholars like Corbera et al. (2020), we posit that the COVID-19 pandemic is a reminder of the importance and applicability of the "ethics of care" (p. 192). This sentiment is especially true for those engaged in leadership.

What is Ethics of Care?

Ethics of care is a moral theory which articulates the moral import of relationships and the interdependence of humanity (Sander-Staudt, 2022). Such an approach requires those engaged in the leadership process to attend to relational maintenance, care for the vulnerable, and the needs of both oneself and others (Sander-Staudt, 2022). These concerns require malleability and adaptability above absolutes and imperatives. Emphasizing adaptation and interdependence points leaders and organizations to adapt to an ever-evolving world and collaborate with other leaders and organizations to generate solutions (Maryland et al., 2020, p. 33). For instance, the availability for remote work provides additional onramps for employment amidst other life responsibilities. Leaders are wise to remember they need not return to old ways of navigating life and work simply because they were the ways of the past. Crisis can drive innovation at the same time grief is honored. Leaders should not rush to find lessons amidst suffering, forcing the tyranny of gratitude upon trauma. At the same time, to work constructively with grief, leaders can invoke the ethics of care by focusing on truth-telling, hopefulness, and joy.

Caring as Truth-Telling

The ethics of care encourages telling the truth about our experiences, particularly painful ones. Swentzell (1997) emphasized the truth-telling about pain that can be born of the realization of our interdependence, saying,

> If we would realize we are all in the same boat, then we would be ahead. I hope we can all realize that we are very sad, blind people right now and that all of us are searching for what we long for–a place, a sense of importance, and love...I would like us to be able to communicate with each other in a

way that we never could before...You are searching for love and I am searching for it, too...We will be able to say *When I cry I know she will understand why I am crying*...Then when you cry in front of me I can say *Go ahead, cry*. At that time we will have peace. (p. 222)

In this sense, those enacting leadership must engage in the rich and challenging work of creating communities in which the truth of community members' experience can be told, honored, and preserved. Truth-telling is an act of trust-building, and as with other instances of mass death, such as the violence of Apartheid-era South Africa, truth-telling will be the pathway to reconciliation and renewal. In this sense, the ethics of care offers leaders a hopeful future.

Caring as Hopefulness

Amidst apathy, loss, and turmoil, the philosophical notion of care and the leadership act of caring serves as a foundation for moving forward with grief rather than dismissing, downplaying, or ignoring it. In a season marked by disconnection and fragmented leadership, the ethics of care provides an innately hopeful and flexible response to ethical deliberation and decision-making. Those who study and practice leadership know that leadership is fundamentally asking and answering questions about what it means to be human and what it means to be human together. The conceptual framework of care ethics provides helpful tools to engage such questions. In particular, Noddings (1984) described,

> The relation of natural caring will be identified as the human condition that we, consciously or unconsciously, perceive as *good*. It is the condition toward which we long and strive, and it is our longing for caring–to be in that special relation–that provides the motivation for us to be moral. We want to be moral in order to remain in the caring relation and to enhance the idea of ourselves as one-caring. It is this ethical ideal, this realistic picture of ourselves as one-caring, that guides us as we strive to meet the other morally. Everything depends upon the nature and the strength of this ideal, for we shall not have absolute principles to guide us. (p. 5)

To view the human condition as good and to view human care as motivation for moral activity is a view that is inherently hopeful, and perhaps restoratively so. As the pandemic contributed to the decline of trust in institutions and one another, a primary strategy for leaders engaging the ethical complexity of grief and loss is to pursue the ethical ideal of mutual care and affection for humanity. As the world continues to change because of the pandemic or new crises, care stands as a grounding force for transformation and steadying joy.

Caring as Transformative Joy

Once the worst of the pandemic is far behind us in the rearview mirror, our communities will continue to grapple with the various losses accumulated throughout the crisis. It remains to be seen, but the collective trauma may drive leaders to "shift expectations about our work, the way we communicate with each other..." (p. 196). Utilizing a care ethics approach, leaders may evaluate the social-political aspects of life through attention to vital biological needs, the development and sustainability of our professional and social lives. Moreover, the ethics of care invites leaders to focus on the fullness of human experience–grief as well as joy. Noddings (1984) explained, "The occurrence of joy is a manifestation of receptive consciousness... Joy's occurrence and recurrence maintains us in caring, and thus, contributes to the enhancement of the ethical ideal" (p. 147). Utilizing an ethic of care, leaders can foster truthfulness, hopefulness, and even joy amidst grief and loss.

Closing Remarks: Bitter, Better, or Beyond?

Without a doubt, leaders and followers alike cannot and should not ignore the pain caused by COVID-19. As meaning-making creatures, we will continue to make sense of our pain and "give it purpose," as Gorman suggested (2021, p. 174). Leadership itself is a meaning-making process, and to address the future with authenticity and respect for humanity, those engaged in leadership must commit to acknowledging and constructively working with grief. Shall we become bitter, better, or something else altogether? Time will tell.

References

Alpert, J. (Director). (2021). *Life of crime: 1984-2020* [Film]. Downtown Community Television Center.

Burke, L. A. & Neimeyer, R. A. (2013). Prospective risk factors for complicated grief: A review of the empirical literature. In M. Stroebe, H. Schut, & J. van den Bout (Eds.), Complicated *grief: Scientific foundations for health care professionals* (pp. 145-161). Routledge/Taylor & Francis Group.

Bowler, K. (2018, January 29). *Before and after* [Video]. Facebook. https://www.facebook.com/katecbowler/videos/before-aftera-tragedy-is-like-a-fault-line-a -life-is-split-into-a-before-and-an-/415096342238061/

Center for Disease Control. (2021, April 29). *Loneliness and social isolation linked to serious health conditions.* https://www.cdc.gov/aging/publications/features/lonely-older-adults.htm

Columbia Broadcasting System. (2022). *The "new normal" according to the CDC* [Video]. https://www.cbsnews.com/video/the-new-normal-according-to-the-cdc/

Corbera, E., Anguelovski, I., Honey-Rosés, J., & Ruiz-Mallén, I. (2020). Academia in the time of COVID-19: Towards an ethics of care. *Planning Theory & Practice, 21*(2), 191–199. https://doi.org/10.1080/14649357.2020.1757891

Edelman, R. (2021, March). *2021 Edelman trust barometer special report: Trust and the Coronavirus.* Edelman. https://www.edelman.com/trust/2021-trust-barometer/trust coronavirus-us

Foster, S. (2020). These are the hands that care. *British Journal of Nursing, 29*(10), 585. https://doi.org/10.12968/bjon.2020.29.10.585

Gorman, A. (2021). *Call us what we carry.* Penguin Young Readers Group.

Griffin, B. J., Purcell, N., Burkman, K., Litz, B. T., Bryan, C. J., Schmitz, M., Villierme, C., Walsh, J., & Maguen, S. (2019). Moral injury: An integrative review. *Journal of Traumatic Stress, 32*(3), 350-362. https://doi.org/10.1002/jts.22362

Han, Y., Millar, K. M. & Bayly, M. J. (2021). COVID-19 as a mass death event. *Ethics & International Affairs 35*(1), 5-17.

Hillis, S. D., Blenkinsop, A., Villaveces, A., Annor, F. B., Liburd, L., Massetti, G. M., Demissie, Z., Mercy, J. A., Nelson, C. A., Cluver, L., Flaxman, S., Sherr, L., Donnelly, C. A., Ratmann, O., & Unwin, H. J. T. (2021). COVID-19–associated orphanhood and caregiver death in the United States. *Pediatrics, 148*(6). doi: 10.1542/peds.2021-053760

Hsu, A. (2021, June 4). *Millions of women haven't rejoined the workforce — and may not anytime soon* [Radio broadcast]. NPR. https://www.npr.org/2021/06/03/1002402802/there-are-complex-forces-keeping-women-from-coming-back-to-work

Mayland, C. R., Harding, A. J. E., Preston, N., Payne, S., & Harding, A. J. (2020). Supporting adults bereaved through COVID-19: A rapid review of the impact of previous pandemics on grief and bereavement. *Journal of Pain & Symptom Management, 60*(2), e33–e39. https://doi.org/10.1016/j.jpainsymman.2020.05.012

Moore, B. (2020). Dying during Covid-19. *Hastings Center Report, 50*(3), 13–15. https://doi.org/10.1002/hast.1122

Murthy, V. H. (2020). *Together*. Harper Collins Publishers.

Noddings, N. (1984). *Caring: A relational approach to ethics & moral education*. University of California Press.

Nuland, S. B. (1994). *How we die: Reflections of life's final chapter*. AA Knopt: Distributed by Random House.

Parker, K., & Horowitz, J. M. (2022, March 10). *Majority of workers who quit a job in 2021 cite low pay, no opportunities for advancement, feeling disrespected*. Pew Research Center. https://www.pewresearch.org/fact-tank/2022/03/09/majority-of-workers-who-quit-a-job-in-2021-cite-low-pay-no-opportunities-for-advancement-feeling-disrespected/

Sander-Staudt, M. (2022). Care ethics. In C. B. Wrenn (Ed.) *The internet encyclopedia of philosophy*. https://iep.utm.edu/care-ethics/

Selby, J. (1998). *Solitude: The art of living with yourself*. Heartsfire Books. Sheposh, R. (2022). Coronavirus disease 2019 (COVID-19). *Salem Press Encyclopedia of Health*.

Swentzell, R. (1997). *Hearing with our hearts*: Interview with Lois Crozier-Hogle and Ferne Jensen. In *Surviving in two worlds: Contemporary Native American voices*. University of Texas Press.

Trump White House. (2022). *15 Days to slow the spread.*
    https://trumpwhitehouse.archives.gov/articles/15-days-slow-spread/

Turkle, S. (2017). *Alone together: Why we expect more from technology and less from each other.* Basic Books.

PART TWO
Social (in)justice

VALUE-BASED INTEGRATED CARE: THE FOUNDATIONS OF A GLOBAL HEALTH ETHICAL APPROACH TO IMPROVING COVID-19 VACCINATION READINESS IN LOW-AND-MIDDLE-INCOME COUNTRIES

Benjamin Roth[1] and Max Alexander Matthey[2]

Abstract: During the COVID-19 pandemic, it proved extremely difficult to achieve a high vaccination rate in the global south. The reasons for this are complex - too little vaccine was supplied by the donor countries and, in addition, not all of the doses supplied could be used due to logistical problems and / or regional skepticism against the vaccines. As a consequence, people in poor countries of the world have a much worse chance to be supplied quickly with effective vaccine, prevailing inequalities are manifested, and people are denied their right to health. From a Global Health Ethics perspective, it is therefore imperative to address the problem to ensure better vaccine management for future pandemics: the goal should be to ensure that everyone who wants to be vaccinated - no matter what region of the world she lives in - has access to vaccine. To achieve this goal, we propose an approach that focuses on suffering reduction as the central normative aspect. At the operational level, this should be achieved by organizing vaccine delivery around the patient's treatment pathway in the spirit of Value-Based Integrated-Care. This requires a precise analysis of the respective situations on the ground in order to establish social institutions and economic incentives that will lead to rapid and comprehensive vaccine distribution.

Keywords: Global-Health-Ethics, LMICs, Suffering, Vaccination, Value-Based Healthcare, Integrated Care

---

[1] Research Associate, Center for Health Ethics, Hannover, Germany
[2] Director of Communication, Incentives for Global Health, USA

Introduction: Vaccine distribution problems in Low-and-Middle-Income Countries

Lower Middle-Income Countries are those whose annual GNP is $4,095 or less. By contrast, the GNP of Low-Income Countries (LICs) is only $1,045 or less (World Bank, 2020). The widespread poverty in these societies is also accompanied by numerous health-related problems at the individual and population level - which were particularly evident during the COVID-19 pandemic: both Low-Income Countries and Lower Middle-Income Countries (LMICs) - usually have very low vaccination rates for COVID-19. With an African vaccination rate below 30% in April 2022, it is still below 10% in seven African countries and even below 1% in two of them (Statista, 2022). One significant reason for this is the low supply of vaccines from high-income nations – some "have hoarded vast quantities of doses" (Jerving, 2021, p. 827) – but there also is a variety of problems on the ground as even delivered doses are not being completely inoculated locally. The reason for this often lies in a combination of exceeding the expiration date, "access" issues, e.g., "logistical barriers" (Saso et al., 2020, p. 1) and vaccine skepticism. In some African countries "hesitancy is high [and] trust low" (Seydou, 2021, p. 1). The reasons for this also have a historical background – Flint (2020) notes that Africa long served as a 'living laboratory' for colonial powers. The last known clinical trial conducted illegally in Africa was in 1996. There, 100 children were given a new, not yet approved meningitis drug without informing the parents or obtaining their consent (Lenzer, 2006; Wise, 2001).

These long-cultivated practices are one reason why there is little trust in vaccination campaigns or vaccines coming from the United States or Europe today. In addition, interventions in LMICs are often done ad hoc and do not take into account local conditions such as poverty and poor infrastructure (Kim, Farmer, et al., 2013) or other cultural concepts of illness, death, or healing; these interventions are often paternalistic "top-down approaches" (Martins, 2021, p. 101).

The vaccination-problem in LMICs has so far received insufficient attention from the scientific community. Thus Simas & Larson (2021, p. 1) mention that vaccine skepticism "remains vastly understudied in low-income and middle-income regions." Without understanding the regional conditions and the wishes, expectations and fears of local populations and their economic and material realities, neither the existing nor the COVID-related problems will be solved. Therefore, the purpose of global health ethics is to address the complete social structures that cause health-related suffering and death and transform them "into structures that give life and life in abundance" (Daly, 2021a, p. 94). It is crucial for the challenge of vaccinations that solution strategies are holistic and take into account "regional, cultural, and economic factors" (Simas & Larson, 2021, p. 2).

To meet this ambitious target, a comprehensive ethical approach to Global Health is developed in the following that combines two approaches:

(1) The ethical premise of minimizing suffering (negative consequentialism).

(2) A value-based healthcare approach adapted to the problem at hand.

The result is a value-based concept explaining how to foster COVID-19 vaccination readiness and furthermore, how future pandemics in LMICs could be countered more comprehensively, faster and - above all - more ethically.

Suffering, Vulnerability and negative ethics

Hunger, poor medical care, lack of sanitation, and poor hygiene are sadly commonplace in many LMICs. Especially on the African continent, the situation is sometimes dramatic - not only regarding vaccine distribution. For example, 96 percent of all malaria deaths in 2020 occurred in Africa with children under five accounting for an estimated 80 % of all malaria deaths in the Region (World Health Organization, 2022). Further, HIV/AIDS is still a leading cause of morbidity and mortality in sub-Saharan Africa (Dwyer-Lindgren et al., 2019). All these conditions are associated with great suffering for those affected. However, the concept of suffering of medical ethics and palliative care neglects these systemic and structural conditions - it focuses solely on the suffering of a sick patient (Martins, 2021, p. 100).

Svenaeus's Phenomenological concept of suffering can be considered a good example here. For him, suffering is "an alienating mood overcoming a person and engaging her in an embodied struggle to remain at home in the face of the loss of meaning and purpose in life" (Svenaeus, 2014, p. 413). Specifically, suffering manifests itself in physical and psychological states and conditions: "Intolerable pain. Not being able to breathe. Constant nausea. Leaking urine and faeces. Not being able to do basic things, such as eating, going to the toilet, reading, and moving around. Becoming dependent upon or a burden to close others. Not having a place and purpose in the world anymore. Losing one's memory and sanity. No longer being in control" (Svenaeus, 2020, p. 336). However, suffering is not limited to one phase or area of life, but can occur at any time in any person – as part of the 'conditio humana'.

Nevertheless, suffering occurs more frequently in old age - where palliative institutions try to minimize the suffering of those affected as much as possible. The concept of suffering in palliative care focuses not only "on the physical dimension of pain, but also addresses the dying patient's psychological, social, and spiritual suffering" (Streeck, 2020, p. 343). This has also been referred to as the 'total-pain' approach since as early as 1964 (Saunders, 1964). For individual ethical questions, this is also sufficient and appropriate - but global health is particularly concerned with the structural conditions of suffering. This requires an extension of the definition of suffering to the supra-individual structural level.

This extension is partly covered by the concept of vulnerability, which is also widely discussed in medical ethics: it describes the broader scope of health care that extends beyond the individual context; families, groups, communities, populations, and countries can be described as vulnerable (Clark & Preto, 2018). This makes it quite clear that the health and well-being of an individual depend to a large extent on the structural conditions for self-care. The Report of the International Bioethics Committee of UNESCO illustrates how broad these conditions can be. There, poverty, discrimination, environmental catastrophes, and many others are mentioned under the term social vulnerability (UNESCO, 2013).

However, it is not entirely clear what the vulnerability discourse ultimately refers to; it could either be about stigmatized groups, or about a concept of protection in medical ethics that takes effect when the classic four principles[3] are no longer sufficient to protect the person concerned. Perhaps it also directly addresses the structures of illness and poverty and would thus be located more on the socio-ethical level. Vulnerability would thus come very close to a structural concept of suffering. Nevertheless, it is not advisable to adopt the vulnerability concept for global health and especially vaccination issues. As outlined above, western people and their concepts are often met with skepticism in LMICs - too often, supposedly well-intentioned interventions have been perceived as paternalistic or even exploitative. Also, the concept of vulnerability is therefore accompanied by an implicit paternalism - which was also partly evident in the Corona crisis when dealing with at-risk groups (Egeolu et al., 2021). This is because the concept of vulnerability usually – as during the COVID-19 pandemic - refers to groups. However, it does not reflect whether the possible members of this group agree with the attribution: not every old person, every African woman or poor worker considers himself vulnerable. On the contrary, mastering one's personal lives under deficient conditions can rightfully be understood as an expression of significant personal strength and autonomy. While this does not change the critical nature of the structures in question, it also shows that people have their own experiences that should be respected. In this sense, Martins (2021) emphasizes that Global North aid workers and scientists can also learn by listening to the voices and experiences of the poor.

Therefore, a concept that is understood from a holistic socio-ethical analysis of suffering is to be preferred. Suffering is not a paternalistic concept, but the expression of a self-experience that is rooted in the natural constitution of the human body. However, this self-experience can also have its causes in extracorporeal - namely in structural - problems and dysfunctionalities and thus are to be interpreted in socio-ethical terms. If suffering is to be the starting point of our investigation, however, the next step is to ask what ethical value can be ascribed to suffering.

---

[3] The four principles of Beauchamp and Childress are autonomy, non-maleficence, beneficence and justice (Beauchamp & Childress, 2001) – they "have been extremely influential in the field of medical ethics, and are fundamental for understanding the current approach to ethical assessment in health care" (Page, 2012, p. 1)

Suffering as a negative moral value

Since suffering is a negative moral value (Lowry & Schüklenk, 2009) from a normative perspective, it seems appropriate to assume an ethical obligation to eliminate or at least minimize suffering. When the reduction or avoidance of a negative value rather than the increase of a positive one is the focus of moral action or normative deliberation, we can speak of 'negative ethics' (Guseinov, 2014). The best-known variation of this school of thought is negative utilitarianism.

Academic reflection on the negative ethics tradition does not play a central role and is also frequently rejected (Griffin, 1979; Smart, 1958). This is not self-evident, since the oldest ethical rules, e.g. the 10 commandments of the Bible, are mostly (8 of 10) formulated negatively (e.g. *You **shall not** kill).* However, formulations alone are not yet the decisive factor. The crucial question is why negative normative statements should be more recommendable for global ethics than positive ones. Popper (1966, p. 284) was one of the first to introduce the concept of negative utilitarianism to the world. He claims that the reduction of "human suffering" – in contrast to the increase of happiness - "makes a direct moral appeal, namely the appeal for help." Furthermore, negative statements are mostly unambiguous: I don't want to be beaten, killed, starved or kidnapped - these are clear interests that formulate precise expectations for action (Ropohl, 1996). In a positive sense, I expect my counterpart to respect me, treat me according to my dignity and help me in problematic situations. This is all true, but highly open to interpretation and my counterpart cannot be sure what my actual expectations and interests are. As the decision makers in politics and economies may have quite different ideas about what "the greatest happiness of the greatest number" or "good and desirable actions" may be, the structural and systemic level of this problem is even bigger. In the end, states may "fall into a paternalism that degenerates too easily into tyranny" (Griffin, 1979, p. 47).

Starvation, however, is a clear negative value that calls everyone to action - even if they have opposing concepts of happiness, prosperity, or economics. The reason why all people can recognize hunger as a universal negative value is that it is rooted in the immediate basic physical needs of every human being; unlike experiences of happiness, which often cannot be shared intersubjectively. The thought of having children represents for some the very essence of their life's, while others see having children as the destruction of their careers. Between these two poles, there is little room for shared positive experiences. Nevertheless, even those who do not want offspring would recognize that it would surely be something negative if someone else's child were to starve. Thus, suffering-oriented ethics can show particularly clearly that all people - regardless of their socioeconomic status, religion, race, origin, age or sexual identity - have the same moral status, which rests on the intersubjective experience of the satisfaction or non-satisfaction of basic needs.

The suffering of unsatisfied basic needs

But before we can go in praxis, a precondition must be explained: which kind of suffering should be the focus of consideration? After all, even a billionaire can *suffer* from the fact that his neighbor has been to space. With a negative-utilitarian approach, which would only be a reversal of classical utilitarianism, one would risk that this suffering of 100 or 1000 millionaires could weigh more heavily than the suffering of a starving person. This objection is to be taken very seriously, since in such a case, the suffering focus could even lead to a worse position of poor people compared to rich ones. Thus, a suffering-centered ethics cannot always be about the suffering of all people - it requires a concretization of the concept of suffering. This is to be achieved by interpreting the concept of suffering in a preferential-utilitarian way and by linking it back to Maslow's (1943) hierarchy of needs.

On the left, we can see Maslow's stages of needs in pyramid form. "Immediate Physiological Needs" and "Safety" are the first two and basic levels. For a person to freely develop and self-actualize, these must be fulfilled. Unlike growth needs, the individual is not able to satisfy its basic needs alone. Without cooperation, she cannot build a sewerage system, establish a police force, or introduce a constitutional state - all this and much more can only be realized in community. Thus, the responsibility for creating structures that best prevent or minimize suffering rests with society and its institutions. Negative ethics approaches are thus no substitute for positive ethics concepts, but necessary supplements.

Fig. 1: *Own representation*

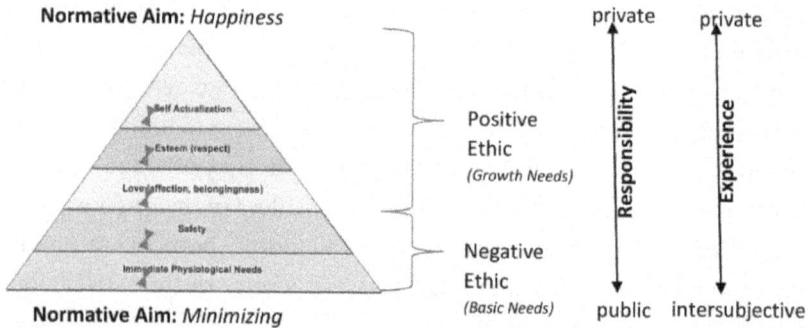

Regarding the question of what kind of suffering should be the focus of global health efforts, the ethical answer can only be the kind of suffering that relates to basic needs. Ethically permissible, suffering can be set off against each other only if it is suffering of the same level: during a famine, it may be ethically legitimate to follow a negative utilitarian approach in the distribution of food aid. One can make an argument to focus the delivery of aid to populations easier to reach if also helping populations in areas difficult to reach would be accompanied by significant spoilage of restricted food resources. In contrast, offsetting between different levels is not ethically permissible: physiological needs thus can't be offset with needs of 'self-actualizing' or 'esteem'.[4] So, some rich people may intersubjectively feel the suffering of not having been in the universe; nevertheless, this suffering - even if thousands may feel so - cannot outweigh the hunger of a single person. Basic needs have not only descriptive but also normative priority over all other needs.

The normative basis: suffering-based preference utilitarianism

This approach is therefore a variant of preference utilitarianism - however, in the concept of suffering presented here, we assume that certain needs are not only expressions of subjective, personal interests/preferences, but

---

[4] Little noted in research so far is that Bentham already designed a hierarchy of pleasures and sufferings that should be used to measure happiness and suffering. Here, too, food and drink are at the top of the list (Bentham, 2000).

intersubjectively shared, objective needs of the human body. These basic needs are grounded on physicality and thus on human nature, which is the starting point of all kinds of needs and ethics.

Value-Based-Healthcare: Incentives as tools and institutions as addressees of global health ethics

Reducing fundamental suffering – and not just collecting and shipping vaccine doses is thus the overarching normative goal of holistically designed vaccination campaigns in resource-poor settings. Suffering reduction in this context presupposes that the sick person feels perceived as a self-responsible, serious and thus sovereign subject. Therefore, suffering reduction cannot be achieved by a paternalistic top-down approach. From an ethical perspective, the goal regarding vaccination should rather be that the person can make an informed decision to be vaccinated and that the necessary resources are available to do so. The bioethical autonomy principle is therefore also crucial for global health ethics.

In summary, it can be concluded that this is an integrative approach that understands the suffering of the sick person as an objective expression of her personhood and corporeality, which thus represents a call for help to the entire global community: considered are not only singular interventions, but the entire vaccination process from first patient contact to monitoring – with individual patients in focus. The Value-Based-Healthcare-Approach (VBHC) of Porter and Teisberg serves as a model for the further procedure (Porter, 2010; Porter & Teisberg, 2006).

Value-Based-Healthcare: The Concept of Porter and Teisberg

Modern health care systems are characterized by a high degree of complexity and hence partly contradictory target dimensions. Since we understand global-health ethics methodologically as social ethics, we need to look as closely as possible at how global care structures work before practical recommendations: "Just as one cannot make a cogent moral claim about abortion before one knows what a fetus, zygote, or blastocyst is, one cannot make strong socioethical claims if one does not know what a structure is and how structures and agency relate" (Daly, 2021b, p. 63).

The basis for a comprehensive structural analysis is that economic efficiency and medical progress are in a state of tension - in addition, different interests clash, which can only be realized at the expense of the other side. Porter calls this a "zero-sum-competition" (Porter & Teisberg, 2006): individual commercialization interests of service providers, for example, are opposed to the economic interests of payers. VBHC tries to overcome these tensions by combining medical and economic rationality to one holistic target point: the patient value. 'Value' represents here the quotient of outcome (O) and cost (C); the lower the cost and the higher the outcome, the better the 'value' (Tunder & Ober, 2020). The value does not refer to a single intervention or the sum of different interventions, but to the entire 'care cycle' of a specific patient. This care cycle also includes personal wishes and needs, as well as her quality of life. In a broad VBHC approach, the beginning of a care cycle lies in the causes that lead to a disease, i.e. poverty, poor infrastructure or lack of health education and awareness (Kim, Farmer, et al., 2013; Kim, Porter, et al., 2013). Thus, the VBHC approach embeds the individual care cycle in the regional and economic treatment context. The entire process is always guided by the basic idea of "value for money " (Jackson, 2011). This means that the number of services provided, or the mere maintenance of specific infrastructure is no longer decisive for funding, but only the benefit ('value') that patients derive from the treatment or the treatment pathway. The phrase 'value for money' represents the actual core idea, but in practice people tend to talk about 'pay-for-performance' (Engineer, 2015) or 'performance-based payment' (Mousaloo et al., 2021). However, this is rather a financing principle for individual interventions and actions than a comprehensive system. The VBHC approach therefore represents the first holistic cross-system pay-for-performance approach to establishing and managing a complete health care system, which puts the patient-needs at the center.

Pay-for-Performance schemes in the healthcare sector

In the following it will be shown how pay-for-performance (P4P) works. P4P represents a concept for financing physician and medical services. In contrast to the still predominant fee-for-service, it does not reward the number of services provided, but their 'quality'. Here, 'quality' must not be understood as a defined quantity - rather, it is an intervention-specific criterion that is first defined and then to be achieved, minimized or maximized. Examples of such a criterion might include treatment time, mortality rate, quality of life, or sequelae. Through predetermined measurement procedures, the final impact of the intervention is measured retrospectively (Veit, 2012) and assigned a monetary value. If the impact is worse than initially expected, money is deducted or less is transferred to the provider. If, on the other hand, the provider meets or exceeds the targets, he receives a bonus. Thus, remuneration is always dynamic and depends on the success of the service provided. This shows that P4P usually only covers one component of the total payment amount. As a definition, we therefore propose:

*P4P in health care are **criteria-based**, **dynamic** billing models for physician (treatment) or medical (drugs, medical devices) services, the monetary amount of which depends on the actual, **retrospectively determined** success of the service provided and usually concerns a part of the negotiated or ensued total amount in the form of surcharges or discounts.*

In addition, P4P can take place at any of the three levels of intervention (micro, meso, and macro levels). The micro-level is the societal level where – 'face-to-face' – individual actions take place. The meso level already belongs to the collective level. Here, institutions and collective actors, such as companies, public authorities, hospitals or NGOs act and communicate. Accordingly, the macro level is the system level where societal subsystems such as the economic, legal or health care systems meet. This also includes the sum of nation-state rules, laws, and institutions (Figure 2).

Fig. 2: *Own representation*

Individual	Micro Level: Patient, Physician…	P4P-Mechanism: P4P for individual remuneration; P4P for patients (e.g. compliance)
Collective	Meso Level: Hospital, Medical office…	P4P-Mechanism: P4P in health maintenance organizations; 'integrated care'
	Macro Level: Health Care System…	P4P-Mechanism: Health Impact Fund (HIF)

There are already P4P models at all three levels. Micro-level programs are well studied for both HICs and LMICs. In contrast, the 'Health Impact Fund' (HIF), launched by philosopher Thomas Pogge and economist Aidan Hollis, focuses on the macro level. Its goal is to make medicines affordable for poor populations in LMICs (Pogge, 2012). But the situation is different at the meso level. There are P4P programs here as well, for example at the Health Maintenance Organizations (Rosenthal et al., 2006) in the United States. However, there are hardly any programs or studies concerning LMICs. This is especially true for health care ethics. At the same time, we know very well that local institutions are particularly important for the reduction of suffering, for subsidiary participation and thus also for the acceptance of those affected locally (Daly, 2021a; Farmer & Vicini, 2021; Putera, 2017). Strengthening these institutions not only helps the sick and suffering, but can also help to overcome the vicious circle of poverty and disease, since functioning institutions are also the basis for sustainable, prosperity-enhancing economic growth (Clark, 2007; Mokyr, 2009).

Value Based-Healthcare and integrated care – practical perspectives to improving COVID-19 vaccination readiness in LMICs

A broad VBHC approach that also considers the conditions and preconditions of illness and suffering must also be based on a comprehensive concept of health. Poor nutrition, lack of access to clean water, unemployment, housing, and inadequate public infrastructure are thus part of global health (Kim, Farmer, et al., 2013). Thus, these issues must also become part of the care cycle. After all, patients living in rural areas can only see a doctor if public transportation exists. Poor people can only leave their jobs for medical treatment if they are compensated for lost wages, and treatment against bacterial diseases can only be sustainable if patients have access to clean water. De Campos (2017) distinguishes between availability issues and access issues in the context of global drug supply. In addition, there are also challenges in patient information. Applied to the vaccination problem, this means that vaccination readiness in resource-poor settings will only occur on a larger scale if the following aspects are taken into account.

Availability issues

(a) Vaccines and vaccination personnel are available.

Access issues

(b) People know when and where they can get vaccinated.

(c) People can get to immunization sites by bus, train, or other means of public transport.

(d) People are compensated for lost work time and other costs incurred.

Information issues

(e) People are informed about benefits and risks.

(f) Information about vaccine damage and adherence problems is provided openly and transparently.

According to the VBHC approach, all these points are part of the Care Cycle and must therefore be considered. To date, the various issues have often been addressed in isolation. This is however not unexpected; as an example, there are different responsibilities for public infrastructure than for vaccine acquisition. In addition, funding budgets in healthcare are usually earmarked and do not take account actual needs; the money can often only be used to fund drugs, medical devices or to reimburse physicians for their services. Delivery- or travel costs are not reimbursed.

To overcome this fragmented system (Porter & Lee, 2018) and thereby increase vaccination readiness, a transformation of health care delivery into an integrated system is needed (Kim, Farmer, et al., 2013). Since 'integrated care is "intersectoral, networked and collaborative" (Tunder & Ober, 2020) and "focuses on reducing the fragmentation of care, thereby improving outcomes for [...] patients by coordinating care providers along a patient's pathway" (Busink et al., 2019, p. 157). The idea is to assemble all stakeholders involved in a care pathway - whether they are part of the healthcare system or not – in the form of an 'Integrated Care Unit' (Porter & Lee, 2018) which is not based on their interests, but solely in terms of their responsibility for improving the patient value. It is therefore also referred to as "value-based integrated care" (Valentijn et al., 2016). Such a process is, of course, characterized by a high degree of complexity - if it is to succeed, it requires targeted and, above all, locally accepted incentives and institutions. Ideally, they form a VBHC-framework that can be adapted regionally and that must be filled with life by the local people, NGOs, government authorities and other stakeholders, depending on the regional characteristics (Fig. 3).

Fig.3: *The model was taken from the WHO working document "Integrated care models: an overview" (Satylganova, 2016) and slightly modified.*

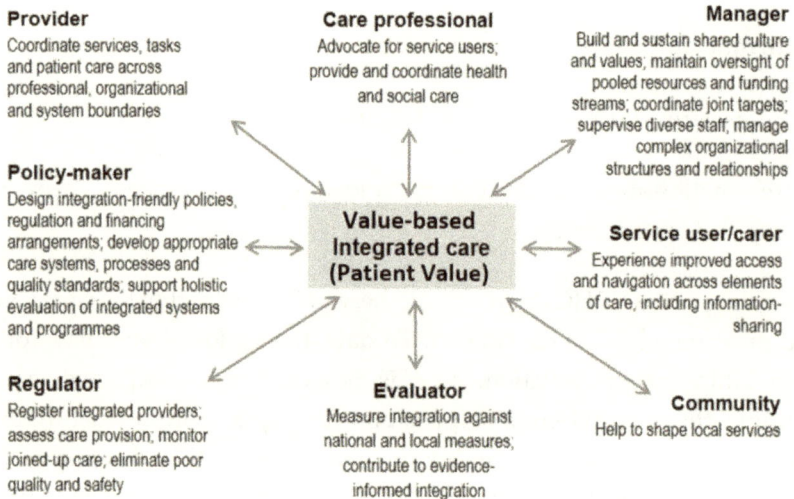

In order to make this complexity operationalizable, it must be limited to one aspect - such as kidney disease (Busink et al., 2019), chronic disease (Ouwens et al., 2005), or even pandemic vaccination in LMICs.

Thus, a vaccination system functionally integrated around the care cycle is at the heart of a VBHC approach. The vaccine-related value (V$_{fac}$) is thus the quotient of the total patient outcome (O) and the total costs of points (a) to (f).

$$Vfac = \frac{O(a \to f)}{C(a \to f)}$$

5. Findings and Recommendation

With this essay, we try to reflect on the problem of missing vaccinations in LMICs on a fundamental basis. The approach of focusing on suffering reduction rather than the maximation of happiness requires further elaboration - especially in the field of applied ethics. Regarding basic needs such a change in perspective is associated with the hope of achieving concrete improvements for the world's poor more quickly. It should not be decisive whether ethical or health-scientific concepts and theories are critical of the state or the economic system, or whether they correctly address guilt and responsibility in the abstract. What matters in the end is whether the approaches help in practice to improve people's situation - as the business ethicist Pies (2019, p. 12) also noted with regard to the ethical methodology: "The proof of the pudding is in the eating."

Nevertheless, the VBHC system also comes with some weaknesses: it has not yet been applied on a larger scale in LMICs. Though conversions of health systems to VBHC models are already underway in many countries, these are almost always high-income countries. For example, the *Cleveland Clinic* in the United States and the *Schön Clinics* in Germany have switched to VBHC (Porter & Lee, 2018) - and the pricing of new drugs in Germany has also been value-based since 2011 (Tunder & Ober, 2020). Here, it has been positively demonstrated that the costs saved far exceed the costs incurred by VBHC - such as administrative and organizational costs. Nevertheless, many LMICs and especially LICs will not be able to cover the costs and organization from their own resources. Ongoing international assistance from donors, NGOs, and other forms of transnational development aid will be and are needed. A major advantage of the integrated VBHC approach is that it is explicitly linked to existing institutions. At this point, ethics plays a special role yet again - it has the task of offering principles that can help to ensure that this encounter of non-regional structures with regional institutions takes place respectfully and on an equal footing. Economic incentives play an important role here. If, for example, horse-drawn carts or oxen are still an important means of transport in a country, there is nothing to stop VBHC from paying coachmen to transport patients. Certainly, this may not be a solution for acute emergencies - but for transports of patients willing to be vaccinated, it may be an efficient, quickly implemented, and regionally accepted solution. Regional healers without academic medical training play a major role in many African countries and can also be offered incentives to support regional vaccination campaigns - they enjoy the trust of local people and can therefore have a positive influence on their vaccination decisions. They can then accompany this vaccination with alternative medical methods, such as the "Covid Organics" (Richey et al., 2021). Finally, the vaccinated patients must be compensated for the costs incurred by the vaccination to maximize the incentive for vaccination. Since this concept relates the maximum possible outcome in relation to its costs, its aim is to ensure that the scarce financial resources available in LMICs are used efficiently without losing sight of the patient or focusing one-sidedly on the costs. Initial studies also show that such concepts have great prospects of success. In Nigeria, for example, outcome-based structures that directly addressed institutions were introduced in three regions. As a result, "the average coverage for fully vaccinated children increased from 1.4% to 49.2%" (Odutolu et al. 2016, p. 297) in just two years. Finally: As a positive side-effect, this way it also strengthens the regional economy and thus comes closer to the ultimate goal of breaking the vicious circle of poverty and disease in LMICs.

References

Beauchamp, T. L., & Childress, J. F. (2001). *Principles of biomedical ethics* (5. Aufl.). Oxford University Press.

Bentham, J. (2000). *An introduction to the principles of morals and legislation*. Batoche Books (eBook).

Busink, E., Canaud, B., Schröder-Bäck, P., Paulus, A. T. G., Evers, S. M. A. A., Apel, C., Bowry, S. K., & Stopper, A. (2019). Chronic kidney disease: Exploring value-based healthcare as a potential viable solution. *Blood Purification, 47*(1-3), 156–165.

Clark, B., & Preto, N. (2018). Exploring the concept of vulnerability in health care. *Canadian Medical Association Journal, 190*(11), 308–309. https://doi.org/doi: 10.1503/cmaj.180242

Clark, G. (2007). *A farewell to alms. A brief economic history of the world*. Princeton University Press.

Daly, D. J. (2021a). Social structures and global public health ethics. In *Ethical challenges in global public health. Climate change, pollution, and the health of the poor* (S. 85–96). Pickwick Publications.

Daly, D. J. (2021b). *The structures of virtue and vice.* Georgetown University Press.

de Campos, T. C. (2017). *The global health crisis. Ethical responsibilities.* Cambridge University Press.

Dwyer-Lindgren, L., Cork, M. A., Sligar, A., Steuben, K. M., Wilson, K. M., Provost, N. R., Mayala, B. K., VanderHeide, J. D., Collison, M. L., Hall, J. B., & Biehl, M. H. (2019). Mapping HIV prevalence in sub-Saharan Africa between 2000 and 2017. *Nature, 570*(7760), 189–193.

Egeolu, M., Stoff, B. & Blalock, T. W. (2021). *The Effects of Paternalistic Policies During COVID-19 on Vulnerable Populations. Journal of the National Medical Association, 113*(3). https://doi.org/10.1016/j.jnma. 2020.11.013

Engineer, D. H., C. Y., Dale, E., Agarwal, A., Agarwal, A., Alonge, O., Edward, A., Gupta, S., Schuh, H. B., Burnham, G. & Peters, D. H. (2015). Effectiveness of a pay-for-performance intervention to improve maternal and child health services in Afghanistan: A cluster-randomized trial. *International Journal of Epidemiology, 45*(2), 451–459.

Farmer, P., & Vicini, A. (2021). An ethical agenda for global public health. In *Ethical challenges in global public health. Climate change, pollution, and the health of the poor* (S. 193–198). Pickwick Publications.

Flint, C. (2020). "Africa isn't a testing lab": Considering COVID vaccine trials in a history of biomedical experimentation and abuse. *Journal of West African History, 6,* 126–140.

Griffin, J. (1979). Is unhappiness morally more important than happiness? *The Philosophical Quarterly, 29,* 47–55.

Guseinov, A. A. (2014). Negative ethics. *Russian Studies in Philosophy, 52*(3).

Jackson, P. (2011). *Value for money and international development: Deconstructing myths to promote a more constructive discussion.* Directorate, OECD Development Co-operation. https://www.oecd.org/development/effectiveness/49652541.pdf

Jerving, S. (2021). The long road ahead for COVID-19 vaccination in Africa. *The Lancet World Report, 398,* 827–828.

Kim, J. Y., Farmer, P., & Porter, E. M. (2013). Redefining global health-care delivery. *Lancet*, 1060–1069.

Kim, J. Y., Porter, M., Rhatigan, J., Weintraub, R., Basilico, M., Hoof Holstein, C., & Farmer, P. (2013). Scaling up effective delivery models worldwide. In *Reimagining global health: An introduction* (1. Edition, S. 184–211). University of California Press.

Lenzer, J. (2006). Secret report surfaces showing that Pfizer was at fault in Nigerian drug tests. *BMJ, 332*, 1233.

Lowry, C., & Schüklenk, U. (2009). Two models in global health ethics. *Public Health Ethics, 2*(3), 276-284.

Martins, A. A. (2021). Ethics and equity in global health: The preferential option for the poor. In *Ethical challenges in global public health. Climate change, pollution, and the health of the poor*. Pickwick Publication.

Maslow, A. (1943). A theory of human motivation. *Psychological Review, 50,* 370–396.

Mokyr, J. (2009). *The enlightened economy. An economic history of Britain 1700-1850*. Yale University Press.

Mousaloo, A., Amir-Behghadami, M., Janati, A., & Gholizadeh, M. (2021). Exploring the challenges and features of implementing performance-based payment plan in hospitals: A protocol for a systematic review. *Systematic Reviews, 10*, 1–7. https://doi.org/10.1186/s13643-021-01657-x

Odutolu, O., Ihebuzor, N., Tilley-Gyado, R., Martuf, V., Ajuluchukwu, M., Olubajo, O., Banigbe, B., Fadeyibi, O., Abdullhai, R. & Muhammad, A. J. G. (2016): Putting institutions at the center of primary health care reforms: Experience from implementation in three states in Nigeria. *Health Systems & Reform 2*(4), 290-301.

Ouwens, M., Wollersheim, H., Hermens, R., Hulscher, M., & Grol, R. (2005). Integrated care programmes for chronically ill patients: A review of systematic reviews. *International Journal for Quality in Health Care, 17*(2), 141–146. https://doi.org/10.1093/intqhc/mzi016

Pies, I. (2019). *Interview: Innovationen und institutionen: über markt, moral und moderne*. Lehrstuhl für Wirtschaftsethik an der Martin-Luther-Universität Halle-Wittenberg.

Pogge, T. (2012). The health impact fund: Enhancing justice and efficiency in global health. *Journal of Human Development and Capabilities, 13*(4), 537–559. https://doi.org/10.1080/19452829.2012.703172

Popper, K. (1966). *The open society and its enemies.*

Porter, M. (2010). What is value in health care? *The New England Journal of Medicine, 363*, 2477–2481.

Porter, M. E., & Teisberg, E. (2006). *Redefining health care. Creating value-based competition on results.* Harvard Business School Press.

Porter, M. E. & Lee, T. H. (2018). The strategy that will fix health care. In M. E. Porter & T. H. Lee (Hrsg.), *On strategy for healthcare* (S. 229–262). Harvard Business Review Press.

Putera, I. (2017). Redefining health: Implication for value-based healthcare reform. *Cureus, 9*(3).

Richey, L. A., Gissel, L. E., Kweka, O. L., Bærendtsen, P., Kragelund, P., Hambati, H. Q., & Mwamfupe, A. (2021). South-South humanitarianism: The case of Covid-organics in Tanzania. *World Development, 141*, 105375. https://doi.org/10.1016/ j.worlddev.2020.105375

Ropohl, G. (1996). *Ethik und technikbewertung.* Suhrkamp.

Rosenthal, M. B., Landon, B. E., Normand, S. T., Frank, R. G., & Epstein, A. M. (2006). Pay for performance in commercial HMOs. *New England Journal of Medicine, 355*, 1895–1902.

Saso, A., Skirrow, H., & Kampmann, B. (2020). Impact of COVID-19 on immunization services for maternal and infant vaccines: Results of a survey conducted by imprint— The Immunising Pregnant Women and Infants Network. *Vaccines, 8*(3), 556.

Satylganova, A. (2016). *Integrated care models: An overview.* World Health Organization. https://www.euro.who.int/__data/assets/pdf_file/0005/322475/ Integrated-care-models-overview.pdf

Saunders, C. (1964). The symptomatic treatment of incurable malignant disease. *Prescribers' Journal, 4*(4), 68-73.

Seydou, A. (2021). *Who wants COVID-19 vaccination? In 5 West African countries, hesitancy is high, trust low.* https://media.africaportal.org/documents/ad432-covid 19_vaccine_hesitancy_high_trust_low_in_west_africa-afrobarometer-8march21.pdf

Simas, C., & Larson, H. J. (2021). Overcoming vaccine hesitancy in low-income and middle-income regions. *Nature Reviews Disease Primers, 7,* 41. https://doi.org/10.1038/s41572-021-00279-w

Smart, R. N. (1958). Negative utilitarianism. *Mind, 67,* 542–543.

Statista. (2022, April 23). *Number of administered coronavirus (COVID-19) vaccine doses per 100 people in Africa as of April 23, 2022, by country.* https://www.statista.com/statistics/1221298/covid-19-vaccination-rate-in-african-countries/

Streeck, N. (2020). Death without distress? The taboo of suffering in palliative care. *Medicine, Health Care and Philosophy, 23,* 343–351. https://doi.org/10.1007/s11019-019-09921-7

Svenaeus, F. (2014). The phenomenology of suffering in medicine and bioethics. *Theoretical Medicine and Bioethics, 35*(6), 407–420. https://doi.org/doi:10.1007/s11017-014-9315-3

Svenaeus, F. (2020). To die well: The phenomenology of suffering and end of life ethics. *Medicine, Health Care and Philosophy, 23,* 335–342. https://doi.org/10.1007/s11019-019-09914-6

Tunder, R., & Ober, J. (2020). Value-based health care—Impulse und implikationen für den deutschen arzneimittelmarkt. In *Market Access Management für Pharma- und Medizinprodukte* (S. 103–123). Springer Nature.

United Nations Educational, Scientific and Cultural Organization (UNESCO) (Hrsg.). (2013). *The principle of respect for human vulnerability and personal integrity. Report of the International Bioethics Committee of UNESCO (IBC).* https://unesdoc.unesco.org/ark:/48223/pf0000219494

Valentijn, P., Biermann, C., & Bruijnzeels, M.A. (2016). Value-based integrated (renal) care: Setting a development agenda for research and implementation strategies. *BMC Health Service Research, 16*(330), 1–11. https://doi.org/DOI 10.1186/s12913-016-1586-0

Veit, Ch., Hertle, D., Bungard, S., Trümner, A., Ganske, V., & Meyer-Hofmann. (2012). *Pay-for-performance im Gesundheitswesen: Sachstandsbericht zu Evidenz und*

Realisierung sowie Darlegung der Grundlagen für eine künftige Weiterentwicklung. Ein Gutachten im Auftrag des Bundesministeriums für Gesundheit (BQS-Institut, Hrsg.).

Wise, J. (2001). Pfizer accused of testing new drug without ethical approval. *BMJ, 322,* 194.

World Bank (Hrsg.). (2020). *The World Bank in middle income countries.* https://www.worldbank.org/en/country/mic/overview#1

World Health Organization (Hrsg.). (2022). *Malaria. Key facts.* https://www.who.int/news-room/fact-sheets/detail/malaria

EQUITABLE ALLOCATION, DISTRIBUTION, AND UPTAKE OF VACCINES FOR COVID-19: MITIGATION OF HEALTH INEQUITIES

Helene Gayle[1] and James Childress[2]

Abstract: This chapter examines the disparities in impact associated with the SARS-CoV-2 virus, which causes COVID-19, in the United States, and the need to equitably allocate and distribute vaccines. Early pandemic data revealed that people of color were up to four times more likely to require hospitalization from COVID-19 than the White population and nearly three times more likely to die of the disease. Once a vaccine became available, the numbers were reduced but disparities persisted. These disparities were not due to biologic susceptibility of racial and ethnic minority groups; they were caused by racism and inequity. In order to reduce severe morbidity and mortality and negative societal impacts due to SARS-CoV-2, the National Academies of Sciences, Engineering and Medicine devised foundational principles relevant to this pandemic. They included: recognizing the immense health and economic impact of SARS-CoV-2; affirming that everyone has equal value; and addressing the disproportionate impact of COVID-19 on communities of color. As such, barriers to vaccination for people of color needed to be clearly understood and addressed. This attentive process can ascertain unrecognized or ignored barriers, hidden disincentives to vaccine uptake, sources of mistrust/distrust and measures to enhance trustworthiness, and effective ways to motivate vaccine uptake, perhaps including positive incentive rewards. Equitable allocation of vaccines to the most vulnerable is essential, where vulnerability includes heightened risks of infection, serious disease, hospitalization, and death. Additionally, disproportionately affected communities and populations must have meaningful access to vaccines as well as the means to receive them.

---

[1] President, Spelman College, Atlanta GA, USA. Former President and CEO, Chicago Community Trust, Chicago, Illinois, USA

[2] Professor Emeritus, University of Virginia, Charlottesville, Virginia, USA

Introduction: Health Disparities and Inequities in the Pandemic

Among each pandemic's distinctive features is its differential impact among populations. The 1918-1919 influenza pandemic in the United States, the H1N1 virus wreaked its havoc mainly among children under 5, adults aged 20-40, and older adults (CDC, n.d.). A "unique feature" of this pandemic was the high mortality among healthy people ages 20-40 (CDC, n.d.). By contrast, severe illness, hospitalization, and death associated with SARS-CoV-2 virus, which causes COVID-19, has been concentrated among people who are older and/or who have underlying health conditions (CDC, 2022a, 2022b). Other disparities in the impact of SARS-CoV-2 stem from and vividly reflect broader, underlying health inequities. (The term "disparities" denotes inequalities while the term "inequities" adds a moral dimension—that is, disparities that are also considered to be ethically unjustified results of inequitable structures and systems).

Evidence of the disparate impact of COVID-19 was clear by the early days of the vaccine rollout in December 2020 and January 2021. In comparison to White, non-Hispanic persons, American Indian or Alaskan Natives (AI/AN), Latinx, and Black persons were 80%, 70%, and 40% more likely, respectively, to become infected with SARS-CoV-2 (CDC, 2020a). People of color were also more likely to have serious cases of COVID-19, as AI/AN, Latinx, and Black communities were 4 times, 4.1 times, and 3.7 times more likely, respectively, than White people to require hospitalization after a COVID-19 diagnosis (CDC, 2020a). Compared to White people, AI/AN, Latinx, and Black people were 2.6 times, 2.8 times, and 2.8 times more likely to die of COVID-19 (CDC, 2020a).

Just over a year after the vaccine rollout, these disparities persist, although some progress has been made in reducing them. Data updated on February 1, 2022, show that, compared to White people, AI/AN, Latinx (or Hispanic), and Black people are 1.5 times, 1.5 times, and 1.0 times, respectively, as likely to be infected; 3.2 times, 2.4 times, and 2.5 times as likely to be hospitalized; and 2.2 times, 1.9 times, and 1.7 times as likely to die from COVID-19 (CDC, 2022b). The available vaccines effectively reduce the number of serious cases of COVID-19 and hence hospitalizations and deaths even though they are less effective in reducing infections by SARS-CoV-2 (CDC, 2022c). As we will argue, vaccine policies and practices can only achieve or approximate health equity when they increase vaccination uptake through fair allocation and distribution systems.

Disparate impacts of COVID-19 among racial/ethnic groups do not result from a biologic susceptibility of racial and ethnic minority groups to SARS-CoV-2 but rather from the socioeconomic conditions they face as direct and indirect effects of racism and structural injustice (Ogedegbe et al., 2020). The problem, in short, is racism rather than race, inequity rather than biology. Nationally, greater social and economic vulnerability in a particular geographic area strongly correlates with the risk of becoming a COVID-19 hotspot (Dasgupta et al., 2020).

People of color are more vulnerable to SARS-CoV-2 exposure, not because of their race or ethnicity but because they are disproportionately represented among low-paid essential workers who cannot work from home and who regularly lack adequate protection on the job (Hawkins, 2020; McNicholas & Poydock, 2020) and because they disproportionately reside in overcrowded living arrangements that increase the risk of transmission (Ahmad et al., 2020; CDC, 2020a). Communities of color also have higher rates of comorbid conditions that increase the likelihood of poor health outcomes following infection (Quinones et al., 2019).

Tragically, such racial, ethnic, and socioeconomic disparities and inequities in health outcomes are long-standing problems in this country, as diverse health indicators have long revealed disparities and inequities in health care access and outcomes (CDC, 2013). What is new about this moment is the coincidence of the COVID-19 pandemic with unprecedented national attention to the role and impact of racism across multiple domains of American life (Galston, 2020). The arrival of several safe, effective COVID-19 vaccines and planning for their allocation and distribution afforded an opportunity to "get this right" this time—at least to ensure that vaccination reached the most vulnerable communities rather than merely replicating and reinforcing underlying inequities (McClung, 2020).

In our judgment, "business as usual" could not ensure just and equitable access to COVID-19 vaccination (Gayle & Childress, 2021). The simple reason is established by historical experience: too often in the past, new medical breakthroughs exacerbated rather than reduced health disparities (Ganguly et al., 2019; Jung & Feldman, 2017; Kabria, 2019). To take only one among numerous possible examples, even though Black people are eight times more likely to be diagnosed with HIV than White people (CDC, 2019) coverage of highly effective HIV pre-exposure prophylaxis (PrEP) is seven times higher among Whites than among Blacks (Harris et al., 2019).

In that context, we (Gayle & Childress 2021) argued a year ago that commitment, innovation, and political and community engagement and leadership would be needed to ensure that the communities most at risk from COVID-19 had equitable access to vaccination and were also motivated to receive it. We believed then and now that it is crucial to prioritize the most vulnerable communities at each stage of roll-out, and to remove the various barriers that have long impeded robust uptake of new technologies in underserved communities.

Achieving equity in the allocation of vaccines requires a clear, intensive focus on ensuring strong uptake of vaccination in the most socially vulnerable communities. Realizing this goal demands approaches that grapple with the diverse socioeconomic factors that increase vulnerability in these communities and diminish their access to and ability to use essential health services.

Frameworks for Equitable Allocation and Distribution of COVID-19 Vaccines

Even though effective COVID-19 vaccines were developed at an unprecedented pace, it was inevitable that the demand would outstrip supply in the early stages of their roll-out. Anticipating this problem, the Centers for Disease Control and Prevention (CDC) and the National Institutes of Health (NIH) asked the National Academies of Sciences, Engineering and Medicine (NASEM—hereafter National Academies) to convene an ad hoc multidisciplinary committee to "develop an overarching framework" for the equitable allocation of vaccine, a high-priority public health tool, in the context of temporary but severe scarcity while the supply of vaccine could be expanded.[3] The sponsors sought such a framework to "assist" both domestic and global policy makers in their planning and to "inform" decisions by health authorities, including the CDC's independent Advisory Committee on Immunization Practices. The statement of task for the National Academies committee also called for the formulation of "criteria" for use in "setting priorities for equitable allocation of vaccine" and guidance on how these criteria should be applied in "determining the first tier of vaccine recipients" (National Academies, 2020, pp. 20-21). The multidisciplinary committee of experts convened by the National Academies sought to develop a framework to guide policy makers in maximizing the public health impact of COVID-19 vaccination and ensuring that vaccines were rolled out in a way that reduced rather than exacerbated underlying health disparities (National Academies, 2020).

The National Academies committee's statement of task was further elaborated in a virtual meeting with CDC and NIH officials, one of whom, the NIH director Francis Collins, called for the "overarching framework" to include "foundational principles" (National Academies, 2020, p. 91). Accordingly, in seeking to advance the goal of reducing severe morbidity and mortality and negative societal impacts due to SARS-CoV-2, the National Academies committee built its framework on key foundational principles relevant to this pandemic:

1. Maximum benefit: Taking account of the immense health and economic impact of SARS-CoV-2;
2. Equal concern: Affirming that everyone has equal value;
3. Mitigation of health inequities: Addressing the disproportionate impact of COVID-19 on communities of color (National Academies 2020).

---

[3] Both authors served on the National Academies committee—Helene Gayle was co-chair, and James Childress was a member.

In addition, the committee relied on three procedural principles:

1.   Fairness: Seeking and incorporating input from groups affected by vaccine allocations;
2.   Transparency: Communicating with the public openly, clearly, and accurately;
3.   Evidence-based: Basing all decisions on the best available scientific evidence (National Academies, 2020).

Around the same time, other public and private bodies were also formulating principles to guide vaccine allocation. There is substantial overlap but also distinctive features among several major sets of principles.

Principles in Different Frameworks of Allocation of COVID-19 Vaccine[4]

NASEM Committee's Framework (National Academies, 2020)	Johns Hopkins Interim Framework (Toner et al., 2020)	WHO SAGE Values Framework (WHO, 2020)	ACIP's Ethics Principles (McClung et al., 2020)
Maximum benefit	Promote public health & economic & social well-being	Human well-being	Maximize benefits & minimize harms
Equal concern		Equal respect	
Mitigation of health inequities	Address inequities Give priority to the worse off	Global Equity National Equity	Mitigate health inequities

---

[4] This table builds on and substantially updates the table in the National Academies report *Framework for Equitable Allocation of COVID-19 Vaccine* (National Academies, 2020, p. 93)

NASEM Committee's Framework (National Academies, 2020)	Johns Hopkins Interim Framework (Toner et al., 2020)	WHO SAGE Values Framework (WHO, 2020)	ACIP's Ethics Principles (McClung et al., 2020)
Fairness	Respect diversity of views in pluralistic society Engage community members	Legitimacy	Promote justice
Transparency	[Incorporated into previous principles]	[Incorporated into legitimacy above]	Promote transparency
Evidence-based	*[Assumed in other frameworks]*		
	Reciprocity	Reciprocity	

Drawing on the principles it developed, in part in dialogue with these other approaches, the committee formulated allocation criteria based on risks: the risk of acquiring or transmitting the virus, the risk of severe disease or death, and the risk of negative societal impacts. In applying these risk-based criteria, the committee quickly moved away from the conventional language of "tiers" to the language of "phases" to identify and characterize priority groups and to delineate the sequence of vaccine roll-out. The term "tiers" inherently denotes a hierarchy, even a hierarchy of value, in a static structure, whereas the term "phases" captures fluidity in the movement toward the goal of providing the vaccine to everyone. The process involves "phasing in" the vaccine in a time of scarcity but with a commitment to vaccinate everyone who is willing to be vaccinated as soon as possible (National Academies, 2020).

The committee developed a four-phase allocation framework that prioritizes vaccination in the earliest phases for those with the highest risk, starting with frontline health and other emergency workers, the elderly in congregate settings, and people with health conditions that increase their risk for severe disease or death. Subsequent phases prioritize vaccination from highest to lowest risk categories. The final phase includes low-risk people residing in the United States, regardless of their legal status.

Equity as a Cross-cutting Consideration in COVID-19 Vaccine Allocation and Distribution

The National Academies committee recognized that scarcities of supply would probably mark each of the vaccination phases it proposed. If health care delivery systems simply operated as usual, the most vulnerable communities would inevitably be left behind at least for a time. This would delay the benefits of vaccination for the very communities that most urgently needed protection from SARS-CoV-2. The co-chairs of the National Academies committee stressed: "We do far more harm, and kill far more people, by our errors of omission, rather than by our errors of commission" (National Academies, 2020, p. xix). Using COVID-19 vaccination as an opportunity to avoid glaring errors of the past required that our society implement clear, robust, proactive measures to ensure equitable access and just distribution of the benefits of vaccination.

A formal framework and criteria of equitable allocation, however attractive, are insufficient by themselves. Instead, equity must be consciously in each phase of the vaccination process. Thus, when health care workers are prioritized for vaccination—as they were in the first phase of vaccination for COVID-19—it is essential to prioritize not only physicians and nurses but also all others who are involved in patient care, among them other front-line workers responsible providing therapies to COVID-19 patients, bringing food to patients, transporting patients, and deep-cleaning patients' rooms.

For each phase, the committee determined that a systematic approach is necessary to ensure that those who are most at risk have meaningful access to vaccination. The committee grappled with how best to achieve this. As it would have been ethically and legally problematic to focus directly on race and ethnicity (Schmidt et al., 2020) in prioritizing vaccination access, the committee recommended that all phases prioritize vaccine distribution and access within census tracts that are rated high on the Social Vulnerability Index (SVI), used by the CDC and the Agency for Toxic Substances and Disease Registry (ATSDR). This index includes such factors as low socioeconomic status, minority status, crowded households and the like (ATSDR, 2021). In response, some have suggested that the Area Deprivation Index (ADI), which does not explicitly include race as a factor, might be more likely to withstand legal challenges (Schmidt et al., 2020).

From Vaccine Allocation and Distribution to Vaccination: Ensuring Uptake

Removing barriers to access

Early in the vaccine roll-out, we stressed that fair allocations of a vaccine would not on their own ensure robust uptake in the most vulnerable communities (Gayle & Childress, 2021). As vaccines are effective only to the degree with which they are used, it was clear that health equity can only be achieved through actual, equitable uptake of the vaccine. The long record of inequities in the roll-out of new health breakthroughs underscores that communities which experience diminished health care access and bias in health service delivery confront numerous impediments to uptake beyond the limits on the availability of technologies, drugs, and vaccines. These barriers may include medical mistrust (which we examine below), lack of a regular source of care, inadequate access to transportation, the deterrent effects of prior experience of stigma and discrimination in accessing health services, inability to afford out-of-pocket costs for health services, and fear of deportation (including fears of running afoul of the public charge rule in immigration law). To address these and other impediments to vaccination uptake, the committee recommended that the roll-out of COVID-19 vaccines should build on lessons from prior mass vaccination efforts—about what has worked, what hasn't, who has been left behind and why, and which steps have proven most effective in closing vaccination gaps.[5]

---

[5] The language in this paragraph and the next draws heavily on our earlier article (Gayle & Childress, 2021).

The committee recommended that COVID-19 vaccination efforts fully leverage existing resources and infrastructure in high-vulnerability areas, including but not limited to state and local health departments, federally qualified health centers, and tribal health services. Focused, prioritized investments were needed to build the capacity of safety-net providers in high-vulnerability areas to enable the rapid uptake of vaccines. Widespread, rapid, and equitable vaccination could not be achieved unless vaccines were free of charge and did not involve out-of-pocket costs.

In a November 2020 survey, 83% of Asian-Americans, 63% of Latinx, and 61% of White people surveyed in November 2020 indicated that they intended to take a COVID-19 vaccine, but only 42% of Black Americans said they intended to be vaccinated (Funk & Tyson, 2020). In view of these differences in willingness to accept COVID-19 vaccination, several proposals were made to close these gaps. One of the most important was to engage communities in planning for the promotion and delivery of vaccines. Many believed that concerted efforts were needed to cultivate and support high-profile vaccination champions in vulnerable communities, such as opinion leaders, faith groups, and political and civic leaders, among others. Moreover, community-led educators and navigators were needed to educate vulnerable communities and to assist individuals in overcoming practical and attitudinal barriers to vaccination, and these projects required investment and support.

While national and state-level public health campaigns of various kinds were certainly important and even indispensable in the roll-out of COVID-19 vaccines, they were also insufficient. Experience underscored that it is also necessary to develop tailored vaccine promotion campaigns in the most affected communities, use community-agreed messages that resonate locally, address medical mistrust and other issues, and emphasize the benefits of vaccination to specific racial and ethnic communities. This required close interaction with and engagement of the community in whatever ways were appropriate for that community. One of us (JFC) was amazed to observe what both a university healthcare system's clinicians and a local health department's professionals were able to accomplish together in engaging local communities of color, especially by clinicians who were themselves members of communities of color and worked closely with local groups, including religious organizations.

All these and many other efforts (including overcoming mistrust and distrust which we discuss below) paid off in significant ways. As of the first week of February 2022, data from the CDC (2022d) indicated that 75.3% of the U.S. population had received at least one dose of a vaccine for COVID-19. Vaccination uptake remained uneven across the country, even as unvaccinated persons continued to be at the highest risk for severe outcomes, including hospitalization and death. White people constitute two-thirds (66%) of the unvaccinated population. Following is one analysis of the data:

> Over the course of the vaccination rollout, Black and Hispanic people have been less likely than their White counterparts to receive a vaccine, but these disparities have narrowed over time and been eliminated for Hispanic people…Black people make up 10% of people who have received at least one dose of the vaccine compared to 12% of the total population (12%); their share of people who have received a vaccination in the last fourteen days is slightly higher at 14%. Hispanic people make up a larger share of vaccinated people (20%) and people who recently received a vaccination (34%) compared to their share of the population (17%). The share of vaccinated people who are Asian is similar to their share of the total population (7% and 6%, respectively), while they make up a slightly higher share (8%) of people initiating vaccination in the last 14 days. (Ndugga et al., 2022; see also CDC, 2022d).

These data show considerable progress in vaccination among all groups, as well as notable resistance remaining in the White population. And they confirm the relative success of vaccination uptake rates in certain populations. Such data, which we know are not complete, should guide our further efforts to ensure the equitable allocation, distribution, and uptake of COVID-19 vaccination. Data on vaccination uptake in specific states and localities should be timely, transparent, and disaggregated by race/ethnicity, gender, age, and income level. Health officials at the state, local, and federal levels, with support from political leaders, should strengthen the collection of data to ensure its completeness and accuracy and use the data to identify and address bottlenecks and gaps as they develop or persist.

Overcoming mistrust and distrust

Removing barriers to access to vaccination may still be insufficient to ensure robust and equitable uptake, as persistent mistrust and distrust affect both individual and collective decision-making about whether to be vaccinated. Trust is confidence in and reliance upon others to act in certain ways. Not surprisingly trust and mistrust/distrust are central factors in people's decisions whether to comply with public health directives, including vaccinations. International studies have identified the level of trust in the government and in fellow citizens as a key variable in different countries' success in early responses to the pandemic (COVID-19 National Preparedness Collaborators, 2022). Trust is essential for public health—it undergirds people's cooperation in protecting and promoting public health by following recommended or mandated measures. In a sharply divided society, dramatically split along ideological or political lines, as in the United States, trust in general may be scarce. Moreover, there are often specific forms of mistrust/distrust directed, for instance, at health care, science, pharmaceutical companies, or the federal government's "Operation Warp Speed," which rapidly brought the COVID-19 vaccines to fruition. All these may limit acceptance of vaccination for COVID-19.

Caution is needed in framing issues of trust and mistrust/distrust. As Debbie Dada and colleagues (2022) remind us, attributing vaccine hesitancy to the Black community's mistrust of government or distrust of the healthcare system encourages the erroneous conclusion that the central problem in community-level vaccine uptake is the Black community's lack of trust. From that misleading perspective, the apparent solution is to find ways to increase the Black community's trust in the government, in the healthcare system, etc. A different framing recognizes that Blacks' mistrust/distrust is warranted and reasonable based on history and prior experience: "not trusting the 'system' is a healthy response to structural racism. It's the structural inequalities and structural racism that's the problem, not the people" (Dada et al., 2022). A call to "trust more and get vaccinated" will ring hollow when the problem is the system's limited trustworthiness over time, as reflected in history and on-going experience. (While the nouns "mistrust" and "distrust" are generally used interchangeably, there is often a subtle difference, perhaps reflected more clearly in the verb forms. "Distrust" often signals what individuals know or have experienced, while "mistrust" often signals initial suspicions or doubts (See, for example, What's the difference, 2020).)

One crucial response, in both policy and practice, is to recognize that vaccine hesitancy may have a reasonable basis in warranted distrust. With this acknowledgement, it is then possible and important to craft truthful messages to indicate why distrust/mistrust, while reasonable, shouldn't apply to or preclude vaccination for COVID-19. Of course, it is not easy to demonstrate the trustworthiness of different aspects of COVID-19 vaccination programs—the government's role, the quality of the science, the distribution of the vaccine, etc. The content of the message needs to indicate why, despite warranted skepticism, vaccination best enables people to protect both themselves and others within the community and beyond. In addition to crafting messages that resonate with the community, attention must also be paid to the messenger, in order to ensure, to the extent possible, the trustworthiness and perceived trustworthiness of the messenger. Trusted personal health care providers play an important role in providing health information and advice, but not all members of disadvantaged communities have established healthcare relationships or easy, reliable access to them, further underscoring the aforementioned need to engage a broad range of community-centered messengers.

Providing monetary and other incentive rewards

Efforts to remove barriers to access to COVID-19 vaccination (e.g., by providing transportation to a vaccination clinic or establishing a "pop-up" vaccination clinic in the neighborhood) or to reduce disincentives (e.g., by providing compensation for unpaid time off work for vaccination) generally pose few ethical questions. It is not problematic to offset costs to potential vaccine recipients in order to promote vaccinations. More complicated and controversial is the provision of positive monetary rewards or goods with monetary value to encourage or nudge people to get vaccinated. These incentives create an additional motive for vaccination, beyond persuasion about the vaccine's individual or societal value.

Some analysts fail to adequately distinguish (1) financial benefits that remove disincentives—for instance, by offsetting costs for the vaccine recipient—from (2) financial benefits that provide positive incentives. However, the distinction is important, even though it may sometimes be difficult to determine which category applies. While various benefits can be useful motivators, we will here concentrate on monetary incentives, including goods with monetary value.

Solid evidence supports such incentive programs for vaccinations in some contexts. The Community Preventive Services Task Force "recommends client or family incentive rewards, used alone or in combination with additional interventions, based on sufficient evidence of effectiveness in increasing vaccination rates in children and adults" (Community Preventive Services Task Force, 2015).[6] The task force was persuaded by research studies indicating that such incentive rewards increased the rates of vaccination by a median of 8 percentage points. The rewards featured in these studies included food vouchers, gift cards, lottery prizes, and baby products, usually in small amounts. These incentive rewards go beyond "interventions that increase access to vaccination services" by offsetting costs; they are instead designed to motivate vaccination decisions.

There are questions about whether the task force's recommendation can be extended to vaccination for COVID-19. The task force's analysis and recommendation not only predated the pandemic; the studies it drew on focused mainly on parental decision making about vaccination for children. For evidence in regard to COVID-19 vaccines for adults, one large randomized controlled trial in Sweden found that modest monetary payments (equivalent to 24 U.S. dollars) increased vaccination rates by 4.2 percentage points over a baseline rate of 71.6% (Campos-Mercade et al., 2021). It is not clear whether this Swedish study can be generalized to the United States which suffers from widespread mistrust/distrust, sharp

---

[6] The Community Preventive Services Task Force was established by the U.S. Department of Health and Human Services in 1996 and charged with the task of identifying population health interventions that are scientifically determined to save lives, increase lifespans, and improve quality of life; the CDC appoints the fifteen members of this independent task force.)

ideological/political divisions, and pervasive vaccine misinformation campaigns. Some modest studies in the United States have found no effects of monetary incentives (Walkey et al., 2021), while others suggest that such incentives may even backfire and actually lead to fewer vaccinations (Chang et al., 2021).

While apparently simple and straightforward, incentive rewards, especially those with monetary value, may symbolically convey messages that can render them ineffective or counterproductive. As Loewenstein and Cryder (2020) observe, "when people aren't sure whether something is good or bad, the prospect of payment helps them decide, in the negative." After all, if compensation is deemed necessary to motivate people to be vaccinated, this may signify (a) that the vaccination is not itself very valuable to recipients, or (b) that it is risky or dangerous to recipients. Some commentators suppose that financial rewards would be particularly attractive in marginalized, disadvantaged communities (Persad & Emanuel, 2021), but negative symbolic messages may resonate in those communities, which already have understandable reasons for mistrust/distrust, and thereby prevent the intended positive effects.

The symbolic messages conveyed by incentive rewards are heavily context dependent. Who is making the offer to whom in what context and for what purpose can thus significantly affect the success or failure of an incentive program. In 2021 state governments in the United States offered several incentive rewards to their populations in order to promote COVID-19 vaccination uptake. These included free beer, entry in a lottery for large prizes (million dollar awards), a lottery for full four-year scholarships at an in-state college, and cash awards of varying amounts (Roy & LeBlanc, 2021). These state incentive rewards programs were mainly aimed at increasing overall vaccine uptake rather than specifically at vaccine equity; of course, an increase in general uptake can also indirectly improve vaccination equity, but it is not clear that these state-based programs have been studied for their equity effects. Businesses and other organizations also offered employees monetary incentives for vaccination.

By contrast, the Equity-First Vaccination Initiative (EVI), supported by The Rockefeller Foundation, "aims to reduce racial and ethnic disparities in

COVID-19 vaccination rates" in the United States; its longer-term aim is "to strengthen the public health system to achieve more-equitable outcomes" (Faherty et al., 2022). EVI's strategy is to "involve communities in designing incentives that are tailored to the community, have value, and will promote, not hinder, equity" (Faherty et al., 2021). EVI's strategy focuses on incentive rewards that offset the costs of vaccination—and thus remove disincentives to vaccinations—but its recommendation of community involvement in tailoring incentives to the community is also crucially important in designing monetary incentive rewards to encourage vaccination uptake.

Brewer and colleagues (2022) draw on rewards research on health behaviors to formulate three conditions that increase the effectiveness of such rewards. Incentive programs for vaccination for COVID-19 are most likely to be effective when (1) the receipt of the reward is certain, (2) the reward is delivered immediately, and (3) recipients value the reward. The last needs to be determined through community engagement but it also needs to be balanced against the unintended effects of the provision of the reward, which may be more difficult to determine.

Other issues also merit attention in deciding whether to employ incentive rewards. It may be difficult, though not impossible, to combine monetary incentives with social solidarity and mutual responsibility for public health (Loewenstein & Cryder, 2020). Further problems may arise if the goal that is sought through incentive rewards expands, say, from two shots to a booster and even a second booster for full vaccination, or if it incorporates other public health responsibilities such as mask wearing. Moreover, the provision of incentives could establish a costly and unsustainable precedent for subsequent public health policy and practice. Finally, despite some dissent in the ethics literature, the kinds of incentives being proposed are generally deemed not to be coercive.

Conclusion

Efforts in the United States to develop a framework for the equitable allocation of vaccine for COVID-19 coincided with a national reckoning about structural injustice and racism, provoked in part by the murder of

George Floyd. This coincidence offered a historic opportunity to address underlying racial and ethnic health inequities in the roll-out of COVID-19 vaccines. Even though equitable vaccine allocation is the first step in the process of achieving vaccination equity, it cannot be the last step. Other indispensable steps include equitable distribution and access along with equitable vaccine uptake. These steps constitute key elements in what should be an integrated strategy for addressing racial and ethnic disparities and inequities in the pandemic.

To further elaborate, equitable allocation of vaccines to the most vulnerable is essential, where vulnerability includes heightened risks of infection, serious disease, hospitalization, and death. An allocation framework that makes vaccines available to those most at risk because of work conditions, living arrangements, underlying health conditions, and the like, is not sufficient by itself. Concerted efforts are also needed to ensure that disproportionately affected communities and populations have meaningful access to vaccines as well as the means to receive them. This requires ongoing imaginative and thoughtful attention to barriers to access and to distributional efforts that can increase vaccine uptake in at-risk communities and populations. This attentive process can ascertain unrecognized or ignored barriers, hidden disincentives to vaccine uptake, sources of mistrust/distrust and measures to enhance trustworthiness, and effective ways to motivate vaccine uptake, perhaps including positive incentive rewards. Determining the actual barriers to vaccination—and the best ways to overcome them—will require close engagement with local communities about their vulnerabilities and their values. Only then will it be possible to identify and embark on the best paths to vaccination equity and health equity.

References

Ahmad, K., S. Erqou, N. Shah, Nazir, U., Morrison, A.R., Choudhary, G. & Wu, W. (2020). Association of poor housing conditions with COVID-19 incidence and mortality across US counties. *PLoS One, 15*(11), e0241327. https://doi.org/10.1371/journal.pone.0241327

ATSDR. 2021. *CDC/ATSDR SVI Fact Sheet.* https://www.atsdr.cdc.gov/placeandhealth/svi/fact_sheet/fact_sheet.html

Brewer, N. T., Buttenheim, A. M., Clinton, C.V., Mello, M. M., Benjamin, R. M., Callaghan, T., Caplan, A., Carpiano, R. M., DiResta, R., Elharake, J. A., Flowers, L. C., Galvani, A. P., Hotez, P. J., Lakshmanan, R., Maldonado, Y. A., Omer, S. B., Salmon, D. A., Schwartz, J. L., Sharfstein, J. M., & Opel, D. J. (2022). Incentives for COVID-19 vaccination. *The Lancet Regional Health — Americas 8*, 100205. doi: 10.1016/j.lana.2022.100205

Campos-Mercade, P., Meier, A.N., Schneider, F. H., Meier, S., Pope, D., & Wengstrom, E. (2021). Monetary incentives increase COVID-19 vaccinations. *Science, 374*(6569), 879-882. doi: 10.1126/science.abm0475

CDC (n.d.). *Influenza (Flu): 1918 Pandemic (H1N1 virus)*. https://www.cdc.gov/flu/pandemic-resources/1918-pandemic-h1n1.html

CDC. (2013). CDC health disparities and inequalities report — United States, 2013. *MMWR 62*,1–187. https://www.cdc.gov/mmwr/pdf/other/su6203.pdf

CDC. (2019). Diagnoses of HIV infection in the United States and dependent areas, 2018 (preliminary). *HIV Surveillance Report, 30*. http://www.cdc.gov/hiv/library/reports/hiv-surveillance.html

CDC. (2020a). *COVID-19 hospitalization and death by race/ethnicity*. https://www.cdc.gov/coronavirus/2019-ncov/covid-data/investigations-discovery/hospitalization-death-by-race-ethnicity.html. Accessed December 9, 2020.

CDC. (2020b). *Health equity considerations and racial and ethnic minority groups*. https://www.cdc.gov/coronavirus/2019-ncov/community/health-equity/race-ethnicity.html Accessed December 10, 2020.

CDC. (2022a). *Risk for COVID-19 infection, hospitalization, and death by age group*. https://www.cdc.gov/coronavirus/2019-ncov/covid-data/investigations-discovery/hospitalization-death-by-age.html#print Accessed March 22, 2022.

CDC. (2022b). *Risk for COVID-19 infection, hospitalization, and death by race/ethnicity*. https://www.cdc.gov/coronavirus/2019-ncov/covid-data/investigations-discovery/hospitalization-death-by-race-ethnicity.html Accessed March 22, 2022.

CDC. (2022c). *COVID-19 vaccine effectiveness*. https://www.cdc.gov/coronavirus/2019-ncov/vaccines/index.html?s_cid=10496:cdc%20covid%20vaccine:sem.ga:p:RG:GM:gen:PTN:FY21 Accessed March 20, 2022.

CDC. (2022d). *COVID-19 vaccinations in the United States.* https://covid.cdc.gov/ covid-data-tracker/#vaccinations_vacc-total-admin-rate-total. Accessed February 10, 2022.

Chang, T. Y., Jacobson, M., Shah, M., Pramanik, R., & Shah, S. B. (2021). Financial incentives and other nudges do not increase COVID-19 vaccinations among the hesitant. *VOX, CEPR Policy Portal.* https://voxeu.org/article/financial-incentives-and-other-nudges-do-not-increase-covid-19-vaccinations-among-hesitant

Community Preventive Services Task Force. (2015). *Increasing appropriate vaccination: Client or family incentive rewards.* Document last updated July 15, 2015. https://www.thecommunityguide.org/sites/default/files/assets/Vaccination-Incentive-Rewards.pdf Accessed, February 9, 2022.

COVID-19 National Preparedness Collaborators. (2022). Pandemic preparedness and COVID-19: an exploratory analysis of infection and fatality rates, and contextual factors associated with preparedness in 177 countries, from Jan 1, 2020, to Sept 30, 2021. *The Lancet, 399*(10334), 1489-1512. https://doi.org/ 10.1016/S0140-6736(22)00172-6

Dada, D., Djiometio, J. N., McFadden, S. M., Demeke, J., Vlahov, D., Wilton, L., Wang, M., & Nelson, L. E. (2022). Strategies that promote equity in COVID-19 vaccine uptake for Black communities: A review. *Journal of Urban Health, 99*(1), 15-27. doi: 10.1007/s11524-021-00594-3

Dasgupta, S., Bowen, V. B., Leidner, A., Fletcher, K., Musial, T., Rose, C., Cha, A., Kang, G., Dirlikov, E., Pevzner, E., Rose, D., Ritchey, M. D., Villanueva, J., Philip, C., Liburd, L., & Oster, A. M. (2020). Association between social vulnerability and a county's risk for becoming a COVID-19 hotspot — United States, June 1–July 25, 2020. *MMWR 69*(42), 1535–1541. https://www.cdc.gov/mmwr/volumes/69/wr/mm6942a3.htm

Faherty, L. J., Ringel, J. S., Williams, M. V., Kranz, A. M., Perez, L., Schulson, L., Jitters, A. D., Phillips, B., Backer, L., Gandhi, P., Howell, K., Wolfe, R. L., & Adekunle, T. (2021). *Early insights from the equity-first vaccination initiative.* RAND Corporation. https://www.rand.org/pubs/research_briefs/RBA1627-1.html

Funk, C., & Tyson, A. (2020). *Intent to get a COVID-19 vaccine rises to 60% as confidence in research and development process increases.* Pew Research Center.

Galston, W. (2020). *When it comes to public opinion on race, it's not 1968 anymore.* Brookings.

Ganguly, S., Mailankody, S., & Ailawadhi, S. (2019). Many shades of disparities in myeloma care. *American Society of Clinical Oncology educational book. American Society of Clinical Oncology. Annual Meeting, 39,* 519–529. https://doi.org/10.1200/EDBK_238551

Gayle H. D., & Childress, J. F. (2021). Race, racism, and structural injustice: Equitable allocation and distribution of vaccines for COVID-19. Guest Editorial. *The American Journal of Bioethics, 21*(3), 4-7.

Harris, N. S., Johnson, A. S., Huang, Y. A., Kern, D., Fulton, P., Smith, D. K., Vallery, L. A., & Hall, I. (2019). Vital signs: status of human immunodeficiency virus testing, viral suppression, and HIV preexposure prophylaxis— United States, 2013–2018. *MMWR, 68*(48),1117–1123. doi:10.15585/mmwr.mm6848e1

Hawkins, D. (2020). Differential occupational risk for COVID-19 and other infection exposure according to race and ethnicity. *American Journal of Industrial Medicine, 63*(9), 817–820. doi:10.1002/ajim.23145

Jung, J., & Feldman, R. (2017). Racial-ethnic disparities in uptake of new hepatitis C drugs in medicare. *Journal of Racial and Ethnic Health Disparities, 4*(6),1147–1158. doi: 10.1007/s40615-016-0320-2

Kabria, G. (2019). Racial/ethnic disparities in prevalence, treatment, and control of hypertension among U.S. adults following application of the 2017 American College of Cardiology/American Heart Association guideline. *Preventive Medicine Reports, 14,* 100850. doi: 10.1016/j.pmedr.2019.100850

Loewenstein, G., & Cryder, C. (2020). Why paying people to be vaccinated could backfire. *The New York Times,* December 14, 2020, Updated December 15, 2020. https://www.nytimes.com/2020/12/14/upshot/covid-vaccine-payment.html

McClung, N., Chamberland, M., Kinlaw, K., Matthew, D. B., Wallace, M., Bell, B. P., Lee, G. M., Talbot, H. K., Romero, J. R., Oliver, S. E., & Dooling, K. (2020). The advisory committee on immunization practices' ethical principles for allocating initial supplies of COVID-19 vaccine — United States, 2020. *MMWR, 69*(47),1–5.

McFadden, S.M., Demeke, J., Dada, D., Wilton, L., Wang, M., Vlahov, D., & Nelson, L. E. (2021). Confidence and hesitancy during the early roll-out of COVID-19 vaccines among Black, Hispanic, and undocumented immigrant communities: A review. *Journal of Urban Health, 99*(1), 3-14.

McNicholas, C., & Poydock, M. (2020). *Who are essential workers? A comprehensive look at their wages, demographics, and unionization rates.* Economic Policy Institute.

National Academies of Sciences, Engineering, Medicine, and National Academy of Medicine (NASEM). (2020). *Framework for equitable allocation of COVID-19 vaccine*. National Academies Press.

Ndugga, N., Hill, L., Artiga, S., & Haldar, S. (2022). Latest data on COVID-19 vaccinations by race/ethnicity. Coronavirus (COVID-19). *KFF* February 02.

Ogedegbe, G., Ravenell, J., Adhikari, S., Butler, M., Cook, T., Francois, F., Iturrate, E., Jean-Louis, G., Jones, S. A., Onakomaiya, D., Petrilli, C. M., Pulgarin, C., Regan, S., Reynolds, H., Seixas, A., Volpicelli, F. M., & Horwitz, L. I. (2020). Assessment of racial/ethnic disparities in hospitalization and mortality in patients with COVID-19 in New York City. *JAMA Network Open 3*(12), e2026881. doi:10.1001/jamanetworkopen.2020.26881

Quinones, A, Botoseneanu, A., Markwardt, S., Nagel, C. L., Newsom, J. T., Dorr, D. A., & Allore, H. G. (2019). Racial/ethnic differences in multimorbidity development and chronic disease accumulation for middle-aged adults. *PLoS One, 14*(6), e0218462. doi: 10.1371/journal.pone.0218462

Persad, G., & Emanuel, E. J. (2021). Ethical considerations of offering benefits to COVID-19 vaccine recipients. *Journal of the American Medical Association, 326*(3), 221-223.

Roy, B., & LeBlanc, M. (2021). *Memorandum: COVID-19 vaccine incentives.*

National Governors Association. https://www.nga.org/center/publications/covid-19-vaccine-incentives/ Accessed February 04, 2022.

Schmidt, H., Gostin, L. O., & Williams, M. A. (2020). Is it lawful and ethical to prioritize racial minorities for COVID-19 vaccines? *Journal of the American Medical Association, 324*(20), 2023-2024. doi:10.1001/jama.2020.20571

Toner, E., Barnill, A., Krubiner, C., Bernstein, J., Privor-Dumm, L., Watson, M., Martin, E., Potter, C., Hosangadi, D., Connell, N., Watson, C., Schoch-Spana, M., Veenema, T. G., Meyer, D., Daugherty Biddison, E. L., Regenberg, A., Inglesby, T., & Cicero, A. (2020). *Interim framework for COVID-19 vaccine allocation and distribution in the United States*. Johns Hopkins Center for Health Security. https://www.centerforhealthsecurity.org/our-work/publications/interim-framework-for-covid-19-vaccine-allocation-and-distribution-in-the-us

World Health Organization (WHO). (2020, September 14). *WHO SAGE values framework for the allocation and prioritization of COVID-19 vaccination.*

https://www.who.int/publications/i/item/who-sage-values-framework-for-the-allocation-and-prioritization-of-covid-19-vaccination

Volpp, K.G., & Cannuscio, C.C. (2021). Incentives for immunity—Strategies for increasing COVID-19 vaccine uptake. *New England Journal of Medicine, 395*(1), e1. doi: 10.1056/NEJMp2107719

Walkey, A. J., Law, A., & Bosch, N. A. (2021). Research letter: Lottery-based incentive in Ohio and COVID-19 vaccination rates. *Journal of the American Medical Association, 326*(8), 766-767. doi:10.1001/jama.2021.11048

What's the difference between 'mistrust' and 'distrust'? (2020). *Dictionary.com.* July 16, 2020. https://www.dictionary.com/e/mistrust-vs-distrust/ Accessed 7 February 2022.

THE GOVERNANCE ETHICAL CHALLENGE DURING THE COVID-19 PANDEMIC IN DEVELOPING COUNTRIES

Zamumtima Chijere[1]

Abstract: Managing crises like COVID-19 requires proper governance structures in all public agencies because it provides the basis for authority and accountability. Proper governance helps in checking the behaviors of individuals as they discharge their duties. Unethical behaviors flourish where public agencies operational guidelines are not clear or overlooked. One of the pertinent issues during the COVID-19 pandemic is an ethical distribution of resources, especially social cash transfer programs. Many African governments introduced various economic measures like social cash transfer and food assistance in response to the rising poverty due to the pandemic. However, research shows that most households that deserve the support never received it (Oduor, 2021). In essence, corruption through these programs has worsened marginalized people's vulnerability since they can't access any economic support while they are losing jobs or closing their businesses. The occupation-related impact of COVID-19 has also hit hard on the vulnerable groups such as women, children, immigrants, and the poor. While others were working online during the lockdowns, middle- and lower-income earning workers' jobs required that they work in person. The lockdowns meant loss of income for many of these workers. Beyond this, the working conditions were harsh for the lower income earners in many developing countries. For instance, the pandemic has worsened women's working conditions who make up 70 percent of the workforce in the healthcare system. This chapter discusses some of these ethical challenges in the management of the COVID-19 in the public sector in developing countries. It will offer an analysis on how unethical behaviors have hampered the response to the COVID-19 pandemic.

---

[1] Co-founder and Executive Director of Rise Malawi Ministries, Lilongwe, Malawi

Introduction

SARS-Cov-2 has brought in the need for ethical reflection about the guidelines that governments have put in place in managing the pandemic. However, it is important to remember that ethical principles are important in governance of any institution, even countries. The ethical principles address questions about the viability and desirability of action to benefit a society. Most of the ethical conduct in public agencies rests in the governance structure of such institutions.

Governance is central to the ethical standing of any public institution. Governance is regarded as processes and structures through which the institution's assets and activities are overseen towards achieving effectiveness, accountability and ultimately fulfilling the long-term goals of the institution (Erwin et al., 2019; Said et al., 2017). It involves the rules and regulations that provide checks and balances on all activities that a public entity does. One of the central issues during crises is leadership and management of public agencies. In crises such as the COVID-19, there are several elements that are liable to destroy ethical principles that govern institutions and even governments.

This chapter discusses some of these ethical principles. These issues include the state capture, ethics in public procurement, equitable healthcare access, the ethics social cash transfer, and ethics in vaccine distribution.

The State Capture and its influence on ethical behavior

The major problem is that the response to the pandemic has been controlled by the political and economic elites. The gains in African development in the past few decades are threatened by high levels of corruption that emanates from state capture which affect the fundamental rights of people (Jenkins et al., 2021; Lawal, 2007). The effort of individuals or companies to control the operation of governments to their advantage by providing illicit private gains to the public officials has been one of the major challenges in governance for many developing countries. There are high issues of petty bribery which has become a norm in many agencies and governments across the globe, especially in developing countries (Keulder, 2021; Masina,

2021). However, there are bigger issues of state capture and crony capitalism which has resulted in shocking corruption in many sectors of development in developing countries.

Keulder (2021) reports that it is estimated that over US$1.3 trillion is lost per year to corruption and public theft in developing countries alone, and state capture is a major source of corruption. The amount of money that is lost through the economic elites has risen with the coming of the pandemic since many people have taken advantage of the loopholes that have been there for generations. However, corruption has soared during the COVID-19 pandemic (Amundsen, 2022; Goldstein et al., 2020; Masina, 2021).

The management of COVID-19 funds hasn't been spared from the corrupt practices that emanate from the state capture. For instance, there have been reports that one individual in Malawi owned over 10 companies which were all contracted by the government (Masina, 2020). These companies in most cases are selected without proper bidding procedure. In addition, several public contracts related to COVID-19 response in many countries have been offered to politicians and their relatives (Nyasulu et al., 2021). For instance, there have been reports that one individual in Malawi owned over ten companies which were all contracted by the government (Masina, 2020). These companies in most cases are selected without proper bidding procedure. This is a pure indication that the pandemic provided the opportunity for businessmen to defraud the citizens. Due to this, the quality and delivery of services has been affected by the high pricing and unqualified contractors doing the work. The major casualties in this malpractice are the poor citizens and marginalized population.

Since these are economic and political elites, they are rarely investigated or tried for their crimes because of their connection with those in top political leadership. However, there are a few cases where the culprits paid the price for their corrupt dealings. It is reported that in Bolivia the Minister of Health was detained for purchasing 179 ventilators at twice the original price. In Peru, Panama, and Bolivia ministers were forced to resign when they were implicated in COVID-19 related corruption cases (Cuadrado et al., 2020; El Deber, 2020). In the same regard, the political and economic elites in South America, Asia, and Africa have been in the forefront in paralyzing the efforts in dealing with pandemic.

The state capture during the pandemic has been attributed to worsening governance performance in many developing countries during the COVID-19 pandemic. Well governed countries like Uruguay are coping well with the pandemic while others are generally struggling with the virus out of control. Countries like South Africa, Brazil and India stand out as the countries that experience high COVID-19 death rate, these countries also experience COVID-19 corruption at a grand scale (OECD Policy Response, 2021). The state capture has made many people in leadership overlook the impact of their unethical behavior on the marginalized population. The capture by economic elites who shape the rules of the game has compromised the leadership of the public institutions in their response to the pandemic especially on the distribution of scarce resources like vaccines and economic incentive. In most cases, this has affected the COVID-19 testing ability and management of the pandemic in developing countries. In some regard, the high infection rates with little resources to combat the virus have been due to the unethical control of the government operations by some elites (Amundsen, 2022; Goldstein et al., 2020). The state capture in many cases led into unethical procurement of resources in the public sector.

Ethics in the Public Procurement

The substantial share of resources meant for COVID-19 response have been lost to procurement corruption. Public procurement presents a significant opportunity for corrupt practices. Cuadrado et al. (2021) claim that corruption around the healthcare sector has existed for several years. This form of corruption ranges from favoritism, theft, and bribes. In most developing countries, petty corruption exists in all departments. However, the scale of corruption since the outbreak of the COVID-19 pandemic has been worse. It has infiltrated the procurement and purchase of medical supplies beyond the imaginable.

COVID-19 has given several governments in developing countries an opportunity for another level of looting in which public procurement is the epicenter of corruption. Several reports from Malawi, Kenya, and

Zimbabwe portray how the fund has been abused by politicians and their close cronies. Public procurement corruption has been evident in the management of COVID-19 funds. In Kenya only, over US$70 million was spent on irregular expenditure (Seydou, 2021; Uche et al., 2021). In Malawi, the labor minister was fired when he used money that was meant for COVID-19 response to fund his personal trip. The most needed resources in fighting the pandemic have been siphoned off by the political leaders who have taken advantage of the crisis as an opportunity for stealing.

The economic elites have taken advantage of the weak procurement systems to channel taxpayers' money into their own benefits. Due to this grand theft, several hospitals in developing countries lacked basic essential medical supplies to control the spread of COVID-19 and treat those who were chronically ill. There were instances in Malawi where local hospital workers were working without personal protective equipment (PPE) because either were not supplied, or the official overlooked such a need. Malawi has lost many health workers to COVID-19 due the mismanagement of funds during the pandemic (Masina, 2020; Mzumara et al., 2021).

There have been irregularities in procurement in several developing countries, related to greedy government officials trying to enrich themselves, that requires serious action to be taken by both the government and donor community. The pandemic has highlighted the insufficient attention paid to good governance in preventing corruption in the public arena. Inadequate controls on governance of resource procurement which have increased the risk of corruption during the COVID-19 pandemic. In most developing countries, there are reports that even though the money was released by the donor community to the governments, most of the money never achieved the intended purpose. This is termed as 'covidgate' in most African countries. There are reports of widespread corruption and lack of transparency in how African governments have used the funds intended to address the economic impact of the pandemic (Oduor, 2021; Ott et al., 2021; Roope et. al., 2021).

The major problem is that there are no clear guidelines and regulations on how the government should respond to crises such as these in many developing countries, especially in procuring the required resources. Such countries are already struggling in putting up measures to close the loopholes in procuring resources, and the COVID-19 pandemic has seen a major drawback in this condition. For instance, the International Monetary Fund (IMF) in 2021 reported that several African countries have no meaningful oversight and guidelines on public procurement of resources.

In Malawi, several companies contracted by the government were either owned by politicians or their close associates in the private sector. Most of these companies never supplied the material in their contract with the government (Nyasulu et al., 2021). This has affected the quality of the healthcare system and access to healthcare in many developing countries.

The Dilapidated Health Sector and its Impact on Equity Healthcare Access

The other ethical issue in public governance is how unethical behaviors have affected the access to healthcare for marginalized individuals. It should be noted that governments have an obligation under the international human rights law to provide adequate standards of living which include the right to health for citizens including during the times of crisis. However, the COVID-19 pandemic calls for a comprehensive switch from governments across the world on how they have been treating humanity during crises especially in the health care sector.

Most healthcare systems in developing countries were never designed for emergency response especially during the pandemic. The private hospitals are not better and in most cases they are termed as "commercial organizations" which put the life of the patient as secondary (Krachler et al., 2022). Before COVID-19, the rich and politicians accessed healthcare from developed countries leaving the poor with no good medical care. The expenditure on healthcare in most developing countries is static and the governments never thought of improving the healthcare system. This condition never favors the ability to address pandemics like COVID-19. The collapsing healthcare infrastructure has been attributed to corruption and lack of seriousness among politicians to invest in the local healthcare system. Poor governance coupled with corruption in the public sector makes any attempt to improve the healthcare sector futile since it hinders any implementation of changes. As such, when COVID-19 was spread across the globe, most countries were caught underprepared, and they remain in a shock up to date.

Public funds mismanagement and lack of desire from the authorities to develop the healthcare systems has greatly affected the response to COVID-19 in Africa. One Malawian civil rights activist raised an alarm over lack of COVID-19 supplies in one of the major referral hospitals in the country while he was at their isolation center. The hospital had no oxygen flowmeter and other necessary equipment in treating people with COVID-19. Sadly, he died a few days after raising the issue. This was happening after the government of Malawi had released over MKW6.2 billion (approximately US$7.8 million) in response to the pandemic. The audit report later found that over 78% of the total funds were spent on staff allowances or benefits. The misplaced priorities and unrealistic expenditures have crippled the already dilapidated health system in Africa. One of the nurses in Malawi reported that working in COVID-19 isolation center is equivalent to working in a war zone (Kateta, 2021). The hospitals that were lacking basic drugs had to cope with the rising cases of COVID-19. They couldn't keep up.

The reports indicate that despite the low rates of COVID-19 in several African countries, decades of corruption have left the region struggling to cope with the few cases of COVID-19 which led to thousands being deprived of their rights to health. Corruption has led many countries to be ill-prepared for the rising numbers of COVID-19 infections. This led countries to decide on how they could prioritize the insufficient resources for the patients who may need it. The rich and the politically connected become the priority for ventilators and hospital bed allocation. The COVID-19 pandemic is complex and unfolded so fast that it has left several developing countries behind in responding to the pandemic. Funding to local health facilities has been at its lowest point in several countries which has affected the availability of resources (Holtz, 2021; Mansefield et. al., 2020; Mzumara et. al., 2021).

One important aspect in dealing with the virus is through the health insurance schemes as a remedy for supporting vulnerable populations who are at financial risk in acquiring healthcare services. Few countries in Africa are implementing social health insurance schemes. Sadly, many poor populations are not the focus of these schemes. Most of these schemes are a barrier to the poor since they cannot afford the terms that go with these medical cover schemes. As a result, they have to depend on out-of-pocket expenditure before they are provided with the needed medical care. In emergencies like COVID-19, access to testing and treatment was prioritized to the rich leaving out the majority poor because they cannot afford to pay for their medical bills. Since most of these insurance schemes leave out the poor, the poor bear the highest burden of the pandemic and experienced high levels of financial burden due to the healthcare expenditures. The Coronavirus pandemic has exposed huge inequalities, with a greater impact on the marginalized and vulnerable population (Graselli et al., 2020).

The distribution of resources, which was already unequal between the wealthiest and poorest nations, has worsened. The distribution of power and money systematically disadvantages the poor, and this has led to unavoidable income disparity and access basic necessities during the pandemic. The next section will discuss the ethics in social cash transfer programs and how unethical behaviors have affected the access to economic incentive for the poor.

The Ethical Problems in Social Cash Transfer Program

In several developing countries, there are documented job losses, loss of income and hunger among people as a result of COVID-19. The International Labor Organization (ILO) reports that lack of unemployment support and other forms of financial assistance for people who have lost income reflects the weakness of several African governments. It is reported that less than 10 percent of people in southern Africa had access to social protection (Devereux, 2021; Gentilini et al., 2020; ILO, 2020).

The lack of support people received or are receiving tend to bring more questions about how governments are using funds for COVID-19 response. For instance, there have been arrests of top government officials due to mismanagement of funds, but none of them are convicted and are back to their normal work (Kateta, 2021). Politicians have hijacked the response and no clear criterion is used to identify the vulnerable populations. Lack of deliberate economic efforts combined with shortage of funds and corruption has slowed recovery for several African countries.

However, governments all over the world have an obligation under the international human rights law to provide adequate standards of living which include the right to health, food and social security for citizens including during the times of crisis. However, the COVID-19 pandemic calls for a comprehensive approach from the government. One pertinent concern is the public policy challenge in the management of the pandemic is to mitigate the economic impact of the pandemic on the middle and low income households.

Social Cash Transfer Programs are being created and extended in developing countries as an economic response to COVID-19 (Amundsen, 2020). The economic impact of COVID-19 hit harder than the virus itself in many low-and-middle income countries. Ahmed et al. (2022) reported that the developing economies will lose over $220 billion in income and over 207 million people will be pushed into extreme poverty by 2030. This has dragged the already marginalized and vulnerable populations deeper into poverty. Measures to contain the virus included lockdowns which had strong restrictions on movements which drastically lowered the income of the vulnerable families (Mzumara et al., 2021). The lockdowns impacted the poor whose job requires them to be physically on site to make money.

Masina (2021) stated that the poor depend on public spaces and movement for their livelihood. In addition, the poor population depends on seasonal agriculture and traveling to marketplaces to buy and produce inputs. Social protection, which included social cash transfer, was introduced to mitigate the impact of the virus that came with lockdowns and economic meltdowns of many economies. However, the scale and speed of the social cash transfer program intensified the corruption risks, in terms of fraud and embezzlement, this also extends to political abuse, particularism, and clientelism (Tholstrup & Peachey, 2020). Therefore, due diligence and critical oversight of the public funds cannot be overemphasized given the huge amount of money at play in the social cash transfer programs.

The Kenyan government's social cash transfer, just as in many developing countries, failed to protect the vulnerable populations who suffered the economic hardship due to COVID-19. The report by Human Rights Watch indicates that there were huge political manipulations by the local elites who were including or excluding certain populations within the scope of the program due to the political or ethical affiliations. In most cases, the implementation of the program was masked in secrecy which was the breeding ground for corruption. The secrecy gave room for the individuals responsible for the program to register their relatives, friends and even ghost beneficiaries (Gentilini et al., 2021; Gondwe, 2020).

Amundsen (2022) summarizes that the corruption risks are identified at four stages of the process: when funds are allocated to and managed by recipient governments; when decisions are made on who will be the recipients; when funds are handled by the distributing agencies; and when the funds are given to the end users. Research in several African countries reveal that corruption has prevented social and economic assistance from reaching those who need it the most. Audit reports on how the funds were used during the second and third wave of the pandemic show that politicians and their relatives are the major beneficiaries of COVID-19 fund (Herbert & Marquette, 2021; Kateta, 2021). This leaves out the intended beneficiaries to only benefit the relatives and close friends of the local officials and politicians.

Scholars (such as Amundsen, 2022; Kateta, 2021) believe that cash transfers can be very efficient in countries with existing structures and methods to deliver cash to the poor, such as previous social security nets, identified recipient groups, and widespread use of mobile money. However, with the already corrupt systems in developing countries, cash is diverted and embezzled all along the entire cash transfer chain, and the scale and speed of these programs will intensify the corruption risks involved (Amundsen, 2020). Money transfers from international aid to recipient governments, and the recipient governments' financial management, always involve some fiduciary risk.

Addressing corruption challenges in cash transfer programs involves establishing clear, transparent, and efficient targeting mechanisms; choosing reliable and context-specific cash distribution systems; ensuring transparency and participation of beneficiaries; and putting robust monitoring and evaluation systems in place. It is only when countries put a good mechanism of tracking the entire chain of operation from donor to the intended recipient that the social cash transfer programs can be successful. But with the current system, most of the money will continue being lost through corrupt practices while the poor become much poorer.

Vaccine Access and Distribution Ethics

The other important ethical public governance issue during the COVID-19 pandemic is the access to COVID-19 vaccines. The World Health Organization (WHO) report indicates that "the continent's coverage of people over 18 years is estimated at 34%, significantly higher than the 18% full coverage in the general population. Nine countries have fully vaccinated more than 70% of their adult population, while 21 have reached more than 40% of adults" (WHO Africa, 2022). Although the vaccine supplies have risen over the years, the vaccine rollout program is still lagging in many African countries. While other countries such as the United States and the United Kingdom are administering booster doses, millions in Africa have little access to the first dose. The global inequalities in COVID-19 vaccines have been highlighted by several African leaders which in most cases it is rooted in the structural racism, apartheid, and colonialism (Johnson, 2022; Madorsky, 2021).

Access to COVID-19 vaccines is an issue of justice and fairness. Fair vaccine access ensures that everyone has equal access to the vaccine. It reflects the longstanding economic, social and political inequality between the rich and poor nations. Even though the availability of doses is increasing for low earning countries, the disparity with the high earning countries is high which leaves the mandate to have the 49% vaccinated in jeopardy (WHO Africa, 2022). The problem lies in the hoarding of vaccines by rich countries that would go to countries that desperately need them.

The value of realizing that this is a global pandemic – no one is safe until everyone is safe – is very important in protecting the dignity of every human being. Numerous barriers and limited supply of COVID-19 vaccines prevent several governments from taking rapid mass immunization. This brings the question of fairness and justice to the ethical framework to guide the immunization process. This trickles down to how countries are making available vaccines to their citizens. How can governments put in place policies that promote equitable access to vaccination? Developing countries have struggled with the equitable distribution of vaccines which prioritizes the rich over the poor and the marginalized. Health facilities in villages have limited access to the vaccines.

The issue of access to vaccines is further affected by the mistrust that citizens have towards their governments. Nearly 1 million doses have been thrown away in Nigeria alone because they expired before being administered (Mlaba, 2021). Several other African countries have also destroyed the already few vaccines because they expired before administration. This is in part due to the distrust that the masses have on their governments. The response to this problem is to hold public health campaigns and direct outreach to clear the misconceptions that were created by the government itself. The greater value of saving people is overlooked in how high earning countries respond to making vaccines available. The global vaccine distribution has been a major challenge since developed countries want it for themselves (Forman et. al., 2021; Vanderslott et. al., 2021).

There are several frameworks that were recommended on allocation of vaccines. Entities on several occasions have proposed strategic frameworks that promote equitable allocation of limited supplies of vaccines locally and globally. For instance, the ACIP proposed allocation of vaccines in priority phases in which healthcare workers, essential workers and adults who are at high medical risk are given priorities (Dooling, 2021). While the World Health Organization Strategic Advisory Group of Experts (SAGE) on immunization recommended six guiding principles of human wellbeing, equal respect, global equity, national equity, reciprocity and legitimacy, the principle of global equity has been at the center of many discussions on the availability of vaccines in developing world, Africa especially (Dooling, 2021). Reducing barriers in the acquiring of vaccines not just within the country but to developing countries should be regarded as a justice issue.

Reflection and Discussion on Public Governance Ethics

COVID-19 has brought an ethical challenge in the governance of public agencies. In a pandemic like COVID-19, the protection of people cannot be overstated. Therefore, governance of public agencies is central in adherence to the ethical standards in regard to fairness, justice and human protection during the calamities. Injustice and unfairness have a big impact on the vulnerable groups such as women, children, immigrants, and the poor. This calls for strong ethical leadership in the public arena. Ethical leadership with an ethical culture will create an environment of ethical conduct during the emergency response and will help in creating governance systems that curb any malpractice in emergency response.

In most cases, unethical behaviors thrive during emergencies due to fast responses and lax checks and balances. There are issues of structural injustice that manifest itself through corruption during the fast implementation of crisis response. Structural injustice takes center stage during such a response. Structural injustice has been at the center in preventing the potential flourishing of the abstract poor while this in turn enables others to excessively benefit by making available to them more opportunities to develop their own potential. It is important to note that addressing the ethical issues in governance may lead to more vibrant economies and greater social flourishing of several individuals if the issues of structural justice are addressed.

Ultimately, the economic recovery of several countries will depend on how the public servants address issues of ethics in the face of COVID-19 especially in public agencies. The obligation for the government should be to promote equity and moral equality as they adhere to ethical standards. The government has the duty of fairness to relatively distribute the risk and benefits of care as the focus in dealing with the pandemic. This calls for the individuals entrusted with the leadership to be good stewards, to act with transparency and have a sense of accountability. There are high rates of abuse in the social cash transfer programs in many countries. Politicians are on the forefront enrolling the beneficiaries of the economic programs which at most instances ignore the eligibility criteria. It is necessary to note that most of these economic stimulus programs are systematically designed to be implemented by the politician. This benefits the supporters of the party in government while overlooking the real beneficiaries. The governments in developing countries need to identify independent agencies that will be emancipated from the political influence.

In addition, we have noted that the rampant conduct of state capture and weak systems in public procurement have created an environment where ethical principles are overlooked. COVID-19 has given several governments in developing countries an opportunity for another level of looting in which public procurement is the epicenter of corruption. State capture happens when firms make payments to public officials in order to receive business favors. The problem of state capture is rooted in the rule and regulations that govern the government agencies. Top government officials should help to revisit the regulation within their agencies to control the influence of economic elites. Reform programs should be created in order to increase competition in the monopolistic markets and at the same time have proper check and balances on how contracts are awarded. Further to this, the development of a legal structure to regulate political financing, conflict of interest, and assets declaration is critical in curbing state capture.

The world has struggled with the equitable distribution of vaccines which prioritizes the rich over the poor and the marginalized. For decades, developing countries haven't seriously invested in the health sector, leaving a dilapidated healthcare system that couldn't effectively respond to pandemics like COVID-19. This calls for huge investment in the health sector infrastructure as well as adherence to ethical principles in the management of health institutions. Proper investment in the healthcare system will improve equality in the access of healthcare. Vaccine access and distribution couldn't have been a big issue if developing countries had a proper healthcare system.

Finally, the concerns over the management of public funds continues to grow in many countries and it rests within the governance principles of such countries. For instance, Brazil has one of the highest COVID-19 death rates and also performs poorly both on the World Justice Project's index score for fundamental rights and the Corruption Perception Index Ranking (Amundsen, 2022). Many reports recognize that several of these deaths may have been avoided if political officials had not pocketed the COVID-19 funding (Goldstein et al., 2020; Steingruber et al., 2020).

Conclusion

The development agenda for many developing countries, especially in Africa, has been affected by lack of good policies necessary for improving the governance and economic performance along with increased corruption. Poor governance and high levels of corruption affect the equitable distribution of scarce resources which ultimately increase the income inequalities in the society. Corruption to a greater extent distorts the decision-making process in public agencies especially during pandemics.

High to the challenges, in responding to the pandemic, is how ethical/unethical policy makers and decision makers are responding to the pandemic by deliberately overlooking the very basics of governance they have set in place. In developing countries, corruption has hindered the governing institutions to properly protect the vulnerable groups during pandemics. Inadequate governance controls have increased the risk of corruption during the COVID-19 pandemics since there is no meaningful oversight on how public funds are used during the pandemic.

The success in fighting corruption rests in the leadership both in the private and public sector. During crises like the COVID-19 pandemic, countries need clear guidelines and enforcement of those guidelines in protecting the public funds. Good leadership provides a culture that will adhere to ethical principles. However, fighting corruption during the pandemic like COVID-19 requires a coordinated effort by all the players in the society. These include traditional leaders, the media, the nonprofit organization, the law enforcers, and the citizens in acting as whistlers in any malpractice.

Leaders both in public and private institutions should stand guard to defend the very ethical principles that govern societies. This is the political will that is lacking in most leadership in developing countries. This calls for ethical leadership. Ethical leadership will create trust in the governance of the public institutions. Ethical leadership in the governance of public agencies will create an ethical culture that will curb corrupt practices including the cronyism that is so rampant in developing countries.

References

Ahmed, N., Dabi, N., Lawson, M., Lowthers, M., Marriott, A., & Mugehera, L. (2022). Inequality kills: The unparalleled action needed to combat unprecedented inequality in the wake of COVID-19. *Oxfam Policy and Practice.* doi: 10.21201/2022.8465

Amundsen, I. (2020). COVID-19, cash transfers, and corruption: Policy guidance for donors. *Chr. Michelsen Institute, 9,* 15. https://www.cmi.no/publications/7222-covid-19-cash-transfers-and-corruption

Cuadrado, C., Monsalves, M., Gajardo, J., Bertoglia, M., Nájera, M., Alfaro, T., Canals, M., Kaufman, J., & Peña, S. (2020). Impact of small-area lockdowns for the control of the COVID-19 pandemic. *MedRxiv.* https://doi.org/10.1101/2020.05.05.20092106

Devereux, S. (2021). Social protection responses to COVID-19 in Africa. *Global Social Policy, 21*(3), 421–447.

Dooling K, Marin M, Wallace M, et al. (2021) The Advisory Committee on Immunization Practices' updated interim recommendation for allocation of COVID-19 vaccine — United States. *Morbidity and Mortal Weekly Report, 69,* 1657-1660. http://dx.doi.org/10.15585/mmwr.mm695152e2external icon

Forman, R., Shah, S., Jeurissen, P., Jit, M., & Mossialos, E. (2021). COVID-19 vaccine challenges: What have we learned so far and what remains to be done? *Health Policy, 125*(5) 553-567.

Gentilini, U., Almenfi, M., Orton, I., & Dale, P. (2020). *Social protection and jobs responses to COVID-19: A real-time review of country measures.* World Bank. https://openknowledge.worldbank.org/handle/10986/33635

Goldstein, J. R., & Lee, R. D. (2020). Demographic perspectives on mortality of COVID-19 and other Epidemics. *National Academy of Sciences, 117*(36), 22035-22041. doi:10.1073/pnas.2006392117

Herbert, S., & Marquette, H. (2021). COVID-19, governance, and conflict: Emerging impacts and future evidence needs. *K4D Emerging Issues Report, 34.* doi: 10.19088/K4D.2021.029

Jenkins, M., Khaghaghordyan, A., Rahman, K., & Duri J. (2020). *Anti-corruption strategies for development agencies during the COVID- 19 pandemic.* Transparency International Anti-Corruption Helpdesk. https://knowledgehub.transparency. org/helpdesk/anti-corruption-strategies-for-development-agencies-during-the-covid-19-pandemic

Johnson, S (2022). Covid vaccine inequity due to 'racism rooted in slavery and colonialism' The Guardian, *Global Development.* https://www.theguardian.com/global-development/2022/apr/30/covid-vaccine-inequity-due-to-racism-rooted-in-slavery-and-colonialism

Kateta, M. W. (2021). How corruption derails development in Malawi. *Foreign Policy.* https://foreignpolicy.com/2021/05/21/how-corruption-derails-development-in-malawi/

Keulder, C. (2021). Africans see growing corruption, poor government response, but fear retaliation if they speak out *Afrobarometer Dispatch, 488.* https://www.afrobarometer.org/wp-content/uploads/migrated/files/publications/Dispatches/ad488-pap2-africans_see_growing_corruption-afrobarometer_dispatch-4nov21.pdf

Krachler, N., Greer, I. & Umney, C. (2022). Can public healthcare afford marketization? Market principles, mechanisms, and effects in five health systems. *Public Admin Rev.* https://doi.org/10.1111/puar.13388

Lawal, G. (2007). Corruption and development in Africa: Challenges for political and economic change. *Humanity and Social Sciences Journal, 2,* 1-7.

Li, B., Qian, J., Xu, J., & Li, Y. (2020). Collaborative governance in emergencies: Community food supply in COVID-19 in Wuhan, China. *Urban Governance.* https://doi.org/10.1016/j.ugj.2022.03.002

Masina, L. (2020). Malawi politicians ignore COVID-19 measures for elections. *Voice of Africa, 6.* https://www.voanews.com/a/africa_malawi-politicians-ignore-covid-19-measures-elections/6189553.html

Mlaba, K. (2021). Why are African countries throwing away COVID-19 vaccines? *Global Citizen.* https://www.globalcitizen.org/en/content/african-countries-throwing-away-covid-19-vaccines/

Mzumara, G. W., Chawani, M., Sakala, M., Mwandira, L., Phiri, E., Milanzi, E., Phiri, M. D., Kazanga, I., O'Byrne, T., Zulu, E. M., Mitambo, C., Divala, T., Squire, B., & Tam, P. (2021). The health policy response to COVID-19 in Malawi. *BMJ Global Health, 6*(5), e006035. doi:10.1136/ bmjgh-2021-006035

Nyasulu, J. C., Munthali, R. J., Nyondo-Mipando, A.L., Pandya, H., Nyirenda, L., Nyasulu, P. L, & Manda, S. (2021). COVID-19 pandemic in Malawi: Did public sociopolitical events gatherings contribute to its first-wave local transmission? *International Journal of Infectious Diseases, 106*, 269-275. https://doi.org/10.1016/ j.ijid.2021.03.055.

Oduor, M. (2021). Africa's Covid-19 corruption that outweighs pandemic. *Africa News.* https://www.africanews.com/2021/05/25/africa-s-covid-19-corruption-that-outweighs-pandemic//

Ott, J. S., Edwards, F. L., & Boonyarak, P. (2021). Global responses to the COVID-19 pandemic. *Public Organization Review, 21*, 619–627. https://doi.org/10.1007/ s11115-021-00595-5

Roope, L., Candio, P., Kiparoglou,V., McShane, H., Duch, R., & Clarke, P. M. (2021). Lessons from the pandemic on the value of research infrastructure. *Health Research Policy and Systems, 19*(54). https://doi.org/10.1186/s12961-021-00704-2

Steingbruber, S., Kirya, M., & Mullard, S. (2020). Corruption in the time of Covid-19: A double-threat for low-income countries. *U4 Brief 2020, 6.* https://www.u4.no/publications/corruption-in-the-time-of-covid-19-a-double-threat-for-low-income-countries

Tille, F., Panteli, D., Fahy, N., Waitzberg, R., Davidovitch, N., & Degelsegger-Marquez, A. (2021). Governing the public- private-partnerships of the future: Learnings from the experiences in pandemic times. *Eurohealth, 27*(1), 49-53.

Vanderslott, S., Emary, K., te Water Naude, R., English, M., Thomas, T., Patrick-Smith, M., Henry, J., Douglas, N., Moore, M., Stuart, A., Hodgson, S. H., & Pollard, A. J. (2021) Vaccine nationalism and internationalism: Perspectives of COVID-19 vaccine trial participants in the United Kingdom. *BMJ Global Health, 6*(10), e006305. doi:10.1136/ bmjgh-2021-006305

World Bank. (2020). World development indicators. http://datatopics.worldbank.org/ world-development-indicators/

THE ETHICS OF RESOURCE DISTRIBUTION IN THE COVID-19 PANDEMIC

Mark Olaf[1]

Abstract: The COVID-19 pandemic has highlighted previously existing resources disparities in the United States and around the world. Access to masks, testing, medications, vaccines, and accurate information have all influenced the health and outcomes of individuals and communities. The limitations of these resources are discussed. The unequal distribution of resources invokes the ethical principles of nonmaleficence, beneficence, justice, and veracity. Given these limited resources, ethical principles must be invoked to contribute to the decisions of how to allocate those resources which are available. Several fundamental values have been identified and include maximizing the benefit of scarce resources, the equal treatment of people, promoting and rewarding instrumental value, and giving priority to the worst off. Any model that seeks to distribute disparate resources, particularly those which are needed urgently, must be founded in a rational set of ethical principles. Six recommendations have been offered for distributing these important, timely, and limited resources. The distribution of resources must: 1) attempt to maximize benefits, 2) prioritize health workers, 3) not allocate on a first-come, first-served basis, 4) respond to available and accepted evidence, 5) recognize research participation and progress, and 6) apply the same principles to both COVID-19 and non-COVID-19 patients.

Our world is filled with variable risk. Each day we encounter variable situations, and make decisions while accounting for many known factors, some of which are inside and some outside of our control. We consider that smoking may place us at higher risk for cardiovascular disease and make a choice whether or not to smoke. We consider that uncontrolled high blood pressure and diabetes may also increase our risk, though we don't always or often have a choice about developing these conditions. We understand that not wearing our seatbelts places us at higher risk of death and injury in vehicle accidents and also make choices according to

[1] Associate Professor of Emergency Medicine, Geisinger Commonwealth School of Medicine, Danville, Pennsylvania, USA

our values. We also realize there are limitations to our knowledge, our time, and our abilities, but we can rely on our values to guide us through these decisions. It is nearly impossible to perfectly calculate risk or even control risk. We recognize that we cannot control the speed of another driver's car, but as a society we can agree on speed limits and incorporate certain safety mechanisms to mitigate the risk of an accident. To maintain the health and well-being of individuals, we develop programs to ensure opportunities for well-being based upon our societal values. Foundational to these programs are the ethical principles that guide our society. Beneficence, non-maleficence, autonomy, and justice are the four main principles that guide medical decisions. Additional principles may be invoked under circumstances where upholding the primary principles is impossible. We may find ourselves needing to closely examine and consider these principles when encountering a novel societal danger, particularly one like COVID-19. The COVID-19 pandemic brought with it large amounts of incalculable risk that were unexpected, hidden, and beyond our control. When we find ourselves with such a paucity of information, it is our ethical principles that must guide us to make decisions. We are left with few other resources to make important decisions regarding providing care for our society. We must also then maintain those same principles as we do acquire new information and evolve our understanding of a problem.

In the time preceding the COVID-19 pandemic, we certainly relied on ethical principles to provide healthcare. However, even without the acute and severe stressors of a global pandemic, we likely fell short of achieving truly ethical care in our society. When we look more closely at the elements that place us at risk of poor health outcomes, we are sometimes surprised to find that the obvious and known risk factors are not the only determinants of our health. These sometimes "hidden" and often surprising factors may even have more influence than the highly recognized ones and may call into question the ethical foundations of our system of healthcare in the United States.

Equity in health care has multiple dimensions including equitable utilization, distribution, access, and health outcomes (Culyer & Wagstaff, 1993). The United States Centers for Disease Control (CDC) defines health equity as a state in which all individuals have a fair and just opportunity to attain their best health (CDC, 2022). These dimensions and this definition contrasts and also overlaps with the concept of ethical equality. Both equity and equality are bound in the concept of fairness. The principle of equality among individuals suggests uniform opportunity presented to all, while the concept of equality invokes the uneven distribution of our backgrounds and suggests a need for differential resources and opportunities to attempt to level the playing field.

Healthcare disparities within our communities present an ongoing and inherent conflict with delivering ethical medical care to society. Disparities in population resources, including housing, financial, food, medication, medical knowledge, and other resources have impacts on how, when, and why individuals may or may not access medical care (Ahmed et al., 2020; Chong et al., 2020). The unequal distribution of resources primarily challenges the ethical principle of equity, but also invokes concepts of nonmaleficence, beneficence, justice, and veracity, as well as the ethical values that shape the care provided to individuals and groups of patients (Robert et al., 2020; Xafis et al., 2020).

In fact, the problem is so large that a Social Vulnerability Index (SVI) has been developed. The SVI is a tool that quantifies risk based on individual background factors and implemented by the CDC in order to quantify and better understand risks for particular communities (Flanagan et al., 2011). The COVID-19 pandemic has highlighted previously existing resource disparities in the United States and around the world (Xafis et al., 2020). Access to testing, medications, vaccines, and accurate information have all influenced the health and outcomes of individuals and communities (Xafis et al., 2020). The unequal distribution of resources during the COVID-19 pandemic invokes and highlights the same challenges to these ethical principles (Acosta et al., 2020; Wiltz et al., 2020; Xafis et al., 2020).

In addition to the inherent disparities that exist in our communities which impact access to healthcare, disparities in healthcare resources also exist. Healthcare resources are finite and include resources of equipment, time, personnel, medications, and other elements. When distributing these resources to a population of patients, it is critical to consider the ethical implications of how the resources are allocated. Equity in distribution should be a primary goal in an ideal world. However, under emergent, urgent, or other time sensitive circumstances, as was seen during the COVID-19 pandemic, doing the most good for the most people may supersede the goal of equity. These two goals can seem to be in conflict and create tension. Other goals of resource distribution should include beneficence for the population; distributing resources to accomplish the most good, reducing the risk of harm to the population, and ensuring patient autonomy in health care decisions.

Existing disparities in the delivery of medical care and ethical challenges

To understand the impact of disparities in healthcare delivery and their consequences in the COVID-19 pandemic, we must first consider the foundation and existence of these disparities in our healthcare system and in our society. The patterns of disparity that we have seen in the COVID-19 pandemic reflect pre-existing differences in our healthcare system that have likely been unmasked during this challenging time.

Inequalities among individuals and among populations are ever-present concepts and realities in our world. These disparities also have a known influence on our health outcomes. For example, despite declines in preterm birth (babies delivered before 37 weeks of pregnancy) in the United States over the past 100 years, African-American/Black women have disparate rates of preterm birth when compared to White women. Preterm birth rates in African American/Black women are 1.5 to 1.6 times higher (Braveman et al., 2021). Scientists and physicians both agree that the causes of this disparity are complex and multifactorial. In attempting to elucidate a plausible cause or set of causes for these differences, scientists have looked at multiple up-stream and down-stream factors that are known influences on women's and children's health in relation to pregnancy, including not only age, rates of diabetes, or hypertensive disorders, but also factors related to stress, social support, socioeconomic factors, and income and education, among many others. While there is not one singular cause of these differences, there are associations between some of these factors and preterm birth rates. Gestational diabetes, hypertensive disorders, and stress have all exhibited direct links, while age presented no direct link to preterm birth rate discrepancies (Braveman et al., 2021). Socio-economic factors are also indirectly linked to these disparities through other factors and causes. We must therefore accept the plausibility that disparities in our social construct contribute to differences in preterm birth rates. These findings are not unique to preterm birth rates. We also see societal differences linked to disparate health care outcomes in other areas, including rates of overall death, chronic disease, and mental health (Pickett & Pearl, 2001). The link between our socioeconomic status and our health is very clear.

Once we recognize that these differences existed before the COVID-19 pandemic, and have been exacerbated by it, we must then consider the ethical implications of these disparities in healthcare outcomes. The ethical delivery of healthcare demands beneficence, non-maleficence, autonomy, and justice. If we know that disparities in the delivery of care exist, and do nothing to correct them, then we deprive those affected of the justice of ethical healthcare delivery as it relates to our societal systems for the delivery of care. If we can be certain that differences exist and do nothing to correct them, then we cannot guarantee the beneficial and unharmful delivery of care to populations. We sometimes find conflict at the juxtaposition of the delivery of individual care and population care where we try to reconcile differences in populations while caring for a particular individual. It is important to recall that while we may recognize disparities at the population level, we may not see them among smaller groups or among individuals and may not be able to correct these broader issues while caring for one particular individual, even if that individual is in an at-risk group. We should not be paralyzed by the concept of factors beyond our individual control, nor deterred from attempting to achieve justice for each individual's care. Rather, embracing the concept should allow us to consider where our efforts are best directed and to develop better systems of care that can address the underlying societal risks and affect disparities in outcomes.

COVID-19 pandemic exacerbated disparities in healthcare delivery and challenges ethical principles

The COVID-19 pandemic has amplified the long-standing inequities that impact the delivery of healthcare in the U.S., and has resulted in a disproportionate burden of illness among certain disadvantaged groups including ethnic and racial minorities, financially disadvantaged groups, and among certain geographic areas (Acosta et al., 2021; Karmakar et al., 2021; Mackey et al., 2021; Ogedegbe et al., 2020; Price-Haywood et al., 2020; Tipirneni et al., 2022; Wiltz et al., 2022). One study found that Black and Hispanic populations experienced higher rates of COVID-19 infection, hospitalization, and mortality (Mackey et al., 2021). Another study indicated increased COVID-19 incidence and mortality among socioeconomically disadvantaged groups (Karmakar et al., 2021). Additional evidence continues to mount that implicates societal factors, including race, as influential among healthcare outcomes from COVID-19 (Taylor et al., 2022). It has been proposed that a more equitable distribution of resources may have led to improved outcomes and reduced disparities in these groups (Horby et al., 2021; Rainwater-Lovett et al., 2021; Taylor et al., 2022).

In order to further investigate and explain the creation or enumeration of disparities in healthcare resources and outcomes in the COVID-19 pandemic, let us look at a few case examples, including inequities in mask availability, hospital resources, geography, and medical treatments.

Masks

The early phases of the COVID 19 pandemic demonstrated a need to ration N-95 masks for healthcare workers and required the development of protocols for reusing masks that were only ever intended for a single use (Emanuel et al., 2020). The rationing of masks as a healthcare resource both implies and leads to inequitable access to vital healthcare necessities. Though it was unclear early in the pandemic, it later became evident that masks were associated with a reduction in the transmission of COVID-19 (Fischer et al., 2021). Inability to access a mask would then raise the risk of contracting COVID-19 and spreading it in a community. In March 2020, the FDA (2021) issued an Emergency Use Authorization allowing for the import of non-NIOSH approved N-95 respirators (masks that fall below the usual U.S. government benchmarks) and allowed for U.S. standards to be modified to those of other countries. The FDA (2020) also issued a letter to healthcare providers to acknowledge the shortage and recommend conservation strategies for the utilization of masks and gowns. In previous years, the U.S. Department of Health and Human Services (HHS) had indicated in its influenza pandemic planning documents that a pandemic would be likely to place "extraordinary and sustained demands" on multiple aspects of the healthcare delivery system (Emanuel, 2020; HHS, 2017). As we progressed through the pandemic, we saw these likely stressors become reality, in the form of limited medical mask availability, and we have observed differences in COVID-19 illness and mortality likely as a result.

Given the impact of masks, and challenges in equitable access, prior authors have suggested six categories of recommendations for mask conservation based upon a review of interventions during previous epidemics and pandemics (Kirubarajan et al., 2020). Strategies have included decontamination, extended wear of disposable masks, layering of masks, the use of reusable respirators, non-traditional mask replacements and alterations, and stockpiling masks. The most effective strategies were thought to include stockpiling masks, the extended wear of masks, and decontamination, all of which have been used during the COVID 19 pandemic (HHS, 2017). While stockpiling may be an attractive option to some larger systems, it presents a challenge to smaller businesses, healthcare systems, and individuals who may not have the resources to purchase or store masks. Thus, extended wear, and decontamination of masks became common practices in some communities and hospitals but posed some inherent risk in this novel viral pandemic as there was uncertainty about the efficacy of these practices. In addition, the instructions for decontamination included the use of chemicals and processes that laypersons may not have access to, or may have had difficulty implementing given the technical nature of these measures. Thus, even as these practices attempted to do the most good for many people, inherent inequalities were created with these practices.

While the limitations of masks as finite resources leading to shortages and disparities in distribution is an ethical challenge itself, governmental or organizational mandates or recommendations can and have exacerbated these difficulties. One study suggested that a universal mask-wearing policy in China would lead to a facemask shortage, further resulting in panic among citizens, and eventually leading to a substantial surge in demand (Wu et al., 2020). The downstream impacts of such panic and surge demand would then lead to a shortage of resources for healthcare workers and those directly affected by pandemic illness, further exacerbating the spread of the virus and straining resources; a sort of vicious cycle would take hold, compounding the disparity of resources and propagating pandemic illness. The study recommended considering additional public health measures, and the risk of illness transmission in concert with a mask mandate as a way to mitigate these disparities (Wu et al., 2020). The principle of doing the most good for the most people certainly is required in such circumstances as an emerging pandemic when resources are limited, but falls short of the goal of generating justice and equity in healthcare outcomes. The hypothetical scenarios posed by researchers in fact came true and manifested during the COVID-19 pandemic, leading to the hoarding of masks, and limited supplies. In the United States, initial recommendations from public health officials led to an increased demand for masks and an abrupt scarcity of specialized masks. The policy which was instituted was likely intended to do the most good; healthcare workers who would have the highest rate of exposure would be prioritized. However, a consequence of the well-intended policy was an induction of panic among the population, and the buying, hoarding, and price-gouging for the limited supply of masks. The resulting impact on mask demand and availability led health officials to loosen mask guidelines so that front-line healthcare workers might have masks available to them (Sun, 2020). One could postulate that additional measures of preparedness could have mitigated the disparity in access to masks; perhaps an enhanced national stockpile could have been considered, or could be considered in anticipation of another pandemic, or as ways to mitigate the spread of known viral pathogens that exist in our communities already, such as influenza. Prior to the COVID-19 pandemic, such a stockpile may have been seen as excessive, but in hindsight, as perceptions have changed, it may appear to be a wise allocation of resources, particularly to equitably protect our society.

Hospitals

The impact of disparities that we have observed is directly tied to the breadth of the COVID-19 pandemic. Endemic illnesses are those that are expected to occur in a community, either continuously, or in waves during particular time periods. Endemic illnesses are likely to cause local impacts and have minimal or no disruptions to national or international resources. Endemic illness is already incorporated into our usual routines in healthcare. For example, we expect an increased rate of influenza in the United States during the winter months. We prepare and anticipate the needs and adjust our preparedness in light of particular populations who may be at risk. However, a pandemic is an unexpected event, has world-wide impact and implications that exacerbate resource disparities. The HHS developed Pandemic Influenza Plans in 2005, and updated them in 2009, and again in 2017. The plan estimated a moderate pandemic would affect 64 million individuals in the U.S., with about 800,000 requiring hospital beds, and 160,000 requiring ICU beds. A severe pandemic would significantly increase the use of resources (Emanuel et al., 2020). The impact of COVID 19 across the world has been variable. Rates of mild, moderate, and critical illness have varied from country to country. Death rates have varied too. Despite the variability, rates of severe illness and death are far above that of seasonal influenza (Emanuel et al., 2020). Given the severity of illness above that of seasonal influenza, the healthcare system has experienced substantial strain, though not uniformly across our large country. Despite the preparation for an influenza pandemic by the HHS, our healthcare systems have struggled to manage the impact of COVID-19, and would likely fall short of the severe pandemic impact that was projected by the HHS.

In particular, healthcare system capacity is expected to experience strain during a pandemic. A 2018 report from the American Hospital Association (AHA) indicated that there were 5,198 community hospitals, 792,417 community hospital beds, 3,532 community emergency departments, and 96,500 community ICU beds in the United States. Of the ICU beds, under 68,400 were adult ICU beds, while the remainder were for pediatric and neonatal patients (AHA, 2018; Emanuel et al., 2020). It is clear from these reports, and the HHS estimates of resource needs in a moderate or severe pandemic, that disparities in resources will be underscored, and the rationing of resources would be implemented. Where resources could not or would not be rationed, alternative types of treatment would also be initiated, for example providing ICU levels of care in non-ICU designated areas or maintaining patients in rooms or areas where continuous patient care was not originally planned.

And while patient rooms and designated space have been largely overwhelmed during our experience with COVID-19, resources for the delivery of care inside and outside of the ICUs have additionally been limited. Early in the pandemic it was proposed that not only would ICU beds be limited in availability, but ventilator availability and the availability of certified respiratory therapists and appropriately trained clinical staff to operate the ventilators would become scarce resources (Emanuel et al., 2020). We in fact saw these projections come to fruition in some cases as ventilators needed to be shared among patients, and treatment regimens were altered to do the most good with scarce resources. Medical providers were forced to develop strategies to share ventilators, for which there are a limited number of resources and little global experience. Sharing ventilators increases risks to patients as individual patients usually require individualized ventilator settings which correspond to lung capacity and other individual respiratory parameters. Sharing ventilators also risks additional infectious exposure to those sharing those ventilators. While patients on a shared ventilator during the COVID-19 pandemic both presumably would have COVID-19 infections, they risked spreading other viruses or bacteria between them, though ventilator filtering helps mitigate it. The alternative to developing unfounded and novel strategies to share ventilators is to ration the resources. During the pandemic hospital ethics committees were charged with assisting in developing and implementing decision tools and parameters to help clinicians who may be faced with the difficult decision to ration health care resources. We again fall short of equitable care, and the resulting disparities in care provided weigh heavily on patients and healthcare providers who know they fall short of their ethical and moral objectives.

Beyond the ICUs, usual diagnostic, therapeutic and preventative resources were anticipated to be diminished, and this prediction has become reality (Emanuel et al., 2020). Routine screening examinations for various diseases, as well as elective procedures have been delayed for many patients.

Waiting lists have been developed, and stratification techniques implemented. It is expected that delays in screening and routine care may lead to increased deaths that are not the direct result of COVID-19, but rather due to delays in routine care (Larson et al., 2020). Throughout the pandemic individuals have had cancelled appointments for mammography, routine colonoscopies, and other screening diagnostic tests. It is proposed that breast, colon, and other cancers, along with a variety of other diseases, will be detected later that they would have under normal screening protocols as patients had extraordinarily limited access to routine testing. This limited access was due to early concerns about the transmissibility of COVID-19 and mitigating disease spread, as well as staff redeployment to assist with the care of COVID-19 patients. Certain groups already experience challenges in accessing care, and these resource limitations are likely to exacerbate such disparities and lead to reduced equity in the provision of routine care.

Geographic factors

It has been proposed that a moderate pandemic would likely lead to regional differences in the scarcity of hospital beds, ventilators, and even staff. It might seem obvious that large population areas might be overwhelmed with large volumes of patients requiring testing and treatment, but at the same time a small population area might quickly succumb to staffing or medical supply shortages with only a minor deficiency creating a relatively large healthcare delivery problem (Emanuel et al., 2020). The healthcare systems aren't necessarily designed for redundancy or crises, but rather are modeled to be efficient and to respond to population needs as they arise. This leads to lags and inequities in care in geographic regions, which are exacerbated during times of increased need, such as the COVID-19 pandemic. New reports have shown us the impact in large population centers, but small population centers are at equivalent, if not increased, risk. In our demand-based system, where there are smaller populations, there are inherently fewer resources. The disparity in resources again generates risk for inequitable health access and outcomes.

The CDC's SVI has been utilized to better understand the impact of social vulnerability risk factors with COVID-19 outcomes (Tipirneni et al., 2022).

In this study, patients living in high vulnerability ZIP codes who contracted COVID-19 were more often Black or Hispanic, and had more baseline comorbid conditions. These same patients had lower pulse oximetry readings (measurements of available oxygen in the blood), and higher respiratory rates (a sign of respiratory failure) when compared to lower vulnerability ZIP codes. These patients were also more likely to be treated in an intensive care unit, require mechanical ventilation, have acute organ failure or dysfunction, or die in the hospital when compared to low vulnerability patients (Tipirneni et al., 2022). After adjusting for confounding variables in this study, the authors found that lower neighborhood SVI scores were associated with increased risk for mechanical ventilation, acute organ dysfunction, and acute organ failure. The authors concluded that a patient's geographic disadvantage affects hospital outcomes; that is, where a patient resides affects their burden of COVID-19 disease, and outcomes associated with it.

Thus, we must conclude that disparities in healthcare outcomes are influenced and exacerbated by the COVID-19 pandemic based on what would traditionally be considered non-medical factors. That is, the location of a person's residence, including the region, and even neighborhood, is both expected to and does produce a disproportionate outcome. In this case, equity is particularly hard to achieve even in a non-pandemic time period. Healthcare outcomes which are associated with locations may be seen as out of the control of hospital workers or administration, limiting the impact that the healthcare system may have on equitable and ethical care across broader regions.

Monoclonal antibodies

The unequal distribution of resources that existed prior to the pandemic has continued and even been exacerbated by the COVID-19 pandemic. Antibodies help us fight off infections. Certain antibodies are specialized to fight off particular infection; these are known as Monoclonal Antibodies (MABs). These MABs have been shown to be effective in protecting against progression of disease for those with mild to moderate severity COVID-19 illness (Gottlieb et al., 2021). However, these effective medications have been in short supply and not available ubiquitously throughout the world, and within regions and localities or hospital systems in the United States. Given these constraints, federal guidelines have been developed to guide the administration of these medications (National Institutes of Health, 2020). One trial studied how the limited supply of COVID-19 MABs was distributed using a convenience sample of Medicare beneficiaries. Of the nearly 2 million patients studied, only 7.2% received MABs. Of those receiving the medication, there was a higher likelihood of having fewer chronic conditions, and a lower likelihood of being Black (Behr et al., 2022).

An additional study analyzed the delivery of MABs by race and ethnicity. Among patients with a positive COVID-19 test result, MAB use was only four percent or less for all racial and ethnic groups. However Hispanic patients were less than half as likely to receive MAB therapy compared to non-Hispanic patients. Black, Asian, or "Other" race patients received MAB therapy substantially less frequently than did White patients (22%, 48%, and 47%, respectively; Wiltz et al., 2022).

These studies highlight the fact that in the era of COVID-19, beneficial treatments have been distributed inequitably. Moreover, with the overall limited distribution, it is particularly concerning that these effective treatments have been distributed at a reduced level to populations that are at particularly high risk. Though consensus recommendations and regulations exist for the use of MABs, early in the pandemic there was not a singularly identified national strategy with regard to the distribution of COVID-19 MABs. The lack of uniform distribution is likely due to a number of factors, including a limited supply, a lack of a forma network for distribution secondary to the private industry nature of medicine in the U.S., as well as the nuanced needs of each community, which each health system serves. It is obvious from the above studies that the distribution of these MABs has been uneven and thus inequitable, but without a particular and nuanced strategy for distribution it also is apparent that we may not have done the most good for individuals. Individuals with easier access to care may have been more likely to receive the medications. Again, the lack of a systematic approach to account for limited access to care has challenged the ethics of the manner of which our healthcare system has approached our vulnerable populations.

Antiviral therapies

Another class of medications which have demonstrated efficacy against COVID-19 are antivirals. Many individuals will be familiar with antiviral medications used to treat influenza, herpes, and the human immunodeficiency virus (HIV). Similarly, antiviral medications have become available for treating COVID-19. However, because of challenges in coordinating testing results and follow-up care, as well as a limited supply of the medication, the clinical effectiveness of these antiviral medications, and therefore the benefits of them, is diminished substantially. The beneficence of the medications, as well as that of the companies that produce them, the researchers that discover them, and the clinicians who prescribe them, is substantially reduced or eliminated due to a system that does not function as a well-oiled machine, but rather functions to create or propagate pre-existing disparities in accessing healthcare (Borio et al., 2022). When we lack a functioning and effective system of care, we cannot be sure that we are delivering equitable care, or even doing the most good. We can be sure we're doing some good, but those with the easiest access to care may be more likely to be the recipients of those benefits, which is not aligned with our ethical goals. The inequality created by this uneven distribution also calls into question the beneficence and justice in our medical system, particularly under the conditions of the pandemic. Unequal access to care is a contradicting principle to these foundational ethical principles.

Vaccines

COVID-19 vaccines are an effective method to prevent or moderate disease (Higdon et al., 2022). In adult populations, COVID-19 vaccines reduce mortality, hospitalization, and severity of disease related to the COVID illness (Bajema et al., 2021; Borio et al., 2022; Fowlkes et al., 2021; Higdon et al., 2022; Olson et al., 2021). And though they are very effective for these critical outcomes, some side effects of vaccines have been noted, including common ones like headaches, muscle aches, and fevers (Higdon et al., 2022). Among the many millions and billions of doses of vaccines administered, there have also been some significant side effects. There have been 49 cases described in the literature, which demonstrate a risk of clotting disorders (thrombotic thrombocytopenia) with the viral vector vaccines AZD1222 (ChAdOx1 nCoV-19, AstraZeneca) and Ad26.COV2 (Johnson and Johnson). No such disorder has been described in the mRNA vaccines (Sharifian-Dorche et al., 2021). Additionally, among men 18-25, there is a slightly increased and rare risk of inflammation of or around the heart (pericarditis and myocarditis) with the mRNA vaccines mRNA-1273 (Moderna) and BNT162b2 (Pfizer-BioNTech) (Wong et al., 2022). However, the rates of peri- and myo-carditis are still lower than that expected with COVID illness (Boehmer et al., 2021). COVID-19 vaccines have been effective in children above 5 years, though less effective than in adults (Fowlkes, 2022; Klein et al, 2022). In children under the age of five years, early data suggested less immunogenicity, with presumed lower rates of protection in this age group (Pfizer, 2021). Clinical trials for vaccine immunogenicity and clinical efficacy among children six months to five years, support their use as safe and effective, though efficacy has been confirmed to be lower than those vaccines for adults, and trials have had fewer enrollments (Willyard, 2022).

It is important to recall that while one goal of a vaccine is to reduce individual illness, another goal is to create a community of individuals who are less susceptible to illness and less likely to spread it within the community. It has been suggested that achieving 90% immunity, through infection or vaccination, would be sufficient to achieve herd immunity and move the pandemic into a phase where life with COVID-19 will resemble something most individuals would consider "normal" (Borio et al., 2022). It is also suggested that achieving this level of population immunity would require vaccine mandates (Borio et al., 2022). However, a broad vaccination mandate in the U.S. would unmask and perhaps create further disparities and differences in healthcare use and accessibility. Vaccination mandates from the U.S. government would only apply to certain government employees and contractors, health care workers, and perhaps larger businesses. Further, it is widely thought that booster shots will be required on a regular or perhaps annual basis (Borio et al., 2022). Thus, an inherent disparity and burden may be placed on a few select individuals in order for the country to achieve a level of vaccination sufficient to temper down the broad effects that the pandemic has had on our society and health care system. It could be argued that healthcare workers and government employees are servants of society, and through that nature a vaccination mandate is reasonable. However, there are limitations to the degree of service these individuals offer. And it would be presumptive and likely incorrect to assume that all of these individuals would willingly share this burden just by the virtue of being employed in a particular job. Again, an unequal or uneven distribution of resources, this time in the form of vaccine mandates, creates a disparity among individuals living in our society, and with it, brings a degree of injustice.

Ethical principles for more equal distribution of resources

Given the aforementioned evidence of resource disparities, both in the global sense of a lack of universally available resources, and in the uneven distribution of those which are available, we must consider ethical principles as we make the complex decisions of how to allocate those resources which are available. Broad and sweeping decisions will lack the nuance and attention of principles within each community, and individual community decisions may lack a universal perspective that accounts for the needs of other communities. Thus, a standard or uniform set of principles may not be able to achieve the most good, or to generate equity, optimize beneficence, or reduce unintended maleficence of our approaches to COVID-19. Rather, broad agreement upon guiding ethical principles should be the foundation of our efforts.

Fortunately, several fundamental values have been identified based upon work related to prior pandemics, the anticipation of a novel pandemic, and the current COVID-19 pandemic. Four fundamental values have been identified: maximizing the benefit of scarce resources, the equal treatment of people, promoting and rewarding instrumental value, and giving priority to the worst off (Bernheim et al., 2011; Biddison et al., 2014; Centers for Disease Control, 2018; Emanuel et al., 2020; Emanuel & Wertheimer, 2006; Persad et al., 2009; Zucker et al., 2015).

We have already discussed the broad evidence of disparities in accessing care related to COVID-19 based upon a number of different factors. While we cannot change the availability of resources, we can maximize their benefit in the manner in which we distribute them. We can make our best efforts to treat individuals equally regardless of race, gender, ethnicity, or geography, but we need to address these factors when considering how localities and hospital systems make decisions about distribution. Based on the previous examples, we have clearly fallen short of attempting to give priority to the worse off. In particular, those who are lowest on the SVI received disproportionately fewer resources and had worse outcomes than those with better access to care or in more affluent regions. In contrast to our ethical principles, we have seen evidence of giving priority to instrumental value of certain individuals during the pandemic: healthcare workers have been given the priority for masks and vaccines in nearly every community and distribution. We need to revisit and remind ourselves and our communities that these principles should guide differential access to COVID-19 prevention, testing, and treatment. Further, we need to weigh these principles equally, and not just focus or prioritize one sole principle while sacrificing others.

Public health planning

As the United States and the rest of the world move towards a "new normal" of existence with endemic COVID-19 in each of our new communities, new ways of conceptualizing the national approach to public health, and infectious diseases are necessary (Emanuel et al., 2022). Without the implementation of an appropriate plan, health disparities and inequities are at risk of becoming greater (Bernheim et al., 2011). The "new normal" will also likely require increased and ongoing attention to testing and population surveillance, when compared to the time before the COVID 19 pandemic (Michaels et al., 2022). This shift in surveillance may benefit the overall population, but raises the ethical concerns of nonmaleficence and autonomy of the individual. Individual harms from testing and surveillance are uncommon, but the burden placed on individuals to obtain regular testing, or the impact of regular testing on the autonomy of the individual deserve important and dedicated attention. In adjusting to a "new normal," one benefit, with regard to reducing health care disparities, may be the implementation of uniform and standardized COVID 19 and respiratory virus mitigation standards and strategies.

Mitigation strategies, if implemented in the appropriate manner, may help diminish inequities in the transmission of respiratory viruses, including COVID 19, particularly in the workplace. Such mitigation strategies have included and could include mobility restrictions for confirmed or exposed individuals, physical distancing, hygienic precautions including hand sanitizing and face masking, and enhanced communication regarding exposures.

Models for ethical distribution of resources

In order to embrace the foundational ethical principles that should guide our decisions, and achieve equity in our healthcare outcomes, our systems of care must adapt to not only the known and prevalent risks and influence, but also address the underlying socio-economic systems in place that influence them. We must include elements of those most affected in the decision making process, and give them a fair and equitable voice in developing solutions (Stone, 2002).

Any model that seeks to distribute disparate resources, particularly those which are needed urgently, must be founded in a rational set of ethical principles. Six recommendations have been offered for distributing these important, timely, and limited resources. The distribution of resources must: 1) attempt to maximize benefits, 2) prioritize health workers, 3) not allocate on a first-come, first-served basis, 4) respond to available and accepted evidence, 5) recognize research participation and progress, and 6) apply the same principles to both COVID-19 and non-COVID-19 patients (Emanuel et al., 2020; Pandemic Influenza Preparedness, 2007; Toner & Waldhorn, 2020).

These ethical principles call into mind some situations which have been anticipated for the COVID-19 pandemic. Given the relative scarcity of ventilators, decisions may have to be made, or might have been made regarding which patient would receive treatment, and which patient might receive some alternative treatment. The decision to treat a healthcare worker with a ventilator instead of a non-healthcare worker is prioritized in some models, but is opposed by some (Sveen & Antommaria, 2020). Certainly, some questions remain. While the healthcare worker arguably has a likely ability to assist others or has already contributed some extra-ordinary service in the midst of the pandemic, it remains uncertain that, if a healthcare worker requires mechanical ventilation, he or she would eventually be able to return to work, or even willing to return to work. It is also important to consider our definition of equity in this realm. Are all healthcare workers given the same treatment? Who would define their relative values? Is it even ethical to consider these relative values in the healthcare realm, or is the consideration of placing increased value on certain individuals due to their occupations not in line with ethical principles as all? While these are all worthy questions without ready answers, the underlying principle of prioritizing healthcare workers recognizes the value of the high-risk work that they do, and helps to discourage absenteeism, which may contribute to the greater good of the population and society (Irvin et al., 2008).

While healthcare workers are prioritized, we must be careful not to prioritize wealthy, famous, or other powerful individuals. Examples of this disparity have occurred time and time again during the pandemic with respect to COVID- 19 testing, vaccination, and medication availability and access (Biesecker et al., 2020). Arguably, access to vetted information has been prioritized towards healthcare workers in the form of peer reviewed and credible journal publications which require unique access and skills in evaluating such information.

In situations where patients have similar prognoses, the ethical principle of equality must be invoked and operationalized through random allocation of resources, such as a lottery system (Emanuel et al., 2020; FDA, 2021). We have seen this come to life through the distribution of monoclonal antibody administration throughout the pandemic. There has been evidence to demonstrate that MABs reduce the chance of hospitalization or death in some cases, and therefore use in the outpatient setting has been implemented. However, there are not enough MABs to treat all patients with COVID 19 who do not require hospitalization. Particular individuals are at increased risk of hospitalization and death, and therefore, based upon the fundamental principles of treating the worst off, and maximizing benefit, these populations have been prioritized for the MAB treatments; priority guidelines have been developed in line with ethical principles which are specific to the intervention and changing scientific evidence (Emanuel et al., 2020). Yet still the resource is limited even among the highest risk population, and lottery systems have been developed and implemented.

And despite the solutions which have been created to address these disparate resources in specific situations, questions remain regarding the weight given to each factor in determining the distribution. Does being a healthcare worker who is young and healthy outweigh the benefits that an elderly patient with multiple co-morbid conditions would receive from a MAB infusion? The evidence would suggest that it likely does not, however, an ethical conundrum arises regarding the prioritization of these values and factors. Ultimately it is not as critical to assign particular values and weights to these factors, but to maintain a fair and consistent allocation procedure that represents all affected groups. Additionally, it is important to maintain transparency in these procedures (Emanuel et al., 2020).

Conclusion

It is clear that we have faced numerous ethical challenges in navigating the COVID-19 pandemic. It is also clear that inequities and inequalities that existed in our healthcare system prior to the pandemic have continued to exist or have been highlighted by our approach to distributing resources related to the care of COVID-19. Universal solutions for countries or communities are unlikely to be the answer. Rather, guiding ethical principles must help us maximize the benefit of scarce resources, treat individuals equally, promote resource use among individuals with instrumental value, and give priority to the worst off.

References

Acosta, A. M., Garg, S., Pham, H., Whitaker, M., Anglin, O., O'Halloran, A., Milucky, J., Patel, K., Taylor, C., Wortham, J., Chai, S., Daily Kirley, P., Alden, N., Kawasaki, B., Meek, J., Yousey-Hindes, K., Anderson, E., Openo, K., Weigel, A.,... Havers, F. P. (2021). Racial and ethnic disparities in rates of COVID-19–associated hospitalization, intensive care unit admission, and in-hospital death in the United States from March 2020 to February 2021. *Jama Network Open, 4*, e2130479. https://doi.org/10.1001/jamanetworkopen.2021.30479

Ahmed, S., Ajisola, M., Azeem, K., Bakibinga, P., Chen, Y. F., Choudhury, N. N., Fayehun, O., Griffiths, F., Harris, B., Kibe, P., Lilford, R. J., Omigbodun, A., Rizvi, N., Sartori, J., Smith, S., Watson, S. I., Wilson, R., Yeboah, G., Aujla, N. … Improving Health in Slums Collaborative. (2020). Impact of the societal response to COVID-19 on access to healthcare for non-COVID-19 health issues in slum communities of Bangladesh, Kenya, Nigeria and Pakistan: results of pre-COVID and COVID-19 lockdown stakeholder engagements. *BMJ Global Health, 5*(8), e003042. doi: 10.1136/bmjgh-2020-003042

American Hospital Association. (2018). AHA annual survey database.

Bajema, K. L., Dahl, R. M., Prill, M. M., Meites, E., Rodriguez-Barradas, M. C., Marconi, V. C., Beenhouwer, D. O., Brown, S. T., Holodniy, M., Lucero-Obusan, C., Rivera-Dominguez, G., Morones, R. G., Whitmire, A., Goldin, E. B., Evener, S. L., Tremarelli, M., Tong, S., Hall, A. J., Schrag, S. J., McMorrow, M., … Surveillance Platform for Enteric and Respiratory Infectious Organisms at the VA (SUPERNOVA) COVID-19 Surveillance Group (2021). Effectiveness of COVID-19 mRNA vaccines against COVID-19-associated hospitalization - Five Veterans Affairs Medical Centers, United States, February 1-August 6, 2021. *Morbidity and Mortality Weekly Report, 70*(37), 1294–1299. https://doi.org/10.15585/mmwr.mm7037e3

Behr, C. L., Joynt-Maddox, K. E., Meara, E., Epstein, A. M., Orav, E. J., & Barnett, M. L. (2022). Anti-SARS-CoV-2 monoclonal antibody distribution to high-risk medicare beneficiaries, 2020-2021. *JAMA, 327*(10), 980-983. doi: 10.1001/jama.2022.1243

Bernheim, R. G., Crawley, L., Daniels, N., Goodman, K., Kass, N., Lo, B., Rosenbaum, S., Ruger, J., Sankar, P., Wheeler, M. C., & Bayer, R. (2011). *Ethical considerations for decision making regarding allocation of mechanical ventilators during a severe influenza pandemic or other public health emergency*. Centers for Disease Control and Prevention.

Biddison, L. D., Berkowitz, K. A., Courtney, B., De Jong, M. J., Devereaux, A. V., Kissoon, N., Roxland, B. E., Sprung, C. L., Dichter, J. R., Christian, M. D., & Powell, T. (2014). Ethical considerations: care of the critically ill and injured during pandemics and disasters: CHEST consensus statement. *Chest, 146*(4), Suppl: e145S-e155S.

Biesecker, M., Smith, M. R., & Reynolds, T. (2020, March 19). Celebrities get virus tests, raising concerns of inequality. *Associated Press*. https://apnews.com/b8dcd1b369001d5a70eccdb1f75ea4bd

Boehmer, T. K., Kompaniyets, L., Lavery, A. M., Hsu, J., Ko, J. Y., Yusuf, H., Romano, S. D., Gundlapalli, A. V., Oster, M. E., & Harris, A. M. (2021). Association between COVID-19 and myocarditis using hospital-based administrative data - United States, March 2020-January 2021. *Morbidity and mortality weekly report, 70*(35), 1228–1232. https://doi.org/10.15585/mmwr.mm 7035e5

Borio, L. L., Bright, R. A., & Emanuel, E. J. (2022). A national strategy for COVID-19 medical countermeasures: Vaccines and therapeutics. *JAMA, 327*(3), 215-216. doi: 10.1001/jama.2021.24165

Braveman, P., Dominguez, T., Burke, W., Dolan, S., Stevenson, D., Jackson, F., Collins, J. Driscoll, D., Haley, T., Acker, J., Shaw, G., McCabe, E., Hay, W., Thornburg, K., Acevedo-Garcia, D., Cordero, J., Wise, P., Legaz, G., Rashied-Henry, K.,... Waddell, L. (2021). Explaining the Black-White disparity in preterm birth: A consensus statement from a multi-disciplinary scientific work group convened by the March of Dimes. *Frontiers in Reproductive Health, 3*, 2673-3153. https://doi.org/10.3389/frph.2021.684207

Centers for Disease Control and Prevention. (2018). Interim updated planning guidance on allocating and targeting pandemic influenza vaccine during an influenza pandemic.

Centers for Disease Control and Prevention. (2022). Health Equity. https://www.cdc.gov/healthequity/index.html

Chong, Y. Y., Cheng, H. Y., Chan, H., Chien, W. T., & Wong, S. (2020). COVID-19 pandemic, infodemic and the role of eHealth literacy. *International Journal of Nursing Studies, 108*, 103644. https://doi.org/10.1016/j.ijnurstu.2020.103644

Culyer, A. J., & Wagstaff, A. (1993). Equity and equality in health and health care. *Journal of health economics, 12*(4), 431–457. https://doi.org/10.1016/0167-6296(93)90004-x

Emanuel, E. J., Persad, G., Upshur, R., Thome, B., Parker, M., Glickman, A., Zhang, C., Boyle, C., Smith, & M., Phillips, J. P. (2020). Fair allocation of scarce medical resources in the time of COVID-19. *New England Journal of Medicine, 382*(21), 2049-2055. doi: 10.1056/NEJMsb2005114.

Emanuel, E. J., Osterholm, M., & Gounder, C. R. (2022). A national strategy for the "new normal" of life with COVID. *JAMA, 327*(3), 211-212. doi: 10.1001/jama.2021.24282

Emanuel, E. J., & Wertheimer, A. (2006). Public health: Who should get influenza vaccine when not all can? *Science, 312*, 854-855.

Fischer, C. B., Adrien, N., Silguero, J. J., Hopper, J. J., Chowdhury, A. I., & Werler, M. M. (2021). Mask adherence and rate of COVID-19 across the United States. *PLoS One, 16*(4), e0249891.

Flanagan, B. E., Gregory, E. W., Hallisey, E. J., Heitgerd, J., & Lewis, B. (2011). A social vulnerability index for disaster management. *Journal of Homeland Security and Emergency Management, 8*(1). doi:10.2202/1547-7355.1792

Fowlkes, A., Gaglani, M., Groover, K., Thiese, M., Tyner, H., Ellingson, K., & HEROES-RECOVER Cohorts (2020). Effectiveness of COVID-19 vaccines in preventing SARS-CoV-2 infection among frontline workers before and during B.1.617.2 (Delta) variant predominance — eight U.S. locations, December 2020–August 2021. *Morbidity and Mortality Weekly Report, 70*, 1167-1169. http://dx.doi.org/ 10.15585/mmwr.mm7034e4

Fowlkes, A. L., Yoon, S. K., Lutrick, K., Gwynn, L., Burns, J., Grant, L., Phillips, A. L., Ellingson, K., Ferraris, M. V., LeClair, L. B., Mathenge, C., Yoo, Y. M., Thiese, M. S., Gerald, L. B., Solle, N. S., Jeddy, Z., Odame-Bamfo, L., Mak, J., Hegmann, K. T., Gerald, J. K., … Gaglani, M. (2022). Effectiveness of 2-dose BNT162b2 (Pfizer BioNTech) mRNA vaccine in preventing SARS-CoV-2 infection among children aged 5-11 years and adolescents aged 12-15 years - PROTECT Cohort, July 2021-February 2022. *Morbidity and Mortality Weekly Report, 71*(11), 422–428. https://doi.org/10.15585/mmwr.mm7111e1

Gottlieb, R. L., Nirula, A., Chen, P., Boscia, J., Heller, B., Morris, J., Huhn, G., Cardona, J., Mocherla, B., Stosor, V., Shawa, I., Kumar, P., Adams, A., Van Naarden, J., Custer, K., Durante, M., Oakley, G., Schade, A. E., Holzer, T.,... Skovronsky, D. M. (2021). Effect of bamlanivimabas monotherapy or in combination with etesevimab on viral load in patients with mild to moderate COVID-19: A randomized clinical trial. *JAMA, 325*(7), 632-644. doi: 10.1001/ jama.2021.0202

Higdon, M. M., Wahl, B., Jones, C. B., Rosen, J. G., Truelove, S. A., Baidya, A., Nande, A. A., ShamaeiZadeh, P. A., Walter, K. K., Feikin, D. R., Patel, M. K., Deloria Knoll, M., & Hill, A. L. (2022). A systematic review of coronavirus disease 2019 vaccine efficacy and effectiveness against severe acute respiratory syndrome coronavirus 2 infection and disease. Open Forum Infectious Diseases, *9*(6). https://doi.org/10.1093/ofid/ofac138

Horby, P., Lim, W. S., Emberson, J. R., Mafham, M., Bell, J., Linsell, L., Staplin, N., Brightling, C., Ustianowski, A., Elmahi, E., Prudon, B., Green, C., Felton, T., Chadwick, D., Rege, K., Fegan, C., Chappell, L. C., Faust, S. N., Jaki, T.,... RECOVERY Collaborative Group. (2021). Dexamethasone in hospitalized patients with Covid-19. *New England Journal of Medicine, 384*, 693–704. doi: 10.1056/NEJMoa2021436

Irvin, C. B., Cindrich, L., Patterson, W., & Southall, A. (2008). Survey of hospital healthcare personnel response during a potential avian influenza pandemic: will they come to work? *Prehospital Disaster Medicine, 23*, 328-335.

Karmakar. M., Lantz, P. M., & Tipirneni, R. (2021). Association of social and demographic factors with COVID-19 incidence and death rates in the US. *JAMA Network Open, 4*, e2036462. doi: 10.1001/jamanetworkopen.2020.36462

Kirubarajan. A., Khan, S., Got, T., Yau, M., Fryan, J., & Friedman, S. M. (2020). Mask shortage during epidemics and pandemics: a scoping review of interventions to overcome limited supply. *BMJ Open 10*(11), e040547. doi: 10.1136/bmjopen-2020-040547

Klein, N. P., Stockwell, M. S., Demarco, M., Gaglani, M., Kharbanda, A. B., Irving, S. A., Rao, S., Grannis, S. J., Dascomb, K., Murthy, K., Rowley, E. A., Dalton, A. F., DeSilva, M. B., Dixon, B. E., Natarajan, K., Stenehjem, E., Naleway, A. L., Lewis, N., Ong, T. C., Patel, P., ... Verani, J. R. (2022). Effectiveness of COVID-19 Pfizer-BioNTech BNT162b2 mRNA vaccination in preventing COVID-19-associated emergency department and urgent care encounters and hospitalizations among non-immunocompromised children and adolescents aged 5-17 years - VISION Network, 10 States, April 2021-January 2022. *Morbidity and Mortality Weekly Report, 71*(9), 352–358. https://doi.org/10.15585/mmwr.mm7109e3

Larson, D. W., Abd El Aziz, M. A., & Mandrekar, J. N. (2020). How many lives will delay of colon cancer surgery cost during the COVID-19 pandemic? An analysis based on the U.S. National Cancer Database. *Mayo Clinic Proceedings, 95*(8), 1805–1807. https://doi.org/10.1016/j.mayocp.2020.06.006

Mackey, K., Ayers, C. K., Kondo, K. K., Saha, S., Advani, S., Young, S., Spencer, H., Rusek, M., Anderson, J., Veazie, S., Smith, M., & Kansagara, D. (2021). Racial and ethnic disparities in COVID-19-related infections, hospitalizations, and deaths: A systematic review. *Annals of Internal Medicine. 174*(3), 362-373. doi: 10.7326/M20-6306

Michaels, D., Emanuel, E. J., & Bright, R. A. (2022). A national strategy for COVID-19: Testing, surveillance, and mitigation strategies. *JAMA, 327*(3), 213-214. doi: 10.1001/jama.2021.24168.

National Institutes of Health. (2021, October 19). Therapeutic management of non-hospitalized adults with COVID-19. In COVID-19 Treatment Guidelines Panel (Eds.), *Coronavirus Disease 2019 (COVID-19) Treatment Guidelines* (pp. 53-58). https://files.covid19treatmentguidelines.nih.gov/guidelines/archive/covid19treatmentguidelines-10-27-2021.pdf

New South Wales Department of Health. (2010). *Key recommendations on pandemic (H1N1) 2009 influenza.* https://www.health.nsw.gov.au/pandemic/Documents/key-recommendations-pandemic-H1N1-NSW-health-2010.pdf

Ogedegbe, G., Ravenell, J., Adhikari, S., Butler, M., Cook, T., Francois, F., Iturrate, E., Jean-Louis, G., Jones, S., Onakomaiya, D., Petrilli, C., Pulgarin, C., Regan, S., Reynolds, H., Seixas, A., Volpicelli, F. M., & Horwitz, L. I. (2020). Assessment of racial/ethnic disparities in hospitalization and mortality in patients with COVID-19 in New York City. *JAMA Network Open, 3*(12), e2026881. doi:10.1001/jamanetworkopen.2020.26881

Olson, S. M., Newhams, M. M., Halasa, N. B., Price, A. M., Boom, J. A., Sahni, L. C., Irby, K., Walker, T. C., Schwartz, S. P., Pannaraj, P. S., Maddux, A. B., Bradford, T. T., Nofziger, R. A., Boutselis, B. J., Cullimore, M. L., Mack, E. H., Schuster, J. E., Gertz, S. J., Cvijanovich, N. Z., Kong, M., ... Overcoming COVID-19 Investigators (2021). Effectiveness of Pfizer-BioNTech mRNA vaccination against COVID-19 hospitalization among persons aged 12-18 years - United States, June-September 2021. *Morbidity and Mortality Weekly Report, 70*(42), 1483–1488. https://doi.org/10.15585/mmwr.mm7042e1

Pickett, K. E., Pearl, M. (2001). Multilevel analyses of neighbourhood socioeconomic context and health outcomes: A critical review. *Journal of Epidemiology & Community Health, 55*(2), 111-122.

Pandemic Influenza Preparedness Team: Department of Health, United Kingdom. (2007). *Responding to pandemic influenza — the ethical framework for policy and planning.* https://webarchive.nationalarchives.gov.uk/20130105020420/; http://www.dh.gov.uk/prod_consum_dh/groups/dh_digitalassets/@dh/@en/documents/digitalasset/dh_080729.pdf

Persad, G., Wertheimer, A., & Emanuel, EJ. (2009). Principles for allocation of scarce medical interventions. *Lancet, 373*(9661), 423-431. doi: 10.1016/S0140-6736(09)60137-9

Pfizer (2021). Press Release, Dec 17. https://www.pfizer.com/news/press-release/press-release-detail/pfizer-and-biontech-provide-update-ongoing-studies-covid-19

Price-Haywood, E. G., Burton, J., Fort, D., Seone, L. (2020). Hospitalization and mortality among Black patients and White patients with Covid-19. *New England Journal of Medicine, 382*, 2534-2543. doi: 10.1056/ NEJMsa2011686

Rainwater-Lovett. K., Redd, J. T., Stewart, M. A., Calles, N., Cluff, T., Fang, M., Panaggio, M, Lambrou, A., Thornhill, J., Bradburne, C., Imbriale, S., Freeman, J., Anderson, M., & Kadlec. R. (2021). Real-world effect of monoclonal antibody treatment in COVID-19 patients in a diverse population in the United States. *Open Forum Infectious Diseases, 8*, ofab398. https://doi.org/10.1093/ofid/ofab398

Robert, R., Kentish-Barnes, N., Boyer, A. Laurent, A., Azoulay, E., & Reignier, J. (2020). Ethical dilemmas due to the Covid-19 pandemic. *Annals of Intensive Care 10*(84). https://doi.org/10.1186/s13613-020-00702-7

Sharifian-Dorche, M., Bahmanyar, M., Sharifian-Dorche, A., Mohammadi, P., Nomovi, M., & Mowla, A. (2021). Vaccine-induced immune thrombotic thrombocytopenia and cerebral venous sinus thrombosis post COVID-19 vaccination; a systematic review. *Journal of the Neurological Sciences, 428*, 117607. https://doi.org/10.1016/j.jns.2021.117607

Stone, J. (2002). Race and healthcare disparities: Overcoming vulnerability. *Theory of Medical Bioethics, 23*, 499–518. https://doi.org/10.1023/A:1021524431845

Sun, L. (2020, March 10). Face mask shortage prompts CDC to loosen coronavirus guidance. *The Washington Post.* https://www.washingtonpost.com/health/2020/03/10/face-mask-shortage-prompts-cdc-loosen-coronavirus-guidance/

Sveen, W., & Antommaria, A. (2020). Why healthcare workers should not be prioritized in ventilator triage. *The American Journal of Bioethics: AJOB, 20*(7), 133–135. https://doi.org/10.1080/15265161.2020.1779852

Taylor, C. A., Whitaker, M., Anglin, O., Milucky, J., Patel, K., Pham, H., Chai, S., Alden, N., Yousey-Hindes, K., Anderson, E., Teno, K., Reeg, L., Como-Sabetti, K., Bleecker, M., Barney, G., Bennett, N., Billing, L., Sutton, M., Talbot, H. K.,

Havers, F. (2022). COVID-19-associated hospitalizations among adults during SARS-CoV-2 Delta and Omicron variant predominance, by race/ethnicity and vaccination status - COVID-NET, 14 states, July 2021–January 2022. *Morbidity and Mortality Weekly Report, 71*(12), 466-473. http://dx.doi.org/10.15585/mmwr.mm7112e2

Tipirneni, R., Karmakar, M., O'Malley, M., Prescott, H. C., & Chopra, V. (2022). Contribution of individual- and neighborhood-level social, demographic, and health factors to COVID-19 hospitalization outcomes. *Annals of Internal Medicine*. doi: 10.7326/M21-2615

Toner, E., & Waldhorn, R. (2020, Feb 27). *What U.S. hospitals should do now to prepare for a COVID-19 pandemic.* Johns Hopkins University Center for Health Security. http://www.centerforhealthsecurity.org/cbn/2020/cbnreport-02272020.html

U.S. Department of Health and Human Services. (2017, December). *Pandemic influenza plan: 2017 update.* https://www.cdc.gov/flu/pandemic-resources/pdf/pan-flu-report-2017v2.pdf.

U.S. Food and Drug Administration. (2020, April 27) *Surgical mask and gown conservation strategies - Letter to health care providers.* https://www.fda.gov/medical-devices/letters-health-care-providers/surgical-mask-and-gown-conservation-strategies-letter-health-care-providers

U.S. Food and Drug Administration. (2021, November 2). *FAQs on shortages of surgical masks and gowns during the COVID-19 pandemic.* https://www.fda.gov/medical-devices/personal-protective-equipment-infection-control/faqs-shortages-surgical-masks-and-gowns-during-covid-19-pandemic

Willyard, C. (2022, June 17). *FDA authorizes COVID vaccines for the littlest kids: what the data say.* Nature. June 17. ISSN 1476-4687 (online)

Wiltz, J. L., Feehan, A. K., Molinari, N. M., Ladva, C., Truman, B., Hall, J., Block, J., Rasmussen, S., Denson, J., Trick, W., Weiner, M., Koumans, E., Gundlapalli, A., Carton, T., & Boehmer, T. (2022). Racial and ethnic disparities in receipt of medications for treatment of COVID-19 — United States, March 2020–August 2021. *Morbidity Mortality Weekly Report, 71*(3), 96–102. http://dx.doi.org/10.15585/mmwr.mm7103e1

Wong, H. L., Hu, M., Zhou, C. K., Lloyd, P. C., Amend, K. L., Beachler, D. C., Secora, A., McMahill-Walraven, C. N., Lu, Y., Wu, Y., Ogilvie, R. P., Reich, C., Djibo, D.

A., Wan, Z., Seeger, J. D., Akhtar, S., Jiao, Y., Chillarige, Y., Do, R., Hornberger, J., ... Anderson, S. A. (2022). Risk of myocarditis and pericarditis after the COVID-19 mRNA vaccination in the USA: A cohort study in claims databases. *Lancet, 399*(10342), 2191–2199. https://doi.org/10.1016/ S0140-6736(22)00791-7

Wu, H. L., Huang, J., Zhang, C. J. P., He, Z., & Ming, W. K. (2020). Facemask shortage and the novel coronavirus disease (COVID-19) outbreak: Reflections on public health measures. *EClinicalMedicine, 21*, 100329. doi: 10.1016/j.eclinm. 2020.100329

Xafis, V., Schaefer, G., Labude, M. Zhu, Y., Hsu, L. Y. (2020). The perfect moral storm: Diverse ethical considerations in the COVID-19 pandemic. *Asian Bioethics Review, 12*, 65–83. https://doi.org/10.1007/s41649-020-00125-3

Zucker, H., Adler, K., Berens, D., Bleich, J. D., Brynner, R., Butler, K. A., Calderon, Y., Corcoran, C., Neveloff Dubler, N., Edelson, P. J., Fins, J. J., Geer, F. H., Gorovitz, S., Henderson, C. E., Khouli, H., Koterski, J. W., Maynard-Reid, H. H., Murnane, J. D.,... Gutmann Koch, V. (2015, November). *Ventilator allocation guidelines.* New York State Department of Health Task Force on Life and the Law.

PART THREE
Suppression Measures: Costs and Benefits

RISK, PROPORTIONALITY AND NECESSITY: AN EVIDENCE-BASED CRITIQUE OF COVID-19 PANDEMIC MANAGEMENT STRATEGIES

Michael Tomlinson[1]

Abstract: Governments were persuaded to adopt universal strategies to manage the COVID-19 pandemic – effectively to suppress the spread of the virus in an interim period until vaccination would eliminate it. To achieve these goals, it would be necessary to reduce population mobility by 75% and then to vaccinate the entire population once vaccines became available. The rationale for the mandates imposed to implement this strategy derives a form of utilitarian ethics - the contention that these measures were necessary to achieve the desired outcome, that they would result in the greatest good of the greatest number, and it was necessary to override individual rights to impose them. What level of support was there in the scientific literature for this strategy, was there enough reason to believe it would be successful in reducing the burden of disease and especially loss of life? What evidence of effectiveness was available prospectively at the time these decisions were first made, and then retrospectively in the light of the outcomes experienced over the first two years of the pandemic? What decision-making process should be followed to form public policy in a pandemic to ensure that it is ethically justifiable?

Lockdown Outcomes

Selective quarantining of sick people or their contacts has been practised since the plague pandemic of 1347–1352, with weak evidence for effectiveness (Tognotti, 2013; WHO, 2019). At the time the governments decided to go down the path of universal quarantining of the whole population, there was little or no evidence in the scientific literature for its effectiveness, as quarantine had never been used before for entire

---

[1] Chair, Human Research Ethics Committee, National Institute of Integrative Medicine, Hawthorne, Australia

populations of countries. There was also no attempt to undertake a utilitarian calculus and calculate the balance of costs and benefits - there was no consideration of the possible adverse effects that these measures might have on health and wellbeing.

Governments and councils of experts relied on statistical modelling of scenarios to guide them when making decisions about what countermeasures to use against the pandemic. However, in the hierarchy of evidence-based medicine (EBM) there are a number of levels, sometimes represented in the form of a pyramid, with randomised clinical trials (RCTs) and systematic reviews of RCTs towards the top (for example, Murad, 2016). Modelling studies are either placed at the bottom or not included at all, on the grounds that they do not consist of evidence if evidence is conceived to consist of actual data, as it should be.

Comprehensive reviews of the effectiveness of NPIs for respiratory illnesses (for example the Cochrane review by Jefferson et al., 2020 and WHO, 2019) had concluded that the evidence for 'social distancing' in general was limited and of low quality. And these reviews did not specify what form of social distancing should be used. Closure of workplaces was covered, but there was no mention of stay-at-home orders at all (sometimes referred to as 'shelter in place').

Governments were particularly influenced by Imperial College London's COVID-19 Response Team's 'Report 9' (Ferguson et al., 2020), which recommended that Non-Pharmaceutical Interventions (NPIs) such as lockdowns should be imposed for an interim period until effective vaccinations were available. But the suppression strategy recommended in this report was not justified by the report's own results, which showed the best outcomes as resulting from a mitigation strategy consisting of case isolation, home quarantine and social distancing of those aged over seventy. Other modelling studies proliferated, but many of these have been found to be unreliable and inaccurate. For example, Chin et al. (2020) compared different variants of the ICL modelling and concluded that: 'Inferences on effects of NPIs are non-robust and highly sensitive to model specification, assumptions and data employed to fit models' (p. 6).

Modelling studies such as ICL's *Report 9* put forward worst-case scenarios of extreme loss of life in the absence of NPIs, scenarios that cannot be falsified as no governments encountered significant epidemic waves without deploying NPIs of some kind. These counterfactual scenarios supporting the case for the initial imposition of NPIs on the way up the epidemic curve cannot be tested or falsified, so have low status as scientific propositions.

However, the modelling groups also made claims about the factual scenarios that developed after governments lifted their non-pharmaceutical measures (NPIs) on the downward curve of epidemic waves, and these can be tested. For example, in May of 2020, ICL's *Report 20* (Volmer et al., 2020) considered the Italian government's plan to relax restrictions and predicted that this would lead to 'a resurgence in the number of deaths far greater than experienced in the current wave in several regions' (p. 2). In reality, there was no such resurgence, and Italy's mortality curve continued to decline over the period to a low point of 0.10 deaths per million people in mid-August 2020, according to the 'Data Explorer' display at the website *Our World in Data* (https://ourworldindata.org/coronavirus, accessed on 30 June 2022). This was pointed out by the epidemiologists Heneghan and Jefferson (2020).

So, the knowledge base on which governments initially took the decision to reduce general mobility through lockdowns was limited and questionable, constituting a thin basis for the measures taken.

Over the next two years, empirical data built up enabling researchers to try and calculate the effect of lockdowns on outcomes. Many of the published studies focus on possible effects of lockdowns on infection rates over a delimited period, often amounting to a few weeks, sometimes making comparisons between selected countries, or states of federal countries such as the USA or Germany. The beginning and end points of these time periods do not have any consistent relationship with the epidemic curves as a whole. The most important outcomes are severe COVID-19 (often measured through hospitalizations or ICU admissions) and deaths, but the studies often only infer these outcomes.

There is great variability in the findings of the observational studies. For example, Flaxman et al. (2020) found that lockdowns reduced case rates and Hsiang (2020) found that they reduced transmission rates. The effect on mortality outcomes was not directly observed but was dependent on assumptions. By contrast, Chaudhry (2020) concluded that although lockdowns did slow the rate of growth of infections, they only succeeded in deferring mortality somewhat, not preventing it.

Flaxman et al. (2020) and other authors often assume that changes in infection rates result from and are caused by prior interventions, which may indicate that their paper is open to the post hoc fallacy. They calculated that a large number of deaths were averted compared to a counterfactual scenario generated by their model, but as we have seen these are unreliable and unfalsifiable.

In a forceful critique of their work, Homburg and Kuhbandner (2020) found that their methods involve 'circular logic' and that 'the results of Flaxman et al. are artifacts of an inappropriate model.' In relation to the UK as a case study, they point out that, allowing for the lag between imposition of the UK lockdown on 23 March 2020 and the first possible date for an impact on deaths, the declining curve 'does not show the slightest break in mid-April', continuing through to 4 May.

Epidemic curves did eventually go down subsequent to lockdowns being introduced, but it is not clear whether they have demonstrated a causative effect. This is a common issue in these studies, and an important one as it is in the nature of epidemic curves to rise and then decline as immunity increases in the population. Atkeson (2021) found a remarkable consistency in the epidemic curve across all jurisdictions regardless of policy differences: between 20 and 30 days after the 25th death in each case, the growth rate in deaths reduced close to zero.

Mendez-Brito et al. (2021) undertook a systematic review of empirical studies of the comparative effectiveness of NPIs and found that: 'The evidence of the comparative effectiveness of NPIs with respect to mortality-related outcomes is not clear' (p. 288).

Sears et al. (2020) found that mortality rates declined in four U.S. states that implemented stay at home mandates earlier than others, but there was considerable variation within this group and states that never implemented mandates had the lowest mortality (p. 16). Populations had already decreased their mobility before mandates were introduced, so the marginal effect of coercion was limited. Human encounters had already decreased on a voluntary basis by 63% (p. 5).

Herby et al. (2022) conducted a meta-analysis of studies using empirical data based on a 'counterfactual difference -in-difference approach', which excludes papers based on modelling such as Flaxman et al. (2020). They concluded that reliable studies using the Oxford Blavatnik Government Stringency Index found that countries adopting stricter policies had reduced mortality by mid-2020 by only 0.2% on average (p. 33). And studies focussing specifically on stay-at-home ('Shelter-in-Place') orders found that these had reduced mortality by 2.9% on average (p. 34).

No doubt meta-analyses based on different criteria for inclusion or exclusion could come to different conclusions. But the reliance on empirical data is sound – coercive mandates should not be based on hypothetical scenarios -and there is not enough consistency in the findings of the outcomes studies to form a robust basis for public policy.

Allen (2021) went a step further by estimating not only reductions in mortality from the epidemic brought about by lockdowns, but also the increases in mortality from the possible collateral effects, in other words the cost/benefit ratio for mortality overall. By contrast: 'Over the course of the COVID-19 pandemic, there has been no public evidence that governments around the world have considered both the benefit and cost sides of their policy decisions' (p. 3).

On his review of the literature, Allen found there was only a marginal impact of mandatory lockdowns on reducing mortality, placing much weight on those findings of Atkeson (2021) that the epidemic curves declined in the same way regardless of interventions.

Against the marginal positive impact, Allen counterposed the substantial negative effects on mortality that would flow from the known effects of:

- loss of educational opportunities
- increased unemployment

- increased drug overdoses
- loss of medical services.

He supported the effects on mortality of each of these with multiple references. Many more are available from the following website: https://collateralglobal.org/studies/.

The effects of poverty on health are well-known (for example, Mathers 2001) and the World Bank projected that 97 million more people would be thrown into extreme poverty in 2020 (Mahler et al., 2020). Other studies focus on mental health, Owens et al. (2022) concluding (in the abstract): 'The evidence suggests that lockdown has caused a wellbeing crisis in young people'. Other studies focus on the effects of delayed medical treatment during lockdowns, especially in forms of cancer where early diagnosis and treatment greatly improves survival prospects: 'As delays in diagnosis allow tumours to continue to grow and advance, this bottleneck in the diagnostic pathway is likely to have a profoundly detrimental impact on colorectal cancer outcomes in England' (Morris et al., 2021).

Allen concludes that 'even under the assumption that lockdowns were little more than a minor inconvenience on average..., the costs were at least thirty-five times higher than the benefits' (p. 20). Whereas in fact lockdowns did in fact impose a considerable burden on populations, which would make the ratio even more unfavourable.

How could lockdowns have such a small effect on reducing COVID-19 mortality, in contrast to the assumptions made by the ICL team? A study by Kephart et al. (2021) of 314 Latin American cities found that there was indeed a link between reduced mobility and reduced infections (they didn't measure mortality) as summarised in the abstract: '10% lower weekly mobility was associated with 8·6% (95% CI 7·6–9·6) lower incidence of COVID-19 in the following week.' However, the effect was only observed in the short term: 'This association gradually weakened as the lag between mobility and COVID-19 incidence increased and was not different from null at a 6-week lag.'

The modelling scenarios assume that governments need to reduce the mobility of asymptomatic people as much as symptomatic people. Even though people are known to be infectious for a few days in the pre-symptomatic phase, the effects on the epidemic curve of reducing the mobility of all asymptomatic people have not been measured and so the need for it is unknown, especially for the earlier variants. The Omicron variant spread with such rapidity across the world despite all barriers that were in place at the time, so it is doubtful that lockdowns would have any effect on either the symptomatic or asymptomatic groups.

The modelling groups and agencies never considered alternative strategies such as a public health campaign to persuade symptomatic people to stay home or to be sent home by their employers. Governments should have asked the modelling groups and agencies for advice on this, and on other strategies, for example rolling out micro-nutrients such as Vitamin D to the vulnerable groups. Retrospectively, Shah et al. (2022) found that on the basis of a meta-analysis of seven systematic reviews: 'in people receiving vitamin D supplements, the odds of mortality were 52% lower as compared to individuals not receiving vitamin D supplements (OR: 0.48, 95% CI: 0.346–0.664' (p. 5). In a double-blind, randomized, parallel RCT, Villasis-Keever et al. (2022) found, as summarised in the abstract: 'The risk of acquiring SARS-CoV-2 infection was lower in the [verum group] than in the [control group] (RR: 0.23; 95% CI: 0.09–0.55) and was associated with an increment in serum levels of 25-hydroxyvitamin D3 (RR: 0.87; 95% CI: 0.82–0.93), independently of VD deficiency.'

Borsche et al. (2021) undertook a meta-analysis of two independent sources of information on the correlation between COVID-19 mortality rates and vitamin D levels. The further correlation between these two datasets is strongly indicative of a causative link:

> One analysis is based on the long-term average vitamin D3 levels documented for 19 countries. The second analysis is based on 1601 hospitalized patients, 784 who had their vitamin D levels measured within a day after admission, and 817 whose vitamin D levels were known pre-infection. Both datasets show a strong correlation between the death rate caused by SARS-CoV-2 and the vitamin D blood level. At a threshold level of 30 ng/mL, mortality decreases considerably. In addition, our analysis shows that the correlation for the combined datasets intersects the axis at approximately 50 ng/mL, which suggests that this vitamin D3 blood level may prevent any excess mortality.

Seal et al. (2022) also found that continuous blood calcifediol concentrations were independently associated with COVID-19- related hospitalization and mortality in an inverse dose-response relationship in a large racially and ethnically diverse cohort of U.S. Veterans Administration patients.

Agencies recommended the perceived majority view to governments. But they should always alert them to the fact that alternative findings, viewpoints and strategies exist and should clearly explain their reasons as to why they recommend their preferred position, above and beyond the fact that they might have majority support.

While many experts believe that lockdowns were effective, others believe that they were not. Ioannidis (2021) pointed out that more highly cited scientists signed *The Great Barrington Declaration* (Kulldorf et al., 2020 - against lockdowns) than signed the *John Snow Memorandum* (Alwan et al., 2020 - for lockdowns).

This is important because one of the conditions considered necessary in the ethical literature for overriding individual rights is that there should be some kind of consensus that the measures will be effective, or at least a negative consensus – that there are no expert views to the contrary. While the authors of the *John Snow Memorandum* titled their contribution 'Scientific consensus on the COVID-19 pandemic: we need to act now', the existence of these two opposing manifestos is conclusive proof that there was no such consensus.

Vaccination Mandate Outcomes

In the case of vaccination, when the first vaccines were developed in Western countries the evidence for their effectiveness from the clinical trials conducted by the pharmaceutical companies seemed straightforward. But there were significant limitations in the evidence that were not considered by governments or their regulatory agencies and limitations in the capability of the vaccines became evident over time.

For example, Peter Doshi (senior editor of *The British Medical Journal*) repeatedly called for the raw data behind the vaccine trials to be released, to clarify a number of issues that he raised in relation to the Pfizer vaccine trial (Doshi, 2021a) which might dramatically change the results:

- inclusion of patients with 'suspected COVID-19' who were not confirmed by testing
- exclusion of five times more patients in the vaccine group compared to the placebo group for protocol deviations
- possible unblinding of individuals in the groups
- inclusion of individuals who were SARS-CoV-2 positive at baseline.

None of these issues were analysed or discussed in the briefs from the U.S. Food and Drug Administration (FDA) supporting Emergency Use Authorisation. The briefs for both the Pfizer and Moderna vaccines prepared for the advisory committee (FDA, 2020a, 2020b) represented the data from the sponsors at face value, without any critical analysis. This represented a major regulatory failure.

On 23 August 2021, Doshi (2021b) called attention to the evidence that the immunity produced by the vaccines was starting to wane and called for full approval to be withheld. Evidence of waning immunity continued to build through 2021 and 2022 and was compounded by the appearance of the new variant, Omicron, towards the end of 2021.

Based on the UK National Health System records, the UK Health Security Agency (2021) found that:

> In all periods, effectiveness [against infection] was lower for Omicron compared to Delta...Among those who received a Pfizer primary course, vaccine effectiveness was around 70% after a Pfizer booster, dropping to 45% after 10-plus weeks.

Veneti et al. (2022) found that the effectiveness of the Pfizer vaccine against Omicron infection declined to only 25% by 63 days after the second vaccination, in their study of adolescents in Norway.

Based on the health records for the total population of Qatar, Chemaitelly et al. (2022) found that (as summarised in the abstract):

> mRNA vaccines provide comparable, moderate, and short-lived protection
> against symptomatic BA.1 and BA.2 Omicron infections, but strong and
> durable protection against COVID-19 hospitalization and death.

Renewed protection from booster doses was again very short term:
'Effectiveness rapidly rebounded to 59.9%....in the first month after the
booster dose, but then declined to 40.5%....in the second month and
thereafter' (p. 2). Repeated vaccinations using vaccines based on the
original strain but deployed against different variants, may be producing
diminishing returns.

By this stage, it was becoming clear that the vaccines were not capable of
producing herd immunity against COVID-19 through vaccination in the
first place because the immunity provided by the vaccines against
becoming infected was relatively short-term in nature, and they had at best
a weak effect on reducing transmission.

The total potential for transmission arises from the combination of the
number of individuals who become infected and the number of those
individuals who pass the infection on to others. Both are reduced by COVID-
19 vaccination only in the short-term. Eyre et al. (2021) found even in the time
when the Delta variant was dominant that: 'Protection against onward
transmission waned within 3 months post second vaccination' (p. 13).

The evidence does not support the feasibility of building herd immunity
against COVID-19 for a whole population through vaccination in a way
that would prevent future outbreaks, and vaccination of high proportions
of a population in many countries (including Israel) did not in fact do so. If
herd immunity is not possible and the vaccines do not prevent
transmission, then it becomes difficult to justify policies exerting coercive
pressure on groups at low risk from the disease. For example, workplace
mandates are difficult to justify in the case of an illness that predominantly
affects the post-working age population, with a vaccine that has a weak
effect on transmission and so offers poor or fleeting third-party protection.

They have not been demonstrated to provide a safer working environment;
the fundamental justification employers use to bring in mandates.
University campuses are useful delimited environments to test their ability

to achieve this goal. Meredith et al. (2022) used Cornell University as a case study and hypothesized that a combination of vaccination mandates and NPIs 'would limit COVID-19 spread on campus and sought to monitor this with a case-series study of university testing records' (p. 1). But the hypothesis was falsified: 'Based on analysis of routinely collected population surveillance data, Cornell's experience shows that traditional public health interventions were not a match for Omicron' (p. 3).

There is limited evidence to support vaccines producing a temporary reduction in the number of individuals becoming infected and so capable of passing the infection on. But arguably, other individuals are able to protect themselves (also temporarily) by themselves becoming vaccinated. High proportions of them have in fact done so in many countries. The marginal effect of an additional ten percent of people becoming vaccinated as a result of mandates, given the short-term protection achieved by the 90% through themselves becoming vaccinated, is almost impossible to calculate. It is doubtful it would be of a magnitude sufficient to justify the gross infringement of individual rights entailed.

Returning to the utilitarian calculus, governments also need to consider the potential for the vaccines to cause adverse effects. This is generally considered to be low, but there are some warning signs with some of the COVID-19 vaccines.

Fraiman et al. (2022) aggregated the data on serious adverse events from the trials of the Pfizer and Moderna mRNA vaccines and found 'an absolute risk increase of 10.1 and 15.1 41 per 10,000 vaccinated over the placebo baselines' (as summarised in the Abstract). They also found that 'The excess risk of serious adverse events of special interest surpassed the risk reduction for COVID-19 hospitalization relative to the placebo group in both Pfizer and Moderna trials', concluding there was a need for formal cost/benefit studies, stratified according to the risk of serious adverse event outcomes such as hospitalization and death.

Particular attention needs to be given to mortality outcomes. It is necessary to demonstrate that vaccination not only reduces mortality specific to COVID-19 as shown by Bernal et al. (2021) and Scobie et al. (2021), but that it meets the primary test for life-threatening illnesses - that it reduces all-cause mortality.

Classen (2021) makes this point and goes on to reanalyse the published clinical trial data for the endpoint of 'all cause morbidity or mortality' for the three trial reports for the vaccines manufactured by Pfizer-BioNTech, Moderna, and Janssen published in the *New England Journal of Medicine*. He summarised these figures in his Table 1 (p. 3) which shows significantly greater numbers of severe events in the vaccinated groups compared to the placebo groups.

Morris (2022) argues that it would not be feasible to measure all-cause mortality in a COVID-19 vaccine clinical trial as the trial population would have to be very large to ensure that it was sufficiently powered, and so a definitive trial would take too long. While this might be true for all-cause mortality alone, Classen's calculations of combined 'all cause morbidity or mortality' yield higher effect numbers. Even if calculating the relative risk of all-cause mortality through an RCT is not practicable, this still leaves us with the conclusion that the vaccines' ability to reduce mortality is not proven at the highest level of evidence in the EBM hierarchy.

Benn et al. (2022) aggregated the data from the trial reports for mRNA vaccines as compared with adenovirus vector vaccines and found that all-cause mortality was lower for the adenovirus vaccines, but not for the mRNA vaccines.

Observational outcomes studies addressing all-cause mortality have been few and variable over the first two years of the pandemic.

A Brazilian study of Buenos Aires residents aged 60 and above by Macchia et al. (2021) found that all-cause mortality was significantly reduced for these cohorts, but the overall outcomes for lower risk age groups are not clear.

Bardenheier et al. (2021) compared outcomes for large cohorts of nursing home residents who were vaccinated in different weeks. Severe outcomes were only monitored for seven days. Table 3 of their study shows that unadjusted mortality was *higher* in the vaccinated groups than in the unvaccinated groups, but after adjusting the data, they found the reverse to be the case. Adjustment was performed according to the 'inverse probability of vaccination', but it is not explained how this probability was calculated, or why it was necessary since the actual vaccination date of each resident was presumably known and recorded by the single healthcare provider that operates all the nursing homes.

Xu et al. (2021) conducted a cohort study of approximately 11 million individuals enrolled in seven U.S. Vaccine Safety Data Link sites and found that vaccinated individuals had lower risk of mortality from non-COVID-related causes compared with vaccinated individuals. As they observe, this was likely to result from 'healthy vaccinee effects' (i.e., the prior health of vaccinated individuals was already better than the unvaccinated individuals), or it may result from misclassification, so it is difficult to draw any firm conclusions from this study.

Craig et al. (2022) suggest official statistics for England reveal 'systematic undercounting of both COVID and non-COVID totalled deaths occurring within the first two weeks of COVID-19 vaccination', casting doubt on claims made for the effectiveness and safety of vaccination.

Pantazatos and Seligmann (2021) studied variations in mortality over time in two datasets: the U.S. Vaccine Adverse Events Reporting System (VAERS) and the European all-cause mortality monitoring organisation 'EUROMOMO'. They found a positive correlation with mortality in the period up to 6 weeks post-vaccination, and a negative association between six and twenty weeks post-vaccination. There are a few critical comments on the pre-print site with some robust rejoinders from Pantazatos.

There are known limitations to the VAERS database, which relies on passive reporting, but it is significant that rates of reporting to VAERS increased greatly in 2021. The background rate for mortality was established by Moro et al. (2015) as one reported death per million doses, amounting to 100 deaths per year on average. By contrast the U.S. Centres for Disease Control and Prevention (CDC) found that 8,638 reports of deaths were received in the period from 14 December 2020 to 14 February 2022, during which period more than 547 million doses of COVID-19 vaccines were administered (CDC, 2022). This is equivalent to a rate of one reported death per 63,000 doses, which is approximately 16 times higher than the background rate.

It is not possible to determine what the true rate is, but the exceptional increase in reports needs to be explained. No explanation has been offered. So, there is weak evidence that the COVID-19 vaccines improve mortality outcomes overall, and a case has been made out that they may cause a kind of 'dark mortality' that is not immediately evident.

It is not ethically acceptable to disregard indicative evidence of excess deaths without conducting a searching and impartial investigation. CDC does not acknowledge that any of the reported VAERS deaths result from vaccination. But the majority of these deaths were reported by the doctors and nurses on the ground who were responsible for treating these patients (McLachlan et al., 2021). It is hardly credible that thousands of doctors and nurses who were able to directly observe the course of events for these patients were mistaken, and that remote agency doctors were in a position to make a more accurate attribution.

Governments should commission eminent evidence-based medicine experts to review the extent of mortality from all causes especially within the first few weeks immediately succeeding each vaccination, with no exclusion period. This issue must be resolved.

The principle of non-maleficence ('first, do no harm') is one of the cornerstones of health ethics. When imposing mandates, government agencies have an ethical duty to fully investigate the risk that their policies might cause harm, especially when a competent and evidence-based case to answer is placed in the public domain. The onus of proof rests on the governments, agencies and companies that are the proponents of universal vaccination and vaccine mandates to show that there is a net benefit in lives saved for all age levels and preferably no lives lost.

Universal vaccination programs and vaccination mandates (especially those that affect the younger age groups) cannot be justified unless convincing evidence can be produced that they reduce all-cause mortality, both overall and stratified by age-group. There should be no opening for reasonable doubt on this.

Public support would be lost if the measures were conclusively shown to cause a significant number of deaths. The College of American Pathologists released a paper on the autopsy of two teenage males with toxic myocarditis described as 'post vaccine injury' (Gill et al., 2022). While some estimates have been made of the prevalence of post vaccine myocarditis, the same approach has not been taken to post vaccine mortality. The existence of post vaccine mortality in the vulnerable young male group calls into question the universality of vaccine strategies and suggests a differentiated approach should be considered.

The occurrence of post-vaccine myopericarditis in this age group is regarded as mild and it is thought to resolve quickly. However, Schauer et al. (2022) found that there were persistent cardiac abnormalities in a group of adolescents with post COVID-19 mRNA vaccine myopericarditis examined through MRI (magnetic resonance imaging).

A foundational principle of bioethics is that individuals should only be given a treatment after informed consent is obtained (Article 6.1 of the Universal Declaration on Bioethics and Human Rights, UNESCO 2005), and this consent should be freely given.

The risk of dying (however small) is not disclosed to the young male demographic. It is incompatible with any coercive policies that put pressure on them to be vaccinated, such as employment mandates or university campus mandates, especially given that the risk from COVID-19 is low for these cohorts.

The model of vaccination in the ethics literature was based on assumptions that vaccines would minimise transmission, prevent disease and lead to herd immunity, and 'save lives', without causing loss of life. The discussions of NPIs likewise concluded that there was a moral obligation on individuals to contribute to the greater good by complying with them. The available indicative evidence indicates that the NPIs are likely to cost more lives than they save and suggests that there is a risk of the novel mRNA vaccines causing an indeterminate number of deaths especially in the lower age groups, which might again be more than lives saved.

Bardosh et al. (2022) reviewed evidence on the effects of vaccine mandates using 'a broad conceptual framework spanning core aspects of behavioural psychology, politics and the law, the socio-demographic drivers of health inequality, and the integrity of science and public health' (p. 4). They found that the negative consequences outweigh the benefits across this broad front and recommended a return to more 'empowering' strategies.

The findings of the empirical and retrospective research studies into the effectiveness of the strategies are too variable to support the use of government coercive power, and the ability of all the vaccines to stop the spread of the disease too short-term at best. There is too much uncertainty in the findings to base government mandates on them.

Although there is more expert consensus on the benefits of vaccination than there is for lockdowns, consensus is not so evident on the desirability of vaccine mandates, which have not been widely favoured by vaccine advocates previously. And the risks had not been adequately investigated at the stage when governments imposed mandates.

Risk, Proportionality, and Necessity

In considering whether to impose coercive restrictions on a population, governments need to proceed through a decision-making path which contains a number of decision gates. These consist in the first place of consideration of the ethical principles that might be used to justify the need for the measures, then the empirical evidence concerning the effectiveness of them, and also their effect on individual rights.

The final decision gates for governments to negotiate are the common legal tests of risk, proportionality, and necessity. Each of these cuts both ways.

The risk posed by COVID-19 itself was clearly high for the post-working age population which was impacted badly in the urbanised countries of Europe and the Americas, but not so high in the younger age groups in those populations or the countries in Oceania and most of Africa which have a younger age profile (this is evident in the visualisations produced by the COVID-19 Data Explorer made available by *Our World in Data*, when selecting regional mortality relative to population). However, the risk of adverse effects was also high: from lockdowns in general and also from mRNA vaccination of the age groups at lowest risk from COVID-19 but highest risk of adverse effects such as myocarditis.

The 'precautionary principle' was often invoked to justify the need for governments to take protective action in the context of imperfect knowledge. But the precautionary principle should also have been considered to guard against the risk of adverse effects.

In the case of proportionality, the magnitude of the pandemic was great for the high-risk groups in the high-risk countries. But the marginal benefit of coercive lockdown and vaccination policies over and above voluntary compliance may be low compared with the extreme infringement of human rights that they imposed on all risk groups and all countries across the entire world. And the greater the infringements of individual liberties, the higher the evidence requirement to justify their effectiveness. should be. Extreme restrictions can only be justified by strong and consistent evidence.

On the face of it, stringent action might seem to meet the test of necessity given the magnitude of the epidemic. But here governments have to demonstrate that alternative, less onerous strategies have been considered and were found to be not sufficiently effective, and so the additional effect of coercion was necessary. Whereas in fact, less onerous strategies were not even considered.

Conclusion

In adopting drastic measures to suppress and then eliminate COVID-19, governments overrode individual rights in the name of the common good. This was on the basis that the measures taken would achieve the greatest good for the greatest number of people.

An essential test of whether this was justifiable is to investigate the evidence to ascertain whether the measures were, in fact, effective.

The empirical literature contains diverse findings on whether universal restrictions on mobility and universal vaccination against COVID-19 do in fact save more lives than they cost, either overall, or for every risk group.

In the light of this uncertainty, there is insufficient justification to impose coercive measures that take away the individual's rights to pursue their own health objectives in consultation with their health advisors, in the light of their own particular risks and opportunities.

References

Atkeson, A. (2021). A parsimonious behavioral SEIR model of the 2020 COVID epidemic in the United States and the United Kingdom. *NBER WP, 28434.* https://doi.org/10.3386/w28434

Allen, D. W. (2022). Covid-19 lockdown cost/benefits: A critical assessment of the literature. *International Journal of the Economics of Business, 29*(1), 1-32. https://doi.org/10.1016/S0140-6736(20)32153-X

Alwan, N. A., Burgess, R. A., Ashworth, S., Beale, R., Bhadelia, N., Bogaert, D., Dowd, J., Eckerle, I., Goldman, L. R., Greenhalgh, T., Gurdasani, D., Hamdy, A., Hanage, W. P., Hodcroft, E. B., Hyde, Z., Kellam, P., Kelly-Irving, M., Krammer, F., Lipsitch, M.,... Ziauddeen, H. (2020). Scientific consensus on the COVID-19 pandemic: We need to act now. *Lancet, 396*(10260), 671-672. https://doi.org/ 10.1016/ S0140-6736(20)32153-X

Bardenheier, B. H., Gravenstein, S., Blackman, C., Gutman, R., Sarkar, I. N., Feifer, R. A., White, E. M., McConeghy, K., Nanda, A., & Mor, V. (2021). Adverse events following mRNA SARS-CoV-2 vaccination among US nursing home residents. *Vaccine, 39*(29), 3844-3851. https://doi.org/10.1016/ j.vaccine.2021.05.088

Bardosh, K., de Figueiredo, A., Gur-Arie R., Jamrozik, E., Doidge, J. C., Lemmens, T., Keshavjee, S., Graham, J., & Baral, S. (2022). The unintended consequences of COVID-19 vaccine policy: Why mandates, passports, and segregated lockdowns may cause more harm than good. *SSRN.* https://papers.ssrn.com/ sol3/papers.cfm?abstract_id=4022798 (Accessed: 16 February 2022).

Benn, C. S., Schaltz-Buchholzer, F., Nielsen, S., Netea, M. G., & Aaby, P. (2022). Randomised clinical trials of COVID-19 Vaccines: Do adenovirus-vector vaccines have beneficial non-specific effects? *SSRN*. https://papers.ssrn.com/sol3/papers.cfm?abstract_id=4072489

Bernal, J. L., Andrews, N., Gower, C., Stowe, J., Tessier, E., Simmons, R., & Ramsay, M. (2021). Effectiveness of BNT162b2 mRNA vaccine and ChAdOx1 adenovirus vector vaccine on mortality following COVID-19. *medRxiv*. https://www.medrxiv.org/content/10.1101/2021.05.14.21257218v1.

Borsche, L., Glauner, B., & von Mendel, J. (2021). COVID-19 mortality risk correlates inversely with vitamin D3 status, and a mortality Rate close to zero could theoretically be achieved at 50 ng/mL 25 (OH) D3: results of a systematic review and meta-analysis. *Nutrients*, 13(10), 3596. https://pubmed.ncbi.nlm.nih.gov/34684596/

CDC. (2022, February 15). Selected adverse events reported after COVID-19 vaccination. https://www.cdc.gov/coronavirus/2019-ncov/vaccines/safety/adverse-events.html (Accessed: 21 February 2022).

Chaudhry, R., Dranitsaris, G., Mubashir, T., Bartoszko, J., & Riazi, S. (2020). A country level analysis measuring the impact of government actions, country preparedness and socioeconomic factors on COVID-19 mortality and related health outcomes. *EClinicalMedicine*, *25*, 100464. https://doi.org/10.1016/j.eclinm.2020.100464

Chemaitelly, H., Ayoub, H.H., AlMukdad, S., Coyle, P., Tang, P., Yassine, H. M., Al-Khatib, H. A., Smatti, M. K., Hasan, M. R., Al-Kanaani, Z., Al-Kuwari, E., Jeremijenko, A., Kaleeckal, A. H., Latif, A. N., Shaik, R. M., Abdul-Rahim, H. F., Nasrallah, G. K., Al-Kuwari, M. G., Butt, A. A., & Abu-Raddad, L. J. (2022). Duration of mRNA vaccine protection against SARS-CoV-2 Omicron BA.1 and BA.2 subvariants in Qatar. *Nature Communications*, *13*, 3082. https://doi.org/10.1038/s41467-022-30895-3

Classen, B. (2021). US COVID-19 vaccines proven to cause more harm than good based on pivotal clinical trial data analyzed using the proper scientific endpoint, all cause severe morbidity'. *Trends in Internal Medicine*, *1*(1), 1-6. https://www.scivisionpub.com/pdfs/us-covid19-vaccines-proven-to-cause-more-harm-than-good-based-on-pivotal-clinical-trial-data-analyzed-using-the-proper-scientific--1811.pdf

Craig, C., Neil, M., Fenton, N., McLachlan, S., Smalley, J., Guetzkow, J., Engler, J., Russell, D., & Rose, J. (2022). Official mortality data for England reveal systematic undercounting of deaths occurring within first two weeks of Covid-19 vaccination. *ResearchGate*. htttp//doi.org/ 10.13140/RG.2.2.12472.42248

Doshi, P. (2021a). Pfizer and Moderna's "95% effective" vaccines—we need more details and the raw data. *The BMJ Opinion*. https://blogs.bmj.com/bmj/ 2021/01/04/peter-doshi-pfizer-and-modernas-95-effective-vaccines-we-need-more-details-and-the-raw-data/

Doshi, P. (2021b). Covid-19 vaccines: In the rush for regulatory approval, do we need more data? *BMJ*, *373*(1244). http://dx.doi.org/10.1136/bmj.n1244

Eyre, D. W., Taylor, D., Purver, M., Chapman, D., Fowler, T., Pouwels, K., Walker, A. S., & Peto, T. E. (2021). The impact of SARS-CoV-2 vaccination on Alpha and Delta variant transmission. *medRxiv*. https://www.medrxiv.org/content/ 10.1101/2021.09.28.21264260v2

FDA – Pfizer (2020a) *FDA briefing document Pfizer-BioNTech COVID-19 vaccine.* Prepared for Vaccines and Related Biological Products Advisory Committee Meeting December 10, 2020. https://www.fda.gov/media/144245/download

FDA – Moderna (2020b) *FDA briefing document Moderna COVID-19 vaccine.* Prepared for Vaccines and Related Biological Products Advisory Committee Meeting December 17, 2020. https://www.fda.gov/media/144434/download

Ferguson, N., Laydon, D., Nedjati-Gilani, G., Imai, N., Ainslie, K., Baguelin, M., Bhatia, S., Boonyasiri, A., Cucunuba, Z., Cuomo-Dannenburg, G., Dighe, A., Dorigatti, I., Fu, H., Gaythorpe, K., Green, W., Hamlet, A., Hinsley, W., Okell, L. C., van Elsland, S.,... Ghani, A. C. (2020). Report 9: Impact of non-pharmaceutical interventions (NPIs) to reduce COVID19 mortality and healthcare demand. *Imperial College London*, *10*(77482), 491-497. https://www.imperial.ac.uk/media/ imperial-college/medicine/sph/ide/gida-fellowships/Imperial-College-COVID19-NPI-modelling-16-03-2020.pdf

Flaxman, S., Mishra, S., Gandy, A., Unwin, H. J. T., Mellan, T. A., Coupland, H., Whittaker, C., Zhu, H, Berah, T., Eaton, J. W., Monod, M., Imperial College COVID-19 Response Team, Ghani, A. C., Donnelly, C. A., Riley, S., Vollmer, M. A., Ferguson, N. M., Okell, L. C., & Bhatt, S. (2020). Estimating the effects of non-pharmaceutical interventions on COVID-19 in Europe. *Nature*, *584*(7820), 257-261. https://doi.org/10.1038/s41586-020-2405-7

Fraiman, J., Erviti, J., Jones, M., Greenland, S., Whelan, P., Kaplan, R. M., & Doshi, P. (2022). Serious adverse events of special interest following mRNA vaccination in randomized trials. *SSRN*. https://papers.ssrn.com/sol3/ papers.cfm?abstract_id=4125239

Gill, J., Tashjian R, & Duncanson, E. (2022). Autopsy histopathologic cardiac findings in two adolescents following the second COVID-19 vaccine dose. *Archives of Pathology and Laboratory Medicine*. https://doi.org: 10.5858/arpa.2021-0435-SA

Heneghan, C., & Jefferson T. (2020, November 1). The ten worst COVID decision-making failures. *The Spectator*. https://www.spectator.co.uk/article/the-ten-worst-covid-decision-making-failures (Accessed: 17 February 2022).

Herby, J., Jonung, L., & Hanke, S. (2022). A literature review and meta-analysis of the effects of lockdowns on COVID-19 mortality. *Studies in Applied Economics*. Johns Hopkins University. https://sites.krieger.jhu.edu/iae/files/2022/01/A-Literature-Review-and-Meta-Analysis-of-the-Effects-of-Lockdowns-on-COVID-19-Mortality.pdf

Hsiang, S., Allen, D., Annan-Phan, S., Bell, K., Bolliger, I., Chong, T., Druckenmiller, H., Huang, L. Y., Hultgren, A., Kresovich, E., Lau, P., Lee, J., Rolf, E., Tseng, J., & Wu, T. (2020). The effect of large-scale anti-contagion policies on the COVID-19 pandemic. *Nature*, *584*(7820), 262-267. https://doi.org/10.1038/s41586-020-2404-8

Ioannidis, J. P. (2022). Citation impact and social media visibility of Great Barrington and John Snow signatories for COVID-19 strategy. *BMJ Open*, *12*, e052891. https://doi.org:10.1136/bmjopen-2021-052891

Jefferson, T., Del Mar, C. B., Dooley, L., Ferroni, E., Al-Ansary, L. A., Bawazeer, G. A., van Driel, M. L., Jones, M. A., Thorning, S., Beller, E. M., Clark, J., Hoffmann, T. C., Glasziou, P. P., & Conly, J. M. (2020). Physical interventions to interrupt or reduce the spread of respiratory viruses. *Cochrane Database of Systematic Reviews*, *11*. https://doi.org/10.1002/14651858.CD006207.pub5

Kephart, J. L., Delclòs-Alió, X., Rodríguez, D. A., Sarmiento, O. L., Barrientos-Gutiérrez, T., Ramirez-Zea, M., Quistberg, D. A., Bilal, U., & Roux, A. V. D. (2021). The effect of population mobility on COVID-19 incidence in 314 Latin American cities: A longitudinal ecological study with mobile phone location data. *The Lancet Digital Health*, *3*(11), e716-e722. https://doi.org/10.1016/S2589-7500(21)00174-6

Kuhbandner, C., & Homburg, S. (2020). Commentary: Estimating the effects of non-pharmaceutical interventions on COVID-19 in Europe. *Frontiers in Medicine*, *761*. https://doi.org/10.3389/fmed.2020.580361

Kulldorff, M., Gupta, S., & Bhattacharya, J. (2020). Great Barrington Declaration. https://gbdeclaration.org.

Macchia, A., Ferrante, D., Angeleri, P., Biscayart, C., Mariani, J., Esteban, S., Tablado, M. R., & de Quirós, F. G. B. (2021). Evaluation of a COVID-19 vaccine campaign and SARS-CoV-2 infection and mortality among adults aged 60 years and older in a middle-income country. *JAMA Network Open, 4*(10), e2130800-e2130800. doi: 10.1001/jamanetworkopen.2021.30800

Mahler, D., Yonsan, N., Lakner, C., Aguilar, R., & Wu, H. (2021). *Updated estimates of the impact of COVID-19 on global poverty: Turning the corner on the pandemic in 2021?* https://blogs.worldbank.org/opendata/updated-estimates-impact-COVID-19-global-poverty-turning-corner-pandemic-2021 (Accessed: 16 February 2022).

Mathers, C. D., Sadana, R., Salomon, J. A., Murray, C. J., & Lopez, A. D. (2001). Healthy life expectancy in 191 countries, 1999. *The Lancet, 357*(9269), 1685-1691. https://doi.org/10.1016/S0140-6736(00)04824-8

Meredith, G. R., Diel, D. G., Frazier, P. I., Henderson, S. G., Koretzky, G. A., Wan, J., & Warnick, L. D. (2022). Routine surveillance and vaccination on a university campus during the spread of the SARS-CoV-2 Omicron variant. *JAMA Network Open, 5*(5), e2212906-e2212906. https://doi.org/10.1001/jamanetworkopen.2022.12906

McLachlan, S., Osman, M., Dube, K., Chiketero P., Choi, Y., & Fenton, N. (2021). Analysis of COVID-19 vaccine death reports from the Vaccine Adverse Events Reporting System (VAERS) Database: Interim results and analysis. *ResearchGate*. https//doi.org/10.13140/RG.2.2.26987.26402

Mendez-Brito, A., El Bcheraoui, C., & Pozo-Martin, F. (2021). Systematic review of empirical studies comparing the effectiveness of non-pharmaceutical interventions against COVID-19. *Journal of Infection, 83*(3), 281-293. https://doi.org/10.1016/j.jinf.2021.06.018

Mill, J., S. On liberty. (2011). *Project Gutenberg*. (Original work published 1859). https://www.gutenberg.org/files/34901/34901-h/34901-h.htm

Miller, E. R., Moro, P. L., Cano, M., & Shimabukuro, T. T. (2015). Deaths following vaccination: What does the evidence show? *Vaccine, 33*(29), 3288-3292. https://doi.org/10.1016/j.vaccine.2015.05.023

Moro, P. L., Arana, J., Cano, M., Lewis, P., & Shimabukuro, T. T. (2015). Deaths reported to the vaccine adverse event reporting system,

United States, 1997–2013. *Clinical Infectious Diseases, 61*(6), 980-987. https//doi.org/10.1093/cid/civ423

Morris, J. (2022). *Why it was infeasible for the phase 3 vaccine trials to use "all cause deaths" as the endpoint.* COVID-19 Data Science. https://www.covid-datascience.com/post/why-it-was-infeasible-for-the-phase-3-vaccine-trials-to-use-all-cause-deaths-as-the-endpoint (Accessed: 22 February 2022).

Morris, E. J., Goldacre, R., Spata, E., Mafham, M., Finan, P. J., Shelton, J., Richards, M., Spencer, K., Emberson, J., Hollings, S., Curnow, P., Gair, D., Sebag-Montefiore, D., Cunningham, C., Rutter, M. D., Nicholson, B. D., Rashbass, J., Landray, M., Collins, R.,... Baigent, C. (2021). Impact of the COVID-19 pandemic on the detection and management of colorectal cancer in England: A population-based study. *The Lancet Gastroenterology & Hepatology, 6*(3), 199-208. doi: 10.1016/S2468-1253(21)00005-4

Murad, M. H., Asi, N., Alsawas, M., & Alahdab, F. (2016). New evidence pyramid. *BMJ Evidence-Based Medicine, 21*(4), 125-127. http://dx.doi.org/10.1136/ebmed-2016-110401

Owens, M., Townsend, E., Hall, E., Bhatia, T., Fitzgibbon, R., & Miller-Lakin, F. (2022). Mental health and wellbeing in young people in the UK during lockdown (COVID-19). *International Journal of Environmental Research and Public Health, 19*(3), 1132.

Our World in Data. COVID-19 Data Explorer. https://ourworldindata.org/explorers/coronavirus-data-explorer

Pantazatos, S., & Seligmann, H. (2021). COVID vaccination and age stratified all-cause mortality risk. *ResearchGate.* https//doi.org/10.13140/RG.2.2.28257.43366

Schauer, J., Buddhe, S., Gulhane, A., Sagiv, E., Studer, M., Colyer, J., Chikkabyrappa, S. K., Law, Y., & Portman, M. A. (2022). Persistent cardiac MRI findings in a cohort of adolescents with post COVID-19 mRNA vaccine myopericarditis. *The Journal of Pediatrics, 245,* 233-237. https://doi.org/10.1016/j.jpeds.2022.03.032

Scobie, H. M., Johnson, A. G., Suthar, A. B., Severson, R., Alden, N. B., Balter, S., Bertolino, D., Blythe, D., Brady, S., Cadwell, B., Cheng, I., Davidson, S., Degadillo, J., Devinney, K., Duchin, J., Duwell, M., Fisher, R., Fleischauer, A., Grant, A.,... Silk, B. J. (2021). Monitoring incidence of COVID-19 cases, hospitalizations, and deaths, by vaccination status—13 US jurisdictions, April 4–July 17, 2021. *Morbidity and Mortality Weekly Report, 70*(37), 1284. https//doi.org/ 10.15585/mmwr.mm7037e1

Seal, K. H., Bertenthal, D., Carey, E., Grunfeld, C., Bikle, D. D., & Lu, C. M. (2022). Association of Vitamin D status and COVID-19-related hospitalization and mortality. *Journal of General Internal Medicine,* 37(4), 853-861. https://pubmed.ncbi.nlm.nih.gov/34981368/

Sears, J., Villas-Boas, J., Villas-Boas, V., & Villas-Boas, S. (2020) Are we #stayinghome to flatten the curve? *medRxiv*. https://doi.org/10.1101/ 2020.05.23.20111211

Shah, K., Varna, V. P., Sharma, U., & Mavalankar, D. (2022). Does vitamin D supplementation reduce COVID-19 severity?: A systematic review. *QJM: An International Journal of Medicine*. https://doi.org/10.1093/qjmed/hcac040

Tognotti, E. (2013). Lessons from the history of quarantine, from plague to influenza A. *Emerging Infectious Diseases, 19*(2), 254. https://www.ncbi.nlm.nih.gov/pmc/articles/PMC3559034/

UK Health Security Agency (2021) *SARS-CoV-2 variants of concern and variants under investigation in England: Technical Briefing 33*. https://www.gov.uk/government/publications/ukhsa-investigation-of-novel-sars-cov-2-variants-of-concern-england-technical-briefing-33-23-december-2021

Veneti, L., Berild, J. D., Watle, S. V., Starrfelt, J., Greve-Isdahl, M., Langlete, P., Boas, H., Bragstad, K., Hungnes, O., & Meijerink, H. (2022). Vaccine effectiveness with BNT162b2 (Comirnaty, Pfizer-BioNTech) vaccine against reported SARS-CoV-2 Delta and Omicron infection among adolescents, Norway, August 2021 to January 2022. *medRxiv*. https://doi.org/10.1101/2022.03.24.22272854

Villasis-Keever, M. A., López-Alarcón, M. G., Miranda-Novales, G., Zurita-Cruz, J. N., Barrada-Vázquez, A. S., González-Ibarra, J., Martinez-Reyes, M., Grajales-Muniz, C., Santacruz-Tinoco, C. E., Martinez-Miguel, B., Maldonado-Hernandez, J., Cifuentes-Gonzalez, Y., Klunder-Klunder, M., Garduno-Espinosa, J., Lopez-Martinez, B., & Parra-Ortega, I. (2022). Efficacy and safety of vitamin D supplementation to prevent COVID-19 in frontline healthcare workers. A randomized clinical trial. *Archives of Medical Research, 53*(4), 423-430. https://www.sciencedirect.com/science/article/pii/S0188440922000455

Vollmer, M. A., Mishra, S., Unwin, H. J. T., Gandy, A., Mellan, T. A., Bradley, V., Zhu, H., Coupland, H., Hawryluk, I., Hutchinson, M., Ratmann, O., Monod, M.,

Walker, P., Whittaker, C., Carrarino, L., Ciavarella, C., Cilloni, L., Ainslie, K., Baguelin, M.,... & Bhatt, S. (2020). Report 20: Using mobility to estimate the transmission intensity of COVID-19 in Italy: A subnational analysis with future scenarios. *medRxiv*. https://www.imperial.ac.uk/mrc-global-infectious-disease-analysis/covid-19/report-20-italy/

World Health Organization (WHO). (2019). *Non-pharmaceutical public health measures for mitigating the risk and impact of epidemic and pandemic influenza*. World Health Organisation. https://www.who.int/publications/i/item/non-pharmaceutical-public-health-measuresfor-mitigating-the-risk-and-impact-of-epidemic-and-pandemic-influenza

Xu, S., Huang, R., Sy, L. S., Glenn, S. C., Ryan, D. S., Morrissette, K., Shay, D. K., Vazquez-Benitez, G., Glanz, J. M., Klein, N. P., McClure, D., Liles, E. G., Weintraub, E. S., Tseng, H., & Qian, L. (2021). COVID-19 vaccination and non–COVID-19 mortality risk—Seven integrated health care organizations, United States, December 14, 2020–July 31, 2021. *Morbidity and Mortality Weekly Report, 70*(43), 1520. http://dx.doi.org/10.15585/mmwr.mm7043e2

FORCE IS IN THE EYE OF THE BEHOLDER:
An Australian Case Study

Samuel White[1]

Abstract: The laws and policy constraints around the domestic deployment of armed forces has become a central question in multiple jurisdictions. This paper addresses the issue from an Australian perspective, looking at the nebulous test of what constitutes 'a use of force'. This test, relevantly, is suggested to separate deployments in potential legal authorities and has become a touchpoint for strategic communications. This paper questions the viability of this test, and asks the critical question: from whose perspective is force to be assessed? Nestled within this question is a discussion of whether the mere presence of troops, unarmed but supporting civilian police, constitutes a use of force. The paper then concludes with a proposed policy change that more accurately captures the deeply held, if imperfectly understood, reservations around the use of the military domestically.

Introduction

Generally, the use of the Australian Defence Force ('ADF') in domestic security operations has been characterised, as White (2005) notes by 'deeply held, even if imperfectly understood, reservations.' This perhaps reflects the isolated nature of the ADF from civilian society or historical aversion that Anglo-Saxon cultures have held towards the military (Goffman, 1997). Such an aversion, says Babington (1990, p. 2), arises because the military were 'the dregs of society... the rogues and vagabonds, the destitute, the condemned felons and the prisoners from the gaols.'

Increasingly, however, the domestic deployment of the ADF is being considered a viable Commonwealth response to less-than-warlike operations. This does not, in itself, represent a novel development: the military have been used to Keep the Peace of the Realm since time

---

[1] Cybersecurity Post Doc Research Fellow, Adelaide Law School, Australia

immemorial (White, 2021) The Prime Minister of Australia (2020) announced that the ADF would move from a force posture of 'respond to request' to 'move forward and integrate' signalling increased domestic deployments; two months later, Operation COVID-19 Assist was enacted and constituted the largest deployment – internal or external - of the ADF since World War Two (DoD, 2020)

Comprised of seven State and Territory based task groups, the role of the operation was to coordinate and deliver customised ADF support to civilian health and law enforcement agencies (DoD, 2020). As a federal construct, it is convention (if not strictly required in law) for the Commonwealth to only operate in States with consent. (*Defence Act 1903*, s 32). Specifically, Operation COVID-19 Assist saw ADF members engage in providing assistance to Australian State and Territories when requested which was met with polarising responses (The Guardian, 2021).

At its peak, several thousand ADF personnel were deployed in support of Operation COVID-19 Assist (DoD, 2020). The role of each task group varied depending upon individual jurisdictional requirements. However, generally speaking, tasks performed by the ADF included:

- operational planning and risk assessments
- logistic and personnel support
- cyber security advice
- assistance to law enforcement agencies as part of quarantine and isolation compliance activities for international arrivals,
- assistance to law enforcement & health agencies in contact tracing
- assistance to law enforcement agencies at inter-state border control checkpoints,
- assistance to law enforcement agencies at intra-state border control checkpoints, and
- assistance to law enforcement agencies to protect vulnerable communities.

It was stressed by the Minister of Defence (MINDEF) that during all stages of the operation that the policy and legal framework did not permit ADF members to use coercive powers at any time (MINDEF, 2020). This determination, taking into account the assistance given to law enforcement (even though unarmed), is the focus of this chapter.

Within Australia, domestic deployments are regulated by a binary policy construct – Defence Assistance to the Civil Community ('DACC') and Defence Force Aid to the Civil Power ('DFACA'). The dividing line is the nebulous and undefined concept of 'use of force' – DACC deployments involve no use of force, whilst DFACA do (DACC Manual, 2020). It is for this reason that particular emphasis was placed by MINDEF that Operation COVID-19 Assist was a DACC deployment.

Under policy, it is remarked that DFACA operations can only occur under a specific Act of Parliament – Part IIIAAA of the *Defence Act 1903* (Commonwealth). Importantly, for this legislation to be enabled, there must be a rather serious state of affairs occurring (so called 'domestic violence' which reflects the language of the Australian *Constitution*). Domestic violence, in the Australian constitutional sense, is best characterised as a riot or ongoing incident that is beyond the conventional capabilities of State civilian constabulary (White, 2021, p. 133). There are clear legal authorities for the ADF to operate below the threshold of domestic violence but above the policy construct of DACC.

This chapter is not concerned with these legal questions however. It is concerned with the question of *ethics*. Rather than focus on the rather tedious and political question of *should* the military be used domestically, this Chapter focuses on a specific ethical problem. If the policy construct of DACC/DFACA is to remain (as the weight of political and military references to the work would suggest) then **from whose perspective should force be defined by?** Ethically, is force best assessed by the citizen, or the 'citizen in uniform' (White, 2019)? Should the mere presence of ADF troops, even unarmed, be conceptually categorised as a use of force? Utilising the recent ADF support to the Commonwealth Government under Operation COVID-19 Assist, this chapter would look to address the ethical conundrum of the use of military force domestically. Such an analysis has never been conducted, and would offer a new and much required contribution to the field of military legal ethics.

The Policy

Replacing the previous *Defence Instruction (General) OPS 05-1: Defence Assistance to the Civil Community*, the current DACC policy framework is contained within the *DACC Manual*. The policy provides two mechanisms for State and Territory requests for assistance. First, requests can be made to local Unit Commanders or the Senior ADF Officer ('SADFO') in location, with approval authorities including the Chief of the Defence Force ('CDF') and MINDEF (DACC Manual, 2020, p. 48). Secondly, requests can be made through Emergency Management Australia, operated by the Department of Home Affairs in the National Situation Room. Importantly, the Manual does not permit the ADF to provide assistance in the absence of a request, or where 'there is any likelihood of the use of force.' (DACC Manual, 2020, [6.31(a)]) Included in this is an implication that the ADF cannot be used to facilitate the use of force by State or Territory (Saultry & Copeland, 2019, p. 168).

The Prevalence of the Policy Framework

This policy framework has become the model that is employed in civilian government rhetoric and military governance when discussing domestic deployments. It is difficult to ascertain when the policy came into action, noting that the DACC Manual was only released on 11 August 2020. However, open source research has shown the policy framework at the centre of Parliamentary debates in 1989 where the then-MINDEF was asked about the prevalence of ADF assistance to police forces (Hansard, 1989) and was noted in a Parliamentary research paper in 1998 (Ward, p. 31.) It currently forms the core operational foundation for any ADF domestic disaster response under current Emergency Management Australia plans.

Perhaps due to a need for strategic communication, it has also become increasingly prevalent within Ministerial comments about Operation COVID-19 Assist, the ADF's contribution to the public health emergency. In March 2020, the then-MINDEF noted that ADF support to mandatory quarantine measures fell under the DACC framework as ADF members had 'no coercive enforcement powers' (MINDEF, 2020). It is further reflected in the ADF's role statement in support of Emergency Management Victoria, and comments to Senate Committees by ADF members have noted the framework is one of DACC (Hansard, 2020, p. 29).

Notwithstanding its clear importance in planning and domestic responses, the key factor between DACC and DFACA – what constitutes a use of force – has never been publicly discussed. It is important, then, to address it.

What is 'Force'?

As Sir Victor Windeyer has noted (1976, p. 295) force is 'a word of varied and extensive denotation.' It holds international and domestic legal meanings which sometimes differ. From a domestic law perspective, the concept of force litters both the common law (assault, battery, false imprisonment, sexual offences) and statute.

Within the context of DACC and DFACA, the threshold of 'any likelihood' makes it difficult to envisage a situation where there is absolutely no likelihood of force being used by ADF members, including self-defence. Such a problem plagues the use of the ADF in industrial actions, particularly strike substitution, where it is possible that the use of the ADF may aggravate the situation and the ADF member would have to use force in self-defence (White, 2020, p. 423). Indeed, any intelligence reports that even suggested a single individual might have to use force would, under a strict interpretation of DACC/DFACA, result in their deployment as involving a likelihood of force. To avoid the *reductio ad absurdum* arguments, it must be implied within this threshold of 'any likelihood of force' a caveat of 'any likelihood of force' outside of self-defence, necessity or sudden and extraordinary emergency.

The notion of force within the DACC Manual is not defined but includes concepts such as 'intrusive or coercive actions' (DACC Manual, 2020) as well as 'the restriction of freedom of movement of the civil community whether there is physical contact or not'. No examples are given, nor do any other publicly available policy documents help interpret these defining terms. Recourse must be taken, then, to the plain English meaning of the words.

'Intrusive' is defined within the Macquarie Dictionary as being 'characterised by or involving intrusion'; to 'come unbidden or without welcome'; or to violate one's privacy. Equally, 'coercive' is defined as 'to coerce', 'to restrain or contain by force, law, or authority' or 'to compel by forcible action'. The golden thread between the words, then, is that it is an act done to an individual, physical or not, without their consent. This is reflected in the second limb of what force constitutes under the 2020 DACC Manual: restricting the freedom of movement of the civil community. At its core is the lack of consent.

This raises the core question of DACC/DFACA – from whose perspective is force to be interpreted? The plain English reading of the DACC Manual definition, alongside comparative tort law, would suggest that force is in the eye of the beholder; an action that is intrusive or coercive, as a matter of public policy, should not be defined and decided upon by the individual conducting the action. This interpretation towards a victim-centric definition of force is supported by criminal law offences such as assault, where it is the fear of coercive or intrusive conduct that can give rise to the offence; or false imprisonment, where it has been held that the authority of a uniform can give rise to a misapprehension of being detained. It moreover encompasses offences where the victim may not even be aware that coercive or intrusive operations (such as trespass) have occurred.

This raises the complicated question, then, as to whether or not presence of ADF members could constitute force. Examples of DACC, historically, include military aid in bushfires, floods and storms or use of specialist military personnel and equipment for explosive ordnance disposal (DACC Manual, 2020). It has also included helicopters or fighter jets appearing at motorsport events, helicopters or skydivers appearing at football matches, or bands appearing at ceremonial functions. Implicit from this pattern of behaviour is that the ADF does not believe that the mere presence of its members, unarmed, constitutes a use of force.

In a Senate Committee inquiring into the *Defence Legislation Amendment (Enhancement of Defence Force Response to Emergencies) Bill 2020*, Major General Roger Noble – Head of Military Strategic Commitments, which administers the DACC Manual (indeed, it is Noble's signature authorising the 2020 DACC Manual) – responded to a question from Senator Fawcett as to the orders for opening fire. Noble comments that for soldiers:

> …this is not advice to them. This is an order with which they must comply: 'You are to act in a calm and professional manner when performing your duties. You are to apply common sense and adhere to Defence values when interacting with members of the public and assisting authorities. You are only to undertake tasks directed by your chain of command. You are not authorised to undertake law enforcement tasks, including arresting anyone, using intrusive or coercive powers against anyone; issue orders to or demand answers from members of the public.'

Noble continues:

> So the notion that you, as an ADF member, can tackle someone leaving a hotel - you would not be complying with the orders you have been given. People will ask, 'What's the point, then?' The answer is: they've got eyes, ears, legs, brains and they are with the police. Their immediate response would be to inform the police, who have the authority to conduct law enforcement. There's a bit of a misnomer, I suspect, on the limits of their powers. They are very clearly laid out to them.

Now, although the Major General is not a legal officer, he receives legal advice through organic command legal officers within Military Strategic Commitments, and wider Defence Legal (of which the head of, Mr. Adrian D'Amico, attended the Senate Committee with Noble). What is clear from Noble and D'Amico's comments is that the mere presence of ADF troops in hotel quarantine is not viewed, within the Department of Defence, as a use of force.

But the presence of ADF troops can, of course, be a use of force – as the Major General notes, 'they've got eyes, ears, legs, brains and they are with police' all of which can deter. Presence is a recognised use of force and the basis for strategic deterrence theory. In a Military Board Pamphlet of 1964, it was said that 'depending on the circumstances, the minimum force necessary to restore law and order can vary from the mere appearance of troops to the use of all the force at the commander's disposal.' Sir Victor Windeyer, famous Australian jurist and recipient of the Distinguished Service Order for his 'gallant and distinguished service in the Middle East' in World War Two, recognised as such when he noted, with respect to whether or not terrorism could constitute a riot that military personnel were historically called out to aid the civil power against:

> Members of the Defence Force so called out may be required to act in ways and with weapons and equipment that are very different from those of their predecessors who were called upon in past times to put down riots. Tear-gas and smoke missiles were then unknown; and today the mere presence of military vehicles, AFV's [Armoured Fighting Vehicles] and APC's [Armoured Personnel Carriers] may be a deterrent.

Indeed, the use of five AFVs and 200 armed troops to suppress rioting migrants (and to protect Commonwealth property) at Bonegilla in 1952 was predicated on the deterring effect of troops in uniform (Pennay, 2007, p. 16).

Within the Royal Australian Infantry Corps, soldiers are taught the need to escalate and de-escalate force in order to resolve situations. This reflects and mirrors training that civilian police undertake in the use of force continuum (Commonwealth Ombudsman, 2012). This doctrine recognises the gravitas and authority that uniforms (police, medical, military) hold and the psychological effect that it can have. In an oft-cited U.S. government police publication (Garner & Maxwell, 1996, 37), it is stated that:

> … the professionalism, uniform and utility belt of the law enforcement officer and the marked vessel or vehicle the officer arrives in … (results in) a visual presence of authority that is normally enough for a subject to comply with an officer's lawful demands.

Recent and tragic experience in other jurisdictions has demonstrated that often even unlawful demands will be complied with off the authority of law enforcement uniform (The Guardian, 2021).

Whilst the above is about law enforcement, the authority that a uniform offers its wearer has been reflected in open source United States Navy doctrine also promotes presence as the first step in the use of force (DoD, 2016). This is reflected in the tactics, techniques and procedures ('TTPs') of stability operations, where the mere presence of military personnel is the starting point maintaining order. Such TTPs were utilised in Vietnam, on UN peacekeeping missions in Rwanda, peace building operations in Timor

L'Este, and warfighting operations in Iraq and Afghanistan (Fishstein, 2018). It is the basis for stability operations and core to the campaign of building hearts & minds. It is therefore a matter of cognitive dissonance that these TTPs – through unarmed ADF members supporting armed civilian police – can be openly used in domestic operations but sweepingly categorised as a DACC operation.

Force is, of course, a matter of context which requires an assessment of the readiness and capacity to use force. As an example, the presence of a medical facility would be unlikely to constitute an intrusive or coercive presence (indeed, the presence of medical facilities was the basis for 'hearts and minds' operations in Vietnam); so too would the presence of members of the Australian Army Band Corps be likely to not constitute force. In Operation COVID-19 Assist, the use of ADF members to support planning, to provide medical assistance, to provide cyber security advice, or to support logistical movements would not seem to contextually be a use of force from the eye of the beholder. So too does the protection of vulnerable communities, in certain contexts, not amount to a use of force under the current policy construct (although the notion of 'protection' can of course be a two-sided sword for the community in question). This is for the context of dismounted troops. Utilising Sir Victor's example, AFVs and APCs contextually denote a readiness and capacity to use force. So too can it be claimed for supporting individuals (civilian constabulary forces) who are empowered and equipped to undertake intrusive or coercive conduct.

Conclusion

The end result then would seem to be an ethical tension between the accepted need for military deployments, and the awkward question of whether or not the policy test of use of force actually implied that force is in the eye of the beholder. Being policy, there is an easy fix: reform. There are many different, and plausible, fixes. Force can be defined as anything that a civilian cannot do: this would allow ADF members to conduct citizen arrests, act in emergencies and under the lawful authority of necessity. Equally, the binary construct can be removed and a more nuanced test could be implemented, such as that currently used within the United Kingdom. There, the question is asked as to whether or not the operation falls within the concept of 'military work'. This term, says the UK Ministry of Justice (2017) includes:

> where Service personnel have been trained by the military, where Service personnel undertake that work as their 'day job', and for work which traditionally has been seen as military work. This type of work is usually, but not exclusively, requested by law enforcement agencies, most commonly the police, the Border Force and Her Majesty's (HM) Revenue and Customs.

Such a position would appear much more consistent with public opinion about what is, and is not, within the remit of domestic operations. Force is, after all, always in the eye of the beholder.

References

Babington, A. (1990). *Military intervention in Britain: From the Gordon riots to the Gibraltar incident*. Routledge.

Commonwealth Ombudsman (2012, May). *Australian Federal Police – ACT Policing Defence Act 1903* (Cth) *Defence Assistance to Civil Community Manual* (2020, 3rd ed.) 6.13(a) ('DACC Manual')

Department of Defence (2020, October 12). Defence Response to COVID-19. *Defence News*.

Department of Defence (2016, November 18). Directive 5210.56 – *Arming and the use of force*.

Dodd, V., & Siddique, H. (2021). Wayne Couzens used police ID and handcuffs to kidnap Sarah Everard. *The Guardian*. https://www.theguardian.com/uk-news/2021/sep/29/wayne-couzens-used-police-id-to-kidnap-sarah-everard-court-told

Fishstein, P., & Wilder, A. (2012, January). *Winning hearts and minds? Examining the relationship between aid and security in Afghanistan*. Feinstein International Centre, Tufts University.

Garner, J. H., & Maxwell, C. D. (1996). *Measuring the amount of force used by and against the police in six jurisdictions: A report*. US Department of Justice.

Goffman, E. (1997). *Asylums: Essays on the social situation of mental patients and other inmates.* Amorrotu.

Hansard. (2020, October 30). *Senate – Foreign Affairs, Defence and Trade Legislation Committee, 29.*

Hansard. Mr Carlton to Mr Beezley (1989, September 4).

Minister for Defence, (2020, March 23). Defence provides additional assistance in response to COVID-19.

Ministry of Defence. (2017, February). Joint Doctrine Publication 02 – UK Operations – *The Defence contribution to resilience and security* (3rd ed.).

Pennay, B. (2007). *The Army at Bonegilla.* Albury & Wodonga.

Prime Minister of Australia. (2020, January 4). *Bushfire relief and recovery.*

Rachwani, M. (2021). 'We feel intimidated': Residents in south-west Sydney Covid hotspots say police are making things worse. *The Guardian.* https://www.theguardian.com/australia-news/2021/aug/15/we-feel-intimidated-residents-in-south-west-sydney-covid-hotspots-say-police-are-making-things-worse

Saultry, P., & Copeland, D. (2019). Domestic legal framework for operation. In R. Creyke, D. Stephens, & P. Sutherland (Eds.), *Military law in Australia* (pp. 161-168). The Federation Press.

Sir Victor Windeyer's 'Opinion' in Mr Justice Robert Hope. (1979, May 15). *Protective Security Review* (unclassified). (Parliamentary Paper No 397/1979) Appendix 9.

Ward, E. (1998). Call out the troops: An examination of the legal basis for Australian Defence Force involvement in 'non-defence' matters. *Research Paper, 98.* 8.

White, M. (2005). The executive and the military. *UNSW Law Journal, 28*(2).

White, S. (2019). A soldier by any other name: A reappraisal of the Citizen in Uniform Doctrine. *Military Law and War Review, 57*(2).

White, S. (2020). *Keeping the peace of the realm.* LexisNexis.

IS TEMPERATURE SCREENING AN ETHICAL AND VALUABLE RESTRICTION ON PRIVACY AND FREEDOM?[1]

Anne Zimmerman[2]

Abstract: This chapter analyzes temperature screening as a tool to improve public health during the COVID-19 pandemic in light of consumer privacy. While temperature screening under normal circumstances in non-medical settings would pose significant ethical issues, evaluating its ethics in the context of the complexities of the pandemic and the gaps in knowledge especially during the early pandemic calls for some lenience concerning privacy and liberty. Grocery and other stores began temperature screening as a condition of entry early in the pandemic. This chapter highlights the issue of whether temperature testing should be permissible when it is a useful tool and who should share any data collected, especially when it is collected by a business. The cost to privacy is considered under the backdrop of burgeoning consumer privacy protections, liberty, and surveillance. The focus is whether the imposition on liberty was ethically justifiable given the information available about the pandemic at the time.

Before the COVID-19 pandemic, the protection of consumer privacy had reached a milestone with the enactment of the California Consumer Privacy Act (CCPA) (The California Consumer Privacy Act, 2018). Early in the pandemic, some stores in the United States began screening customers for elevated temperatures, an act that challenges the basic ethical underpinning of the evolving privacy frameworks that serve to balance diverse interests: that people should control their personal data. The Health Insurance Portability and Accountability Act of 1996 (HIPAA), is a federal law in the United States that governs the use and disposition of protected health information (Health Insurance Portability and Accountability Act,

---

[1] This chapter is a revised version of Zimmerman, A. (2020). Vigilante grocers: Is temperature screening of customers by retailers an ethical and valuable restriction on privacy and freedom? *Voices in Bioethics*, 6. https://doi.org/10.7916/vib.v6i.5833

[2] Founder, Modern Bioethics

1996). Stores are not subject to HIPAA, which governs certain types of data collected or used by entities including healthcare providers, insurance companies, and clearinghouses that process medical data. While it protects privacy, HIPAA also serves to allow access to records and shareability for specified purposes. Privacy and control over personal data could impede and, in the past, have impeded, public health goals (Tomaszewski et al., 2020). Gavin Newson, the Governor of California, began enforcement of the CCPA on July 1, 2020. According to Milligan, in an email to Forbes, the California Attorney General's office warned California businesses prior to enforcement: "We're all mindful of the new reality created by COVID-19 and the heightened value of protecting consumers' privacy online that comes with it. We encourage businesses to be particularly mindful of data security in this time of emergency" (Milligan et al., 2020).

Yet there is precedent to release personal medical information in other public consumer arenas. "Government has a unique role in public health" which during the pandemic calls for extraordinary means to control the spread of COVID-19 (Childress et al., 2002). In the absence of clear governmental guidance mandating temperature screening at malls and stores, companies had to navigate public health and implement fair policies to promote safety, acting in what is traditionally the government's realm.

During the pandemic, customers were subject to data collection, but an absence of use-based laws left it unclear as to whether temperature data collected could be used for either marketing or public health (Rosenfeld et al., 2020). Subjecting customers to temperature screening arguably violates traditional notions of personal data, data privacy, and freedom. This chapter explores whether temperature screening can be justified as noncoercive, a public health necessity, and as less restrictive than keeping businesses closed. The justification does not necessarily imply that companies should be managing the public health task themselves. Temperature screening is an important public health tool that can keep febrile people out of enclosed public spaces at their most contagious, could couple exclusion for the flu or other viruses as well, and could alleviate the need for COVID-19 tests, which were in short supply for much of the pandemic. During the pandemic, some cities and venues relied on proof of vaccination. The current Omicron variant is leading to widespread positivity rates even among the vaccinated, undermining the protection offered by vaccine passports. Like temperature screening, vaccination passports will be evaluated based on best practices as part of a basket of risk management strategies rather than on exceptional effectiveness. Many public health officials expressed hope that each of the temperature screening and vaccination passports would be the one thing needed to reel in the pandemic. Neither proved true, but the evaluation of the ethics of both relies on contextualization and information availability. Temperature screening may be a valuable part of any store or business's repertoire as more indoor public spaces, malls, retail stores, and service industries can no longer expect proof of vaccination to do the heavy lifting.

Employees and customers call for different treatment: employees rightly subject to some tracking and stored data. There is some government input with respect to employee temperature screening. The American with Disabilities Act (ADA) governs and the Equal Employment Opportunity Commission (EEOC), Occupational Safety and Health Administration (OSHA), some states, and the CDC have given broad guidance urging temperature screening in certain cases but not giving procedural advice (Rosenfeld et al., 2020; see also, Cowie et al., 2021)..

Is temperature screening a public health necessity?

Many countries believed that it was and initiated widespread temperature testing during the pandemic. The possibility that temperature screening for containment of COVID-19 is ethical and valuable depends on considerations including its efficacy. Is temperature testing in fact valuable to pandemic management? A review of preliminary data and articles covering the use of temperature screening in varied settings demonstrates its effectiveness as well as its limitations (Lippi et al., 2021).

In the early pandemic, the majority of COVID-19 patients presented with fever. Data from China from December 2019 through early 2020 showed "common signs and symptoms are fever (83%–98%), cough (76%–82%), and short of breath (31%–55%)" (Wu et al., 2020). South Korea began temperature testing travelers arriving in South Korea (Kim et al., 2021). The first confirmed case in South Korea was confirmed by airport temperature screening (Lee & Lee, 2020). South Korea placed temperature screening devices at all hospital entrances (Jeong et al., 2020). In Singapore, temperature screening was mandatory at airports, schools, workplaces, public buildings, and healthcare settings (El Guerche-Séblain et al., 2021). Israel used thermal cameras to measure temperatures in crowds (Barriga et al., 2020). China and Malaysia considered AI helmets that would monitor temperature along with other data points (El Guerche-Séblain et al., 2021). Italy used temperature testing robots when it reopened after its initial wave of COVID-19 (*Covid-19: Drones take Italian's*, 2020; Meisenzahl, 2020). For air travel, the International Air Transport Association recommended temperature screening (IATA, 2020).

The value of temperature screening may have decreased as public health experts gained a better understanding of asymptomatic spread, and the virus itself underwent various mutations, with Omicron, for example, being somewhat less likely to cause fever. Pre-Delta, fever was a common symptom. Post-Delta, it was less so (Bendix, 2022).

Schools in New York used temperature scanning as did COVID-19 vaccination sites like the Javits Center. Many schools also used apps so that people could record and submit their temperature prior to arrival with the rule that with an elevated temperature, they must stay home. During the reopening process, New York City required restaurants to screen all customers and staff (NYC Health Department, 2021).

While temperature screening would not address asymptomatic or afebrile cases, to many, it was still considered a valuable protection from exposure in cases where fever is apparent. The many papers addressing temperature screening, on balance, seemed to find it a valuable, if limited, tool, especially early in the pandemic, becoming less valuable much later.

Limitations of Temperature Testing

We now have more data about the limitations of temperature testing. One article that found about 20 percent of those testing positive for COVID-19 had a temperature over 100.4 Fahrenheit against temperature screening as the only approach to preventing transmission of COVID-19 (Vilke et al., 2020). Similarly, articles note the different readings based on style of thermometer as well as which body parts temperatures are measured and whether measurements accurately represent core temperature (Buoite Stella et al., 2020). Studies found that manual temperature checking is more effective than infrared scanners that capture many people's temperatures at once (Jung et al., 2020). Another study found that temperature screening was feasible but not determinative enough to be a primary method of detection (Facente et al., 2021). Another concern is that normal body temperature is quite variable. Temperature screening may miss someone whose normal temperature is low for whom 98.6 Fahrenheit may be unusually warm rather than normal (Adams, 2022). Most of the studies concern cases missed by temperature screening. Importantly, more research is needed to demonstrate how many people with elevated temperatures subsequently or simultaneously tested positive for COVID-19 to measure the benefits of temperature screening policies. COVID-19 policy generally is a risk reduction policy, although some countries did aim for complete containment, like China's zero-COVID strategy. While much of the research hinges on finding best practices, one important question is whether there is value in keeping someone known to have an elevated temperature out of a contained or crowded space, and how to measure that value. This chapter looks to temperature screening as a tool, not as the only method to prevent spread, and analyzes the ethics of its use based on knowledge at the time and current information. Much of the research cites the asymptomatic carriers, yet one important question is the likelihood that a person with a fever has COVID-19 at any given time in any jurisdiction, something that would likely change to reflect the local disease prevalence. Caution at a time of huge societal disruption is an important consideration when evaluating the justification of using temperature testing as one tool among many. There were many practical benefits to barring those with an elevated temperature from crowded or intimate spaces while healthcare systems were overwhelmed. The general current complaint about temperature testing is that it allows asymptomatic and afebrile people who are positive for COVID-19 to enter or participate but bars the febrile, regardless of their COVID-19 status. The World Health Organization

(WHO), Centers for Disease Control (CDC), and other public health organizations suggest that people with fevers isolate themselves from others.

Liberty and Surveillance: Must it be a Necessity to be Ethically Justifiable?

Generally free society looks for justifications for public policies that may intrude on rights or even on commonly accepted behaviors. "In a liberal, pluralistic democracy, the justification of coercive policies, as well as other policies, must rest on moral reasons that the public in whose name the policies are carried out could reasonably be expected to accept" (Childress et al., 2002, p. 171). Temperature screening is arguably not coercive: staying home is an option for customers wishing to shop, eat out, or engage in other relevant group or public activities. Another option is to arrive at a store, deny the screening, and be denied entrance to the normally open-to-the-public space, also negating the coercive aspect. The customer, having made the decision, would be free to leave. In certain industries, businesses have rules that more severely restrict people's freedom and include the collection of personal medical information. In most cases, there is a legal requirement for the action. Airport scans, recently adapted to reveal less and preserve more privacy, are TSA-driven and not imposed on customers by airlines themselves. Airlines do have a lot of power to ensure that flights are safe, on balance, giving them power over personal data. Amusement parks are governed by rules and regulations by state, local, and the federal government that include height and weight requirements; they ensure safety by following laws as well as internal and industry guidelines. Even bungee jumping and zip-lining are regulated to promote safety in ways that may require demonstrating an absence of certain medical conditions. Customers must divulge personal information and medical histories. The permitting process in many industries requires proof of safety measures and agreement to hold inspections. From the customer perspective, the laws and regulations matter less than the action. Customers benefit from safe airlines and amusement parks and willingly give medical information in exchange for participation in air travel or amusement park entertainment. Temperature screening is within accepted standards of requirements to participate, justified by the public health it would promote and its non-coercive nature.

While many stores have nondiscrimination policies, the potentially contagious customer does not have any fundamental right to access that would override the public health concern. It is reasonable to accept and even embrace temperature screening knowing others inside the space will also have been screened. Temperatures often indicate the most contagious time in a viral stage and even non-COVID-19 temperatures can indicate contagious conditions. Under normal circumstances, we would assume that people engaged in public activity assume the constant albeit small risk of contracting an infectious disease. Temperature is usually protectable data: it is to be kept private if it is a product of a hospital or doctor's appointment, as both are governed by HIPAA.

COVID-19 disproportionately affects certain populations including, most notably, the elderly. Reopening stores and businesses created an opportunity for those without special vulnerabilities wanting to go back to public space. As with the early pandemic, with the newest variant, immunocompromised individuals may choose to protect themselves by staying home, wearing additional personal protective gear, or avoiding crowds. The immunocompromised may benefit from temperature screening directives because other members of their community or household are less likely to bring the virus home if public spaces are engaging in temperature screening and enforcing social distancing and mask recommendations. Even keeping a few febrile people out of contained spaces can diminish the risks. Early on, stay-at-home orders combined with other nonpharmaceutical interventions like closing schools and wearing masks in crowded spaces to flatten the curve (Markel, 2020). The strain on the economy and on personal liberty makes those approaches unsustainable in the long term. A solution like temperature screening makes public spaces somewhat safer but may work best in conjunction with particularly vulnerable people continuing to avoid crowded spaces.

During the pandemic, in the United States, many states and the federal government used emergency orders. Some were challenged as unconstitutional. Many courts applied a deferential approach to pandemic restrictions, often citing *Jacobson v. Massachusetts*, the seminal case on permitting vaccination mandates. Other courts applied strict scrutiny, citing case law focused on fundamental rights rather than emergency public health law (Zimmerman, 2021). Strict scrutiny requires a compelling government interest and use of the least restrictive means. There must be a strong likelihood that the restriction would further that government interest to justify certain restrictive orders. Notably, among federal courts, actions infringing religious rights were more consistently strictly scrutinized than actions infringing other freedoms like interstate travel, the ability to evict tenants, make contracts, and keep businesses open (*Lawsuits about state action,* 2021). In the United States, state and federal courts applied varied approaches.

To analogize ethics to law, temperature screening would generally be more ethically justified if it meets two criteria: a reasonable expectation that it would be useful to a proper goal like decreasing transmission and a limited degree of bodily intrusion. Furthermore, in analyzing the ethics of an action, it is important to contextualize it. Temperature screening was seen at the time as a way to reintroduce many other much more valuable freedoms like the ability to move about freely, to enter contained spaces normally open to the public beyond those providing essential goods, to operate businesses, earn a living, and in some cases, to travel. The non-invasive nature of temperature screening would lean in its favor, yet the question of stored data and the privacy infringement complicates the issue and may bolster the arguments against it.

Context: Early Pandemic Spring 2020

There was an urgency to addressing the ethical basis for retail stores performing temperature screening. In Connecticut, LaBonne's grocery stores began checking temperatures without recording data early in the pandemic Atlanta's City Farmer's Market chain was also screening its customers (NBC Connecticut, 2020). Walmart chose to stay out of what it considered a public policy issue, refraining from testing customers' temperatures (Meyersohn, 2020). Dr. Luciana Borio, former director for medical and biodefense preparedness at the National Security Council under President Donald Trump and former acting chief scientist at the FDA suggested that "Even a modest benefit can be of value when our public health options are so limited in the absence of diagnostic tests, capacity for large scale contact tracing or a vaccine." Matthew Freeman, associate professor of environmental health and epidemiology at Emory University's Rollins School of Public Health, said it "makes sense for businesses to take the temperatures of shoppers to protect employees and patrons, but what would be the response if someone did indeed have a fever? A plan of action is critical'" (Meyersohn, 2020; see also, CBS Sacramento, 2020).

Greenburgh, New York, a municipality, required grocery stores and pharmacies to check temperatures as early as April, 2020 (Propper, 2020). Greenburgh Supervisor, Paul Feiner said, "Next week, when I extend the order, I intend (unless otherwise directed by the state) to also require the noninvasive taking of temperature of employees and customers. I don't believe that people with temperature should be allowed into the stores --we all worry about the risk of being infected or infecting others. Many people in Westchester are dying from the COVID-19 -partially because people are careless or inconsiderate of others. Although NYS law authorizes me to issue the order - the Town Board unanimously approved a resolution endorsing the contents." (Feiner, 2020; see also, Kimmel, 2021). It is reasonable to have concluded, at the height of the emergency with so many unknowns, that no one should be permitted entry into enclosed spaces with a fever. As discussed above, this chapter assumes enough efficacy to warrant some temperature screening policy -- some benefit or containment would derive from screening those entering public indoor spaces and barring those with a temperature of 100.4 or higher from entrance.

While this chapter concerns the decision by retail establishments to screen absent government mandates, under OSHA, many precautions would be justifiable to protect employees. Temperature screening of customers has two rationales: limiting exposure to customers who are likely at a contagious moment if they have the virus and an elevated temperature; and, the precautions serve the public health goal of transmission prevention. If reporting requirements or tracking ensued, the public health benefits would grow at the expense of control over one's own data. Websites usually offer data restriction choices by using a pop-up. An in-person temperature screening is a new data point that companies (especially small retail companies) were not prepared to deal with. If any data were collected, customers should have been notified about how the temperature would be used, who can access it, and how the customer would remain deidentified. Failing to track the febrile customer who might transmit the virus seems more ethically problematic than the privacy violation. Without government directives, stores would have trouble justifying saving or sharing the data for the sake of public health.

Private Action in the Absence of Government Mandates in the Early Pandemic

Public health initiatives required by law, permitted by law, and ones not addressed by law have different ethical implications. Efficacy alone would not allow stores to impede freedom and privacy more severely. Stores cannot detain those who display a symptom or refuse to wear a mask. Temperature screening must be within reason to be considered permissible. Stores like Walmart used the absence of a governmental directive as an excuse to avoid temperature screening. Walmart was permitted to remain open as essential, a huge economic benefit. Customers may see Walmart's stance as more ethical: valuing customer privacy and freedom. Stores like LaBonne's are managing risk themselves to protect employees and the public. In Greenburgh, store employees can simply argue they are following a local government directive, preventing their need to provide justification to customers, placing power with the government entity as traditionally expected in public health policy. I argue that temperature screening within a rights-driven, liberty-oriented society can be appropriate. It had a reasonable likelihood of preventing a febrile person with COVID-19 from spreading COVID-19 and it was not overly intrusive. As one tool among many, it created the possibility of cautiously reopening many stores and public spaces before widespread testing was available. Based on the information available at the time, and the overwhelming strain on the healthcare system, even preventing a person from spreading a different virus like the flu would arguably have been justifiable. Some freedom is gained and maintained by a small loss of privacy and restrictions on a different freedom. Reopening depended on public health tools.

Bioethics includes a principle of doing no harm. Under a harm avoidance ethic, entering and remaining in contained spaces with those with temperatures has potential for harm. However, the typical analysis would evaluate a public health or medical practitioner's decisions. Here, the ethical obligation of business owners to prevent harm as they see fit, whether motivated by self-preservation or by care for their customers, is different. Business owners act without special knowledge of the biology and virology of COVID-19. Their need to add protections before anyone in an official capacity instructed them propelled their behaviors. It would be difficult to say that prior to public health orders, they had an ethical duty to engage in any particular not-yet-proven but hopefully effective strategy. An ethical obligation may be framed as ethically compelled, permissible, or forbidden. Temperature screening is in murky territory, and permissibility may be the best ethical categorization, especially during the early pandemic.

Privacy in public temperature screening

Privacy in the doctor-patient relationship enhances value by promoting trust. Confidentiality promotes open communication with doctors and healthcare professionals. In COVID-19 customer temperature screening, the person taking the temperature is likely not trained in confidentiality and not HIPAA educated or subject to HIPAA requirements. Customers, traditionally not compared to patients, are operating outside of the traditional scope for the sake of the common good, allowing a non-invasive screening. Stores that screen customers should have a non-invasive thermometer that hovers and does not touch the customer. Evaluated by the principles of efficacy, necessity, and the least restrictive means, temperature screening may allow more freedom to move about and more businesses to remain open, even with changing variants that threaten to call for more shutdowns. Strict stay-at-home orders would prevent the necessity for widespread screening, but they are more intrusive than necessary. The initial reopening of stores created a situation ripe for more pervasive temperature screening.

Companies, stores, the local government, or police have little to no experience with personal medical data collection in the sphere of retail goods and services. In some cases, people might ask for a private space for the temperature screening. Stores should provide such a space but realistically they probably will not, making the screening a public event. Arguably, an elevated temperature would be witnessed by others outside the store who may know the identity of the febrile customer as many shop among their friends and neighbors. Yelling the temperature over to a different employee would be a serious breach of privacy; the employee taking customer temperatures should be trained to be discreet. Largescale temperature checks using thermal imaging systems do not require stopping individuals and do not require diverting employees from other tasks. For companies that can afford them, they may be the best path toward large scale temperature checks, although, as noted above, some technologies are less accurate than others.

An ethical lapse: the failure to record data that could improve public health and the economy

The results (a high or normal temperature) bring up an ethical conundrum: if the customers are asked to leave, the data and the customer are still in limbo. As COVID-19 testing becomes more readily available, the customers could be referred to a COVID-19 testing site. Failure to track them could allow them to try their luck at another store, spreading the virus if in fact they do have it. For privacy, it would be best not to store any temperature data creating no metadata for the event. The right thing for a business to do probably lies in between: for an elevated temperature, recommend an online doctor's appointment or send the customer home to consider seeking medical advice. I argue that a government directive to report elevated temperatures for legitimate public health purposes like tracking is reasonable if there were mechanisms to prevent abuse of power, and would have been an appropriate directive for stores to follow in the early pandemic. Later in the pandemic, as COVID-19 became arguably endemic, the ethical calculus changed, although as seen in hospital settings, temperature checking has a special precautionary benefit for the immunocompromised. Absent government use of the data, companies and stores should not be operating vigilante public health schemes that track and ban certain customers for extended periods, behavior that risks producing scarlet-letter-style stigma.

WHO's early-pandemic goals to find, isolate, test, and treat every case would be furthered by tracking and testing those with elevated temperatures (The Guardian, 2020). South Korea used a mechanism through apps and electronic bracelets to track those who tested positive (Smith et al., 2020). While such policies conflict with privacy and freedom, more businesses could reopen, and more people could go more places while following social distancing and mask-wearing recommendations early in the pandemic when the United States was still experiencing widespread stay-at-home orders. The U.S. population might be amenable to a model like South Korea's when it is key to exercising freedom to move about in public, allowing workers to return to work, and consumers to enjoy stores and businesses. WHO seems not to envision its goals being handled by companies rather than by public health authorities. The return to retail businesses and in-person services in the United States lacked a distinct protocol that fairly applied to all retail establishments. The acceptable tradeoff for forgoing privacy would be allowing stores to open, people to work, and consumers to consume. Instead of through temperature testing, the trade-off became vaccine passport systems, or simply proof of vaccination. While the system of showing restaurants and stores proof of vaccination requires sharing sensitive data and similarly violates privacy, or arguably violates it even more given the politically polarized nature of vaccination status in the United States, it too is no longer as effective at preventing spread of COVID-19 due to the ability of vaccinated people to spread the omicron variant. While asymptomatic spread is a risk that is difficult to control, people with elevated temperatures are a known risk.

Ethical baseline: notice and informed consent

Notice of policies affecting customers is an ethical obligation. Companies wishing to engage in customer temperature screening should make a statement on a website and install signs announcing that temperature screening will begin on a certain date (official notice) and what the screening will entail. Businesses that require temperature taking could provide exceptions based on proof of antibodies or a current negative COVID-19 test (Forgey, 2020). Otherwise, there is no obvious expeditious way to request, accept, or deny an exception if the interaction is taking place outside on the curb instead of online (Tomaszewski et al., 2020).

Kinsa, the thermometer company now well known for gathering temperature data, sells the data to pharmacies who use it for commercial purposes, specifically, to boost sales of products people with an elevated temperature might want (The Economist, 2020).[3] Through a built-in feature, Kinsa avoids any type of consent of the unwitting customer. While no personal data accompanies the temperature data, Kinsa profited from the data in unexpected ways. Stores do not give notice to customers about that type of data collection.

Conclusion

Historically, the government has been the accepted public health authority yet during the pandemic, certain policies and procedures were up for grabs. For example, in New York City, companies made their own rules, until far into the pandemic, about whether to require employee vaccination and how to go about implementing and enforcing vaccination policies. While temperature screening under normal circumstances in non-medical settings would pose significant ethical issues, evaluating its ethics in the context of the complexities of the pandemic and the gaps in knowledge especially during the early pandemic calls for some lenience concerning privacy and liberty. While knowing now that the benefits may have been overstated at the time, temperature screening was an opportunity to add one more level of safety to spaces that are open to the public. Temperature screening had a role in achieving the goal of decreasing risk despite its limitations as unable to single-handedly contain COVID-19. In the future, government entities should weigh in on stores and businesses imposing temperature screening as a condition of entry prior to their undertaking the task. Depending on the nature of a future pandemic, the stores that engage in temperature screening could be furthering employee safety and contributing to public health.

---

[3] Users of Kinsa apps which offer medical advice based on temperature data are likely aware the company stores and sells the data. Thermometer users probably do not realize their temperatures are recorded or that the company can narrow down their location to the zip code (The Economist, 2020).

Absent government directive, companies should agree not to store or use customer medical information, despite the data's valuable role in public health. In circumstances of vast uncertainty and a severe disease, or when the benefit is clear, a government order requiring reporting for the sake of tracking and isolating those with a given communicable and severe disease could be a proper use of government authority, especially if it would ensure standardized, ethical data protocols. Hopefully, in future pandemics or should the COVID-19 pandemic plod on with variants that more often present with elevated temperature, temperature screening can return to the toolkit to make shopping or just being in spaces open to the public safer. In 2020, the government vacuum in temperature screening handed power to retailers and grocers who do not know quite what to do with it.

References

Adams, J. U. (2022, January 16). Body temperature may not be an effective gauge of covid-19. *The Washington Post*. https://www.washingtonpost.com/health/covid-fever-body-temperature/2022/01/14/91a0527c-6d94-11ec-a5d2-7712163262f0_story.html

Barriga, A. do, Martins, A. F., Simões, M. J., & Faustino, D. (2020). The COVID-19 pandemic: Yet another catalyst for governmental mass surveillance? *Social Sciences & Humanities Open, 2*(1), 100096. https://doi.org/10.1016/j.ssaho.2020.100096

Bendix, A. (2022, January 14). 2 charts show how Omicron symptoms differ from Delta and past coronavirus variants. *Business Insider*. https://www.businessinsider.com/omicron-common-symptoms-vs-other-variants-charts-2022-1

The California Consumer Privacy Act of 2018, California Civil Code, Part 4, Division 3, Title 1.81.5 § AB375 (2018). https://casetext.com/statute/california-codes/california-civil-code/division-3-obligations/part-4-obligations-arising-from-particular-transactions/title-1815-california-consumer-privacy-act-of-2018

CBS Sacramento. (2020, April 9). *Why grocery stores could start taking customers' temperatures*. CBS Sacramento. https://sacramento.cbslocal.com/2020/04/09/coronavirus-grocery-stores-taking-temperature-reading/

Childress, J. F., Faden, R. R., Gaare, R. D., Gostin, L. O., Kahn, J., Bonnie, R. J., Kass, N. E., Mastroianni, A. C., Moreno, J. D., & Nieburg, P. (2002). Public health ethics: Mapping the terrain. *Journal of Law, Medicine & Ethics, 30*(2), 170–178. https://doi.org/10.1111/j.1748-720x.2002.tb00384.x

Covid-19: Drones take Italians' temperature and issue fines. thestar.com. (2020, April 11). https://www.thestar.com.my/tech/tech-news/2020/04/11/covid-19-drones-take-italians-temperature-and-issue-fines

Cowie, P., Hensley, K., & Phillips, J. (2021, February 13). *Employee privacy forecast: Temperature checks.* Labor & Employment Law Blog. https://www.laboremploymentlawblog.com/2020/03/articles/coronavirus/employee-privacy-forecast-temperature-checks/

The Economist Newspaper. (2020, March 26). Taking people's temperatures can help fight the coronavirus. *The Economist.* https://www.economist.com/science-and-technology/2020/03/26/taking-peoples-temperatures-can-help-fight-the-coronavirus

El Guerche-Séblain, C., Chakir, L., Nageshwaran, G., Harris, R. C., Sevoz-Couche, C., Vitoux, O., & Vanhems, P. (2021). Experience from five Asia-Pacific countries during the first wave of the COVID-19 pandemic: Mitigation strategies and epidemiology outcomes. *Travel Medicine and Infectious Disease, 44,* 102171. https://doi.org/10.1016/j.tmaid.2021.102171

Facente, S. N., Hunter, L. A., Packel, L. J., Li, Y., Harte, A., Nicolette, G., McDevitt, S., Petersen, M., & Reingold, A. L. (2021). Feasibility and effectiveness of daily temperature screening to detect COVID-19 in a prospective cohort at a large public university. *BMC Public Health, 21*(1). https://doi.org/10.1186/s12889-021-11697-6

Feiner, P. (2020, April 8). *Greenburgh imposes health/safety conditions on supermarkets - next week: Non-invasive temperature of employees to be required before entering store.* LinkedIn. https://www.linkedin.com/pulse/greenburgh-imposes-healthsafety-conditions-next-week-paul-feiner/

Forgey, Q. (2020, April 10). *Fauci:* Coronavirus immunity cards for Americans are 'being discussed'. *POLITICO.* https://www.politico.com/news/2020/04/10/fauci-coronavirus-immunity-cards-for-americans-are-being-discussed-178784

Guardian News and Media. (2020, March 13). WHO urges countries to 'Track and trace' every covid-19 case. *The Guardian.* https://www.theguardian.com/world/2020/mar/13/who-urges-countries-to-track-and-trace-every-covid-19-case

Health Insurance Portability and Accountability Act of 1996, 5 U.S.C. § 553 *et seq.*, 8 U.S.C. § 1481 and 1481, 10 U.S.C. § 1072 (1996).

IATA (International Air Transport Association). (2021, April). *Temperature screening: A public health responsibility existing guidance.* https://www.iata.org/ contentassets/67e015cf3db1410392cd5b5bb5961a16/iata-temperature-screening-public-health-responsibility.pdf

Jeong, G. H., Lee, H. J., Lee, J., Lee, J. Y., Lee, K. H., Han, Y. J., Yoon, S., Ryu, S., Kim, D. K., Park, M. B., Yang, J. W., Effenberger, M., Eisenhut, M., Hong, S. H., Kronbichler, A., Ghayda, R. A., & Shin, J. I. (2020). Effective control of COVID-19 in South Korea: Cross-sectional study of epidemiological data. *Journal of Medical Internet Research, 22*(12). https://doi.org/10.2196/22103

Jung, J., Kim, E. O., & Kim, S.-H. (2020). Manual fever check is more sensitive than infrared thermoscanning camera for fever screening in a hospital setting during the COVID-19 pandemic. *Journal of Korean Medical Science, 35*(44). https://doi.org/10.3346/jkms.2020.35.e389

Kim, J.-H., An, J. A.-R., Oh, S. J. J., Oh, J., & Lee, J.-K. (2021, March 5). *Emerging COVID-19 success story: South Korea learned the lessons of MERS.* Our World in Data. https://ourworldindata.org/covid-exemplar-south-korea

Kimmel, R. (2021, May 20). Strict new rules for groceries and pharmacies in unincorporated Greenburgh to combat covid-19. *The Hudson Independent.* https://thehudsonindependent.com/strict-new-rules-for-groceries-and-pharmacies-in-unincorporated-greenburgh-to-combat-covid-19/

Lawsuits about state actions and policies in response to the coronavirus (COVID-19) pandemic. Ballotpedia. (n.d.). Retrieved from https://ballotpedia.org/Lawsuits_ about_state_actions_and_policies_in_response_to_the_coronavirus_(COVID-19)_pandemic

Lee, D., & Lee, J. (2020). Testing on the move: South Korea's rapid response to the COVID-19 pandemic. *Transportation Research Interdisciplinary Perspectives, 5,* 100111. https://doi.org/10.1016/j.trip.2020.100111

Lippi, G., Nocini, R., Mattiuzzi, C., & Henry, B. M. (2021). Is body temperature mass screening a reliable and safe option for preventing COVID-19 spread? *Diagnosis.* https://doi.org/10.1515/dx-2021-0091

Markel, H. (2020, April 20). *What history revealed about cities that socially distanced during a pandemic.* PBS. Retrieved from https://www.pbs.org/newshour/ health/what-

history-can-teach-us-about-flattening-the-curve?fbclid=IwAR1CQzbfhiLm-
1hmB586kt6RsCBPcI5Q8KwKaOmln_pyN9KKKp OSAsOJvGs

Meyersohn, N. (2020, April 9). *Why stores could start taking customers' temperatures*.
CNN. Retrieved from https://www.cnn.com/2020/04/09/business/walmart-
amazon-home-depot-whole-foods-temperatures/index.html

Milligan, R., Dummit, D., & Tomaszewski, john. (2020, April 7). *The impact
of COVID-19 on the California Consumer Privacy Act*. Seyfarth Shaw.
https://www.seyfarth.com/news-insights/the-impact-of-covid-19-on-the-
california-consumer-privacy-act-2.html

NBC Connecticut. (2020, April 8). *Labonne's markets to take customers'
temperatures*. NBC Connecticut. https://www.nbcconnecticut.com/news/
coronavirus/labonnes-markets-to-take-customers-temperatures/2251765/

NYC Health Department. (2021, February 12). *Reopening New York City: Checklist for
food service establishments offering indoor food service*. https://www1.nyc.gov/
assets/doh/downloads/pdf/covid/businesses/covid-19-reopening-food-
services-indoor-dining-checklist.pdf

Propper, D. (2020, April 9). Supermarkets and pharmacies in Greenburgh could
start taking temperatures of workers, customers. *The Journal News*.
https://www.lohud.com/story/news/coronavirus/2020/04/09/greenburgh-
supervisor-wants-customers-and-workers-get-temperature-taken-before-
entering-store/2974662001/

Rosenfeld, J., Lenzi, M., Stauber, A., Heiple, B., Otum, P., & Schneider, L. (2020,
April 3). *Covid-19: Screening employee temperatures: What employers need to know*.
WilmerHale. https://www.wilmerhale.com/en/insights/client-alerts/20200403-
screening-employee-temperatures-what-employers-need-to-know

Smith, J., Shin, H., & Cha, S. (2020, April 15). *Ahead of the curve: South Korea's evolving
strategy to prevent a coronavirus resurgence*. Reuters. https://www.reuters.com/
article/us-health-coronavirus-southkorea-respons/ahead-of-the-curve-south-
koreas-evolving-strategy-to-prevent-a-coronavirus-resurgence-
idUSKCN21X0MO

Tomaszewski, J., Dummit, D., & Milligan, R. (2020, April 6). *The impact of COVID-
19 on the California Consumer Privacy Act: Seyfarth Shaw*. Trading Secrets.
https://www.tradesecretslaw.com/2020/04/articles/privacy-2/the-impact-of-
covid-19-on-the-california-consumer-privacy-act/

Vilke, G. M., Brennan, J. J., Cronin, A. O., & Castillo, E. M. (2020). Clinical features of patients with COVID-19: Is temperature screening useful? *The Journal of Emergency Medicine, 59*(6), 952–956. https://doi.org/10.1016/j.jemermed.2020.09.048

Wu, Y.-C., Chen, C.-S., & Chan, Y.-J. (2020). The outbreak of COVID-19: An overview. *Journal of the Chinese Medical Association, 83*(3), 217–220. https://doi.org/10.1097/jcma.0000000000000270

Zimmerman, A. (2020). Vigilante grocers: Is temperature screening of customers by retailers an ethical and valuable restriction on privacy and freedom? *Voices in Bioethics.* https://journals.library.columbia.edu/index.php/bioethics/article/view/5833

Zimmerman, A. (2021). Weeding out disingenuous emergency orders: A consistent ethical justification to determine whether to apply Jacobson v. Massachusetts' deferential approach or the tiered scrutiny that would apply absent an emergency. *Voices in Bioethics, 7.* https://doi.org/10.7916/vib.v7i.8037 (Original work published March 12, 2021)

ETHICAL QUESTIONS IN PANDEMIC RESPONSE: DOES SCHOOL CLOSURE SAVE LIVES OR CRUSH LIVES?

Bhaskaran Raman[1]

Abstract: Much of the world's response to the COVID-19 pandemic has been in terms of lockdowns and other such restrictions. Before March 2020, such measures were unthinkable. Initial arguments for the lockdowns were to "flatten the curve" so that hospital systems are not overwhelmed. We look at ethical questions in the context of children and education. Is it ethical to force children to attend online class, without knowing the long-term effects on their education, mental health, and future well-being? When children lose continuity in schooling, there is a learning loss and many children even tend to drop out, especially those from a poor economic background. It is well known that illiteracy and poverty are deeply connected, and both are connected with healthcare. So by closing schools, are we not condemning children to future poor health? Furthermore in India, many schools run a mid-day meal program, to supplement their nutrition. Disruptions to this have affected children's health directly. This raises further ethical questions of school closure. This writeup will touch upon such ethical questions with a focus on India.

Introduction

The declaration of the COVID-19 pandemic in early 2020 brought an extended period of crisis and uncertainty to much of the world. In such times, what does one do? There are some guiding principles of ethics one can use in such situations. The first is the principle of "do no harm" (Finlay, 2006). We can try new steps in a new situation, even without evidence, but we must adhere to this guiding principle. The second is the principle of natural justice: we should prioritize the welfare of children, even in times of distress, especially in times of distress. Prioritizing children is instinct,

---

[1] Professor, Department of Computer Science and Engineering, IIT, Mumbai, India

common to not just humans but all mammals. Have we followed these principles in our response to COVID-19?

"A few weeks to flatten the curve" is how it started (Jenson, 2020). Schools were shut for children. Children were not even allowed to play with one another. After all it was for the noble cause of "saving lives." Over time, various governments have tried various methods to control COVID-19 spread, including harsh lockdowns. But is there scientific evidence that various restrictions on children have had effect? Specifically, is there evidence that school closure is beneficial? Did the world adhere to the principle of "do no harm to children" in its pandemic response?

In India, most schools were closed for nearly two years, since the lockdown started on 25 March 2020. In this writeup, we first examine the risk of COVID-19 for children, comparing it with other risks they face. We then look at the question of whether school closure was a necessary step to control the spread of COVID-19. Did it "flatten the curve" so as to not overwhelm hospitals? Next we example the costs of extended school closure, and which sections of society face these costs the most. This allows us to compare these costs against the risks of school reopening. We then look at whether other countries opened schools amidst the pandemic. While some of the initial panic is understandable, did India consider scientific evidence for course correction later on? India has the ignoble distinction on the global stage among 200+ countries, in terms of the longest school closure (UNESCO, 2021). We look at the various facets of whether this was justified or ethical.

Fear for children, and a common myth

Has the basis for the world's response to COVID been reason or fear? In the context of children, there are two kinds of fears. The first is the fear *for* children: will COVID-19 affect our children? This fear is natural, and was rational in the early period when we did not know much about COVID-19. But over a period of time we need to pause and ask: has COVID-19 affected children? Do we know in our circles of any child who has been affected severely by COVID-19? If we pause and ask ourselves this question, we find that such instances are very rare indeed.

Our own personal experience apart, several careful studies have shown the same conclusion. As early as after the first wave of the pandemic, based on a study of 137 million school-age children in the U.S. and Europe during the period February-May 2020, (Bhopal, 2020) observed that COVID-19 in this age group is less than half as risky as seasonal influenza, and over 20 times less risky than death by "unintentional injury". An analysis of nearly 2 million children in Sweden during the four months of peak pandemic first wave (March-June 2020), found that there was not a single child death due to COVID-19 (Ludvigsson et al., 2021). Notably, Sweden had its schools open for under-16 children throughout during this period. While this analysis has been vehemently critiqued (Vogel, 2021), a quick look at the EUROMOMO website (EuroMoMo, 2022) shows that Sweden had no excess mortality in any age-group under 45 years throughout the pandemic: in 2020 or in 2021.

A later study of German children considered seroprevalence as well as child hospitalization data until May 2021, and showed a similar result: no healthy child in the school age-group died due to COVID-19 (Sorg et al., 2021). In both the Swedish and German studies, even ICU admissions related to COVID-19 were very rare for children.

Another study in the UK examined all deaths and hospitalizations (due to any cause) among children aged 0-17, during the period 1 February 2019 to 31 January 2021, and noted that the risk of severe illness or death from SARS-Cov-2 in children is extremely low; and those at higher risk are also those who are also at higher risk from any winter virus or other illness, i.e., children with other health conditions and disabilities.

Comparison with other risks

Although the concern of children acting as virus carriers was also there, the primary emotional "reason" stated for school closure was to "protect children." For instance, Delhi's Chief Minister on 15 July 2021 said "we would not like to take risk with children" (Outlook, 2021). In mid-May 2021, there was a huge concern in India that there would be a third wave of COVID-19, this time affecting children (NDTV, 2021). Therefore it behooves us to pause a moment and examine this with analogies and comparisons. Suppose the government told that children would henceforth be banned from cars and motorbikes, to protect them, what would our reaction be? Surely, we would consider it absurd. Now, data shows that the risk of COVID-19 for those under 25 years is about ten times *lesser* than that of traffic accident (Fox, 2021)! So school closure to "protect children" is ten times as absurd as banning children from cars.

COVID-19 risk for children is in fact so miniscule that as per U.S. data, it is even less than drowning accidents (Høeg, 2021). Do we spend every day of our life worrying about children drowning? So is fear for children being affected by COVID-19 reasonable?

Let us now turn our attention to a stark comparison in India. The city of Mumbai has had one of the best COVID-19 tracking and management dashboards in India. As per Mumbai's dashboard data (BMC, 2022), the COVID-19 IFR (Infection Fatality Rate) for under-19 is miniscule: about 0.003% (Raman, 2021a). In comparison, the infant mortality rate in India is about 3% (1,000 times greater) and the infant mortality rate in Japan (one of the lowest) is 0.18% (60 times greater).

We must therefore realize, and be grateful that the risk of COVID-19 for children is much lower than for adults, and is also much lower than other (already small) risks children face in daily life anyway.

A common myth

A common myth in this context in India is that *we* have somehow protected children from the virus by shutting schools. However, various sero-surveys shatter this myth. Despite school closure, children in India were exposed as much as adults: as high as 75% even as of June 2021 (Dutt, 2021), likely to be near 100% after Omicron. It is just that we did not even notice it, since children' bodies have had no problem fighting the virus.

Did third-wave concern have a basis?

At the end of the second wave in India, around mid-May 2021, even before the thought of reopening schools could begin, a concern was voiced that a possible third wave involving newer variants could affect children (NDTV,

2021). The concern quickly grew into an overwhelming media talking point. Did the concern have any basis? A careful look at the data told that the age-profiles of those affected in the second and first waves are similar (Pandit, 2021). There was thus no scientific basis for this fear. Yet it had the effect of prolonging school closure for another nearly nine months, beyond the already long closure of around fifteen months.

Is paediatric COVID-19 case-count meaningful? Is zero-COVID-19 possible?

A common refrain is that even children can get infected with COVID-19. What does such an infection mean? Does it have clinical significance? Paediatric "case" reporting arises from a misplaced zeal for zero-risk and zero-COVID-19, a scientific impossibility. A clear fact which has been lost amidst the fear-ridden pandemic response is the *age-differential* risk of COVID-19. While COVID-19 is deadly for old/comorbid people, it is literally a thousand times less risk for children (Kulldorff et al., 2020). Despite this, surely every parent would say "my child should not face *any* risk, however small." This is natural and emotional, but irrational on three counts.

- First, zero risk is an impossibility. A UK study concluded that children under 10 are 20 times more likely to die of accidental injury, compared to COVID-19 (Chalmers, 2020). Surely, we wouldn't shut schools or children' play to avoid accidents. So how is it reasonable to shut schools to supposedly reduce COVID-19 risk?
- Second, staying at home away from schools has *not* protected children from exposure to COVID-19. As cited earlier, sero-surveys in India have shown that a majority of children were already exposed and had antibodies even as of June 2021, despite almost continuous school closure. What has protected these children from any severe outcome is their own natural immune system (for which we should be thankful), not school closure.
- Third, school closure *increases* health risk for children: causing great psychological harm, even suicides (NYT, 2021), alongside increasing manifold other severe problems like child labour (Iyer, 2021), child marriage (Rose & Goverde, 2021), malnutrition (Shukla, 2021), etc. We detail these in a later section.

The fact that children are at negligible risk from COVID-19 immediately raises a plethora of ethical questions on school closure as a pandemic response measure. What about children's right to education and a normal childhood? Such questions become sharper as we delve into further details of ostensible reasons for school closure.

Fear *of* children: are schools super-spreaders?

While the first element of fear is fear *for* children, a second element of fear and anxiety in COVID-19 times has been that of fear *of* children. We have been told that children could carry the virus from school to elders at home. What is the scientific evidence for schools as COVID-19 hotspots? Let us now examine this.

There have been several careful scientific studies across various parts of the world, measuring the role of in-person classes in COVID-19 spread (Raman, 2021b). The overwhelming conclusion has been that the risk of COVID-19 spread in schools is minimal compared to other locations.

As early as June 2020, a comparison of Sweden (schools open) vs. Finland (schools closed) showed no statistical difference in paediatric cases, and no increased risk to teachers compared to other professions (Carlson, 2020). A later more detailed study across Sweden concluded that schoolteachers in fact faced less risk compared to other professions (Ludvigsson et al., 2021).

In the United States, the issue of school closure during the pandemic has been a politically charged issue, with schools open in some states/counties while closed in others. The state of Florida has kept its schools open since September 2020, and did not have worse COVID-19 outcomes compared to other states which had schools closed. A USA-wide study conducted between March and December 2020 concluded "no increase in COVID-19 hospitalization rates associated with in-person education" (Leidman et al., 2021). Another USA-wide scientific study of 57,000+ child-care providers, published in the journal of the American Academy of Pediatrics concluded "no association was found between exposure to child care and COVID-19" (Gilliam et al., 2021).

A detailed study in Spain looked at data from over 1 million children of all ages in schools, and found that the R-factor (rate of virus spread) is well less than one for all school-age children (Alonso et al., 2021). Furthermore, the R-value is lower for lower ages, as low 0.2 for pre-primary children. In other words, children are neither affected severely by COVID-19, nor contribute significantly to community spread of the virus (Lee & Raszka, 2020).

Does school closure help reduce hospitalization?

Many schools did open in several parts of the world, many even at the peak of the COVID-19 curve. But reports of COVID-19 outbreaks in schools have been few and far between. Let us look rationally at a few such recent reports from India as well as abroad, to gauge the level of concern warranted.

After the second wave in India, the state of Punjab opened schools from 02 August 2021. It was reported that "infection" was high among children in Punjab following school reopening (News18, 2021a). The state of Tamil Nadu opened schools for classes 9-12 on 01 September 2021. By mid-September, a total of 117 paediatric cases were reported in that state (*The Times of India*, 2021). Toward the end of August 2021, a report of a COVID-19 outbreak in California, USA made waves in the media (News18, 2021b).

To a layperson, such reports painted a picture that schools are dangerous places, hospitals may crumble if schools are opened. Is this picture accurate, or is it a gross exaggeration? It is important to note that none of the media reports say anything about the *severity* of the "cases." Have there been any severe cases? Any hospitalizations? None reported on this. Taking "no news" as "good news," perhaps we can conclude that there have been no severe cases or hospitalizations. Indeed the original CDC report of the California outbreak says "No persons infected in this outbreak were hospitalized" (Lam-Hine et al., 2021). Another report from the U.S. CDC in January 2021 cited a study which found "no increase in COVID-19 hospitalization rates associated with in-person education" (Leidman et al., 2021).

While there were certainly reports of COVID-19 hospitalization of children during the Omicron wave (Schreiber, 2022), a large fraction of it was reported as being hospitalization *with* COVID-19 as opposed to *because of* COVID-19. That is, people hospitalized for other reasons just happened to test positive on the RTPCR test, which can give a positive result up to twelve weeks after infection (Smith-Schoenwalder, 2021). Importantly in our context, reports of any hospitalization *due to* schools were markedly absent.

In other words, there was *no curve to flatten* through school closure.

Does case-counting serve a useful purpose?

Thus even the rare reports of supposed COVID-19 spread in schools report only "cases." Does this serve any purpose? But as mentioned earlier, in children, an "infection" or a "case" does not mean much. Indeed, COVID-19 is mild for the vast majority of healthy adults as well. It would do good to remind ourselves what the abbreviation SARS-Cov-2 stands for. The first "S" stands for "severe" and the "A" stands for "acute." "Cases," or PCR positive results can happen among children too. But the risk of *severe* outcomes is very rare (Ludvigsson et al., 2021). The human body has hundreds of different kinds of viruses: if we test for them, we will find them, but there is no clinical relevance since the body is able to fight off the bad ones. For most children, SARS-Cov-2 is just one other such virus with severe outcomes being very rare: ICU admission rate about 1.7 per 10,000 as per the German study (Sorg et al., 2021), and just about 0.07 per 10,000 as per the Swedish study (Ludvigsson et al., 2021).

Therefore counting "cases", especially in children, serves only the negative purpose of increasing anxiety. In September 2021 it was reported that the Supreme Court of India had said that it would hold the state of Kerala accountable "if even one case is reported" during conduct of class-11 exams (Express, 2021). Is this level of containment humanly possible? That too against a respiratory virus spreading through airborne aerosols? When the harshest of military enforced lockdowns have not contained the virus in much more sparsely populated countries like Australia (Sky, 2021)? Instead of seeking the impossible, should we not be celebrating the fact that the virus has spared children and young people from severe outcomes? In the above pronouncement, did the Honourable Supreme Court show balance, or hurt the cause of childrens' education?

Is fear of children natural or ethical?

Fear of children being virus vectors has not been restricted to schools. There have been extreme instances around the world. In the United States, a mother in Texas placed her 13-year old son in the trunk of her car, to "avoid being exposed" after her son tested positive (Sutton & Dominguez, 2022). Is this level of fear *of* children acceptable? We cannot write off the mother as a "bad-apple", as the episode turned for the worse: the concerned judge found "no reason to charge" the mother (Sutton & Dominguez, 2022). How is this justifiable?

In many parts of the world, including in India, children' playgrounds were closed; many housing societies placed arbitrary rules against children playing, for several months. Even where governments have been willing to open schools, teachers' unions have lobbied against the same (Tareen, 2022). At one point, innocent children were even blamed for the death of old people (Lin & Money, 2021). Are these ethical? What about childrens' well-being, their right to a normal and enjoyable childhood? Is this not society devouring its young, consumed by fear of COVID-19. Is this even human?

Did India follow scientific evidence?

Even as various experts and international bodies were saying that "schools should be the last to close and the first to reopen" (Fore & Azoulay, 2021), unfortunately various Indian governments did the exact opposite. Even as most other venues opened, schools were kept shut. At that point, one did not need careful studies, but only plain common sense. How can schools be super-spreaders when every other place in India was crowded: banks, markets, buses, trains, airports, and even malls and theatres?

Furthermore, in various Indian states, even where schools opened, *anganwadis* (day-care centers for pre-school children) and primary classes were the last to open. This is in sharp contrast to the Spanish study which said that younger children spread COVID-19 even less (Alonso et al., 2021)!

The ethics behind such fear *of* children becomes highly questionable especially when it is not even backed by scientific evidence. We now look at the costs borne by children, due to such fear.

What are the costs of school closure?

With school closure as a component of pandemic response, children have been forced into "online education". But does "online" constitute education? Early on in the pandemic, whether children would be affected by COVID-19 may have been an unknown. But it was always known that "online" is a poor replacement for in-person education. Experience since about 2013 with MOOCs (Massively Open Online Courses) in college education has shown that learner engagement and student retention are huge practical issues (Alemayehu & Chen, 2021). This issue is even more stark among children. Children, especially those in primary and pre-primary classes, can achieve their learning as well as social and emotional development only through human interaction: with teachers and peers. A study from the Netherlands, which has among the best broadband Internet connection rates, looked at student learning during the first wave lockdown period, and concluded that student learning had pretty much stagnated in this period (Engzell et al., 2021). Thus, despite knowing that online learning for children is ineffective, we shut schools, experimenting with childrens' lives in an attempt to achieve "zero-COVID-19," a scientific impossibility in itself.

The results of this extreme experimental intervention are devastating. Even pre-pandemic, online learning was at best a supplement, and that too for older children and college students. Younger children absolutely cannot learn online, and in fact they even forget skills. More significantly, for children and young adults, the mental health issues arising from lockdown and loss of social contact is much more concerning than COVID-19 itself. We detail these aspects below.

Despite a shorter school closure than India, the UK has reported alarming increases in mental health issues among children (Walderman, 2021). It reported a 40% rise in the number of children taking antidepressants (Donnelly, 2021). Scotland reported rising numbers of children reporting to hospital for self-harm (Grant, 2021). In the USA, the American Academic of

Paediatricians called the mental health crisis among children a national emergency (Shivaram, 2021). In the 15-19 age-group, U.S. statistics from the CDC reveal a 14% increase in *non-COVID-19* deaths in 2020 (Raman, 2022). Since the COVID-19 deaths in this age-group is much rarer, the likely cause of this excess death is the lockdown related mental health issues. In Las Vegas (USA), a surge of student suicides forced schools to reopen in January 2021 (NYT, 2021). A systematic review across 36 studies from 11 countries affirmed the obvious: that school closures and lockdowns were associated with adverse mental health symptoms in children and adolescents (0-19 years) (Viner et al., 2022).

In India, aside from mental health issues, there have been other severe consequences of school closure. A detailed survey report from September 2021 shows the tip of the iceberg in terms of the catastrophic consequences (Khera, 2021). Reading and writing levels of children have declined, with nearly half the children unable to read more than a few words. A mere 8% of children in rural areas were studying online regularly. This was due to a mix of issues arising out of poverty: unavailable of devices, unavailability of Internet access, lack of technical knowhow, etc. More than a third of the children were not studying at all.

A study by Azim Premji University among children of classes 2-6 across 5 states of India, undertaken in January 2021, found that as much as 82% *lost* at least one mathematical skill and 92% lost at least one language skill, compared to the previous year (APF, 2021). This is catastrophic, but not surprising given that children do not make learning progress even with high speed Internet availability, as found by a methodical study in Netherlands (Engzell et al., 2021). Doctors in the city of Bengaluru in India reported that among children under the age of 5, there has been over a 10-fold increase in those with speech disorders, due to lack of social stimulation and increased screen time (Suraksha, 2021). Thus a loss of 1.5 years for a child can cause long-term harm. How is this ethical? Has there been any sense of balance in the pandemic response?

Another detailed study by Pratham, a non-governmental organization in India, conducted across 7000 government schools in 25 states during the period September-October 2021 found that nearly two-thirds of teachers reported that children were unable to cope with grade level curriculum due to the extended school closure (ASER, 2022). Even in the relatively well-off California (United States), students in grade-8 in 2021 showed math skills expected of those in grade-5 (Fensterwald, 2022).

People in the middle and lower economic strata in India make considerable investments in their childrens' education, as a way toward a better living standard. Even prior to the pandemic, there was a huge attainment gap across students, especially in higher grades. The bottom half of children passing 10th grade are 2+ years behind in terms of skills. Prolonged school closure has widened this gap. What will this do to their future? Does it not push the next generation deeper into poverty? Ironically, the poorest families living in dense urban slums, who bore the brunt of the first wave and largely immune from the virus itself as early as August 2020 (as shown by serosurveys), are the ones who suffered the most from school closures. A survey conducted in early 2022 in India's capital city New Delhi showed that school closure affected the urban poor severely: as many as one in five households reported that their children completely stopped studies due to lack of access to an Internet-enabled device (Attri, 2022).

Even as early as November 2020, a survey across 10 states estimated that nearly two-thirds of children in rural India may drop out of school, a staggering statistic which likely worsened with continuing closure (Agrawal, 2021).

Unfortunately, the costs of school closure do not end with loss of education. The charade of "lives versus education" could not be more stark than in India. In every single day, nearly two-thousand children in India die of malnutrition related preventable causes (Banerjee, 2021)! The malice of malnutrition has been so severe over the decades that schools served a crucial role toward alleviating the problem: by providing supplemental nutritional meals, commonly known as the mid-day meal program. By shutting schools, India neglected the mid-day meal scheme, and worsened the far bigger problem of child malnutrition. Even as early as June 2020, it was estimated that about 800,000 additional children would face underweight and wasting (Rajpal et al., 2020). So was the closure of schools a "life vs. education" issue?

Aside from malnutrition, decades of progress against the severe malice of child labour in India has been reversed due to extended school closure (Parth & Pierson, 2021). A report titled "Without food, without jobs and without education" was released in April 2022, by non-governmental organizations ActionAid Association and Slum Mahila Sanghatane (Express, 2022). The report documented drastic increase in the number of children who had turned to child labour for their survival. As per the 2011 census, India had an estimated 10.1 million children in child labour (Iyer, 2021). This number is staggering: we should be asking as to how many lives were saved by school closure, to justify the worsening of the lives of these many children? Child labour not only condemns that child to poverty, but subsequent generations too.

Yet another social malady in India is that of child marriage, especially a problem for girl children. Prolonged school shutdown has severely set back India's fight against this social ill of child marriage (Bahl et al., 2021).

If we had a daily updates on malnutrition or child labour or child marriage cases, like COVID-19 case counts, would we have closed schools this long? Would we not have paid attention to the plight of India's children?

In an attempt to justify lockdown and school closure , the Prime Minister of India famously remarked "जान है तो जहान है" : life is more valuable than anything else. Given the costs of school closure, the statement is not just banal, it is a cruel twist. Children are clearly not in danger from COVID-19, but have suffered extreme harms due to school closures and other restrictions. Not only is the mental health of children in tatters, but their future is bleaker than ever due to extended school closure. The link between illiteracy and poverty is well known, as is the link of both with health-care. It is especially known that literacy of girls is extremely important for the health of the subsequent generation. Therefore we need to ask: has school closure achieved the stated aim of "protecting children," or the exact opposite? If these children fall further into poverty, how will they earn or access healthcare? How will it affect their lifespan and future generations?

Are COVID-19-19 jabs necessary for children?

Yet another myth in India, in the context of schools has been that schools are safe only after children can be vaccinated against COVID-19. This defies logic, as schools have been open in tens of other countries even before adults' jabs. An opinion piece in October 2021 by two medical professionals argued that COVID-19 jabs for children are necessary, as otherwise children may carry the infection from school back home to adults (John & Seshadri, 2021). Aside from the obvious ethical question of jabbing children for the benefit of adults, such a stance is also quite unscientific, as it is known now that the current COVID-19 vaccines (even boosters) do not prevent infection or transmission (Levine-Tiefenbrun et al., 2022). Indeed, Omicron cases have been reported predominantly in double jabbed people. While jab-induced protection against severe disease and hospitalization lasts longer, even this has been found to be waning in about six months (Katikireddi et al., 2022); hence the push for boosters (The Daily, 2021). While no one can be against a children' vaccine shown to be safe and effective after rigorous trials, where was the case for linking schools and education to a vaccine still under clinical trial? How can there be emergency authorization of the jabs for children, when there has been no COVID-19 emergency for children? This was indeed the position of the National Technical Advisory Group on Immunisation (NTAGI) (Chandna, 2021); the Indian government's nod for jabbing children in the 15-18 age group defied explanation (Bureau, 2021).

Conclusion

So why did we shut schools as part of the pandemic response? The saying goes: "the road to hell is paved with good intentions". We shut schools to keep children safe. Or to keep parents safe. Or to keep grandparents safe. Or to keep society safe from the COVID-19 curve. All well intentioned perhaps, but there is now significant evidence that none of these are remotely true. Were children not exposed to COVID-19? No, they were exposed (but safe) despite school closure. Were parents or grandparents safe due to school closure? India has its tall second wave to answer that. There have been several self-evident contradictions in India that any layperson can see: how can schools be viewed as super-spreaders when everything else including malls, theaters, markets, banks, post-offices, public buses, etc. are open?

Worldwide, children' education has suffered the worst since World War 2. Even as of September 2020, UNICEF estimated that 24 million children will never return to school (UNICEF, 2020). In India, 260 million children face an education emergency (Education Emergency, 2021), due to 700+ days of school closure, the longest on the planet, surpassing 200+ other countries (UNESCO, 2021).

So did school closures flatten the COVID-19 curve, or flatten childrens' futures?

References

Agrawal, S. (2021). 64% kids in rural India fear they have to drop out if not given additional support: Survey. *The Print.* https://theprint.in/india/64-kids-in-rural-india-fear-they-have-to-drop-out-if-not-given-additional-support-survey/625146/

Alemayehu, L., & Chen, H.-L. (2021). Learner and instructor-related challenges for learners' engagement in MOOCs: a review of 2014–2020 publications in selected SSCI indexed journals. Routledge. https://doi.org/10.1080/10494820.2021.1920430

Alonso, S., Alvarez-Lacalle, E., Català, M., López, D., Jordan, I., García-García, J. J., Soriano-Arandes, A., Lazcano, U., Sallés, P., Masats, M., Urrutia, J., Gatell, A., Capdevila, R., Soler-Palacin, P., Bassat, Q., & Prats, C. (2021). Age-dependency of the propagation rate of Coronavirus Disease 2019 inside school bubble groups in Catalonia, Spain. *The Pediatric Infectious Disease Journal, 40*(11), 955–961. https://doi.org/10.1097/INF.0000000000003279

APF. (2021). The loss of learning for children during the pandemic. *APF Magazine.* https://azimpremjiuniversity.edu.in/publications/2021/report/loss-of-learning-during-the-pandemic

ASER. (2022). Annual Status of Education Report (Rural) 2021. http://img.asercentre.org/docs/schoolsurveymajorfindings.pdf

Attri, V. (2022). Online schooling hit urban poor the hardest, 1 in 5 homes say kids missed a year. *The Indian Express.* https://indianexpress.com/article/cities/delhi/delhi-schools-aap-model-online-schooling-lokniti-csds-study-7871406/

Bahl, D., Bassi, S., & Arora, M. (2021). *The impact of COVID-19 on children and adolescents: Early evidence in India.* Observer Research Foundation. https://www.orfonline.org/research/the-impact-of-covid-19-on-children-and-adolescents-early-evidence-in-india/

Banerjee, A. (2021). Good science also needs a thriving democracy. *National Herald India.* http://epaper.nationalheraldindia.com//imageview_2498_181263_4_71_10-10-2021_i_1_sf.html

Bhopal, R. S. (2020). COVID-19 zugzwang: Potential public health moves towards population (herd) immunity. *Public Health in Practice, 1,* 100031. https://pubmed.ncbi.nlm.nih.gov/34173570

BMC. (2022). STOP CORONAVIRUS in Mumbai. https://stopcoronavirus.mcgm.gov.in/

Bureau. (2021). PM Modi announces Covid-19 vaccination for children aged 15-18 from Jan 3. *Hindu Business Online.* https://www.thehindubusinessline.com/news/pm-modi-announces-covid-19-vaccination-for-children-aged-15-18-from-jan-3/article38038722.ece

Carlson, J. (2020). *Covid-19 in schoolchildren; A comparison between Finland and Sweden.* Public Health Agency of Sweden. https://www.folkhalsomyndigheten.se/contentassets/c1b78bffbfde4a7899eb0d8ffdb57b09/covid-19-school-aged-children.pdf

Chalmers, V. (2020). Children under 10 are 20 TIMES more likely to die in an accident than of Covid-19 - and even flu is twice as deadly to them, study reveals. *Daily Mail.* https://www.dailymail.co.uk/news/article-8685159/amp/Children-10-20-times-likely-die-injury-Covid-19.html

Chandna, H. (2021). *No need to vaccinate kids against Covid right now, centre informed about decision: NTAGI member.* News18. https://www.news18.com/news/india/no-need-to-vaccinate-children-against-covid right-now-centre-informed-about-decision-ntagi-member-4577267.html

Donnelly, L. (2021). Number of children taking antidepressants hits all-time peak during pandemic. *The Telegraph.* https://www.telegraph.co.uk/news/2021/06/23/number-children-taking-antidepressants-hits-all-time-peak-pandemic/

Dutt, A. (2021). Kids, adults have similar antibodies: AIIMS Sero Survey. https://www.hindustantimes.com/india-news/kids-adults-have-similar-antibodies-sero-survey-101623953000262.html

Education Emergency. (2021). *Education Emergency: A silent and invisible emergency in education*. https://educationemergency.net/

EuroMoMo. (2022). EuroMoMo: Graphs and maps. https://www.euromomo.eu/graphs-and-maps

Express. (2022). Report: Pandemic forced students to drop out of school, turn to child labour. *The Indian Express*. https://indianexpress.com/article/cities/bangalore/report-pandemic-forced-students-to-drop-out-of-school-turn-to-child-labour-7880744/

Express. (2021). 'Situation alarming': SC stays Kerala plan to conduct offline exams for Class 11. *The Indian Express*. https://indianexpress.com/article/india/kerala/sc-stays-kerala-govt-decision-to-hold-offline-class-11-exams-covid-alarming-7487380/

Fensterwald, J. (2022). Student math scores touch off 'five-alarm fire' in California. *EdSource*. https://edsource.org/2022/student-math-scores-a-five-alarm-fire-in-california/669797

Finlay, I. (2006, May). 'First do no harm'--a clear line in law and medical ethics. *Journal of the Royal Society of Medicine, 99*(5), 214-215. https://doi.org/10.1258/jrsm.99.5.214

Fore, H., & Azoulay, A. (2021). *Reopening schools cannot wait*. Unicef. https://www.unicef.org/press-releases/statement-reopening-schools-cannot-wait

Fox, J. (2021). *How Covid's toll compares with other things that kill us*. Bloomberg. https://www.bloomberg.com/opinion/articles/2021-03-01/covid-19-s-death-toll-compared-to-other-things-that-kill-us

Gilliam, W. S., Malik, A. A., Shafiq, M., Klotz, M., Reyes, C., Humphries, J. E., Murrar, T., Elharke, J. A., Wilkinson, D., & Omer, S. (2021). COVID-19 Transmission in US Child Care Programs. *Pediatrics, 147*(1). https://doi.org/10.1542/peds.2020-031971

Grant, A. (2021). Rising numbers of children attending hospital for self-harm in Scotland. *The Herald*. https://www.heraldscotland.com/politics/19510415.rising-numbers-children-attending-hospital-self-harm-scotland/

Høeg, T. (2021). Putting kids first: Addressing COVID-19's impacts on children. https://docs.house.gov/meetings/IF/IF02/20210922/114054/HHRG-117-IF02-Wstate-BethHegT-20210922.pdf

Iyer, K. (2021). *As extreme poverty returns, India sees surge in child slavery.* Aljazeera. https://www.aljazeera.com/amp/news/2021/9/2/as-extreme-poverty-returns-india-sees-surge-in-child-slavery

Jenson, H. B. (2020). How did "flatten the curve" become "flatten the economy?" A perspective from the United States of America. *Asian Journal of Psychiatry, 51.* https://doi.org/10.1016/j.ajp.2020.102165

John, J., & Seshadri, M. (2021). Why we need to vaccinate our kids against Covid. https://www.newindianexpress.com/opinions/columns/2021/oct/23/why-we-need-to-vaccinate-our-kids-against-covid-2374571.html

Katikireddi, S. V., Cerqueira-Silva, T., Vasileiou, E., Robertson, C., Amele, S., Pan, J., Taylor, B., Boaventura, V., Werneck, G. L., Flores-Ortiz, R., Agrawal, U., Docherty, A. B., McCowan, C., McMenamin, J., Moore, E., Ritchie, L. D., Rudan, I., Shah, S. A., Shi, T.,… Sheikh, A. (2022). Two-dose ChAdOx1 nCoV-19 vaccine protection against COVID-19 hospital admissions and deaths over time: A retrospective, population-based cohort study in Scotland and Brazil. *The Lancet, 399*(10319), 25-35. https://doi.org/10.1016/S0140-6736(21)02754-9

Khera, R. (2021). *Locked out: Emergency report on school education.* Road Scholarz. https://roadscholarz.net/locked-out-emergency-report-on-school-education/

Kulldorff, M., Gupta, S., & Bhattacharya, J. (2020, 10). Great Barrington Declaration. https://gbdeclaration.org/270 Ethical questions in pandemic response

Lam-Hine, T., McCurdy, S., Santora, L., Duncan, L., Corbett-Detig, R., Kapusinszky, B., & Willis, M. (2021). Outbreak associated with SARS-CoV-2 B.1.617.2 (Delta) variant in an elementary school — Marin County, California, May–June 2021. *Morbidity and Mortality Weekly Report, 70*(35), 1214-1219. http://dx.doi.org/10.15585/mmwr.mm7035e2

Lee, B., & Raszka Jr, W. (2020, 8). COVID-19 transmission and children: The child is not to blame. *Pediatrics, 146*(2). https://doi.org/10.1542/peds.2020-004879

Leidman, E., Duca, L., Omura, J., Proia, K., Stephens, J., & Sauber-Schatz, E. (2021). COVID-19 Trends Among Persons Aged 0–24 Years — United States, March 1–December 12, 2020. *Morbidity and Mortality Weekly Report, 70*(3), 88-94. http://dx.doi.org/10.15585/mmwr.mm7003e1

Levine-Tiefenbrun, M., Yelin, I., Alapi, H., Herzel, E., Kuint, J., Chodick, G., Gazit, S., Patalon, T., & Kishony, R. (2022). Waning of SARS-CoV-2 booster viral-load

reduction effectiveness. Nature Communications, 13(1237). https://doi.org/
10.1038/s41467-022-28936-y

Lin, R.-G., & Money, L. (2021). Children apologize to their dying elders for
spreading COVID-19 as L.A. County reels. Los Angeles Times.
https://www.latimes.com/california/story/2021-01-12/children-apologizing-to-
parents-grandparents-spreading-coronavirus-into-families- as-l-a-county-reels

Ludvigsson, J., Engerström, L., Nordenhäll, C., & Larsson, E. (2021). Open schools,
Covid-19, and child and teacher morbidity in Sweden. New England Journal of
Medicine, 384(7), 669-671. https://doi.org/10.1056/ NEJMc2026670

NDTV. (2021). "Third Covid Wave To Hit Children More": Dr Devi Shetty to NDTV.
https://www.ndtv.com/video/news/the-news/third-covid-wave-to-hit-
children-more-dr-devi-shetty-to-ndtv-586079

News18. (2021a). As schools reopen, states witness rise in Covid-19 infection among kids;
highest in Punjab. https://www.news18.com/news/education-career/as-schools-
reopen-states-witness-rise-in-covid-19-infection-among-kids-highest-in-
punjab-4152029.html

News18. (2021b). Unvaccinated teacher spreads Covid to 26 people in California, including
12 students. https://www.news18.com/news/world/pakistan-detects-2nd-polio-
case-in-a-week-triggers-concern-over-possible-spike-during-eid-holidays-
5084977.html

NYT. (2021). Surge of student suicides pushes Las Vegas Schools to reopen. The New
York Times. https://www.nytimes.com/2021/01/24/us/politics/student-suicides-
nevada-coronavirus.html

Outlook. (2021). Delhi schools to remain closed as Kejriwal says no plans to reopen.
Outlook India. https://www.outlookindia.com/website/story/india-news-delhi-
schools-to-remain-closed-as-kejriwal-says-no-plans-to-reopen/388309

Pandit, A. (2021). Covid-19: Data dispels myth of young people being more at risk
during 2nd wave. Times of India. https://timesofindia.indiatimes.com/india/
covid-19-data-dispels-myth-of-young-people-being-more-at-risk-during-2nd-
wave/articleshow/83558847.cms

Parth, M., & Pierson, D. (2021). A lost generation: India's COVID crisis reverses
decades of progress for children. Los Angeles Times. https://www.latimes.com/
world-nation/story/2021-09-14/india-covid-children-lost-generation

Engzell, P., Frey, A., & Verhagen, M. D. (2021). Learning loss due to school closures during the COVID-19 pandemic. *Proceedings of the National Academy of Sciences, 118*(17). https://doi.org/10.1073/pnas.2022376118

Rajpal, S., Joe, W., & Subramanian, S. (2020, 12). Living on the edge? Sensitivity of child undernutrition prevalence to bodyweight shocks in the context of the 2020 national lockdown strategy in India. *Journal of Global Health Science, 2*(2). https://doi.org/10.35500/jghs.2020.2.e19

Raman, B. (2021). Mumbai and USA: Age-wise risk of Covid-19. https://docs.google.com/presentation/d/1LfowuS-r7NuA6WIMqVP55dTDy YTdf3LHPNK0RDyy9rU/ edit#slide=id.gd889e83e74_0_0

Raman, B. (2021). Schools and Covid-19 questions and answers. https://tinyurl.com/ schoolsc19

Raman, B. (2022). Excess deaths in US: 15-19 years age group. https://docs.google.com/presentation/d/1KKpKcZCfJaYAtErcWX8EdCFEfURR jphfrLeXvQBXlkQ/edit?usp=sharing

Rose, C., & Goverde, R. (2021). INDIA: Girls in India facing greater online risk of child marriage and trafficking during pandemic. https://www.savethechildren.net/news/india-girls-india-facing-greater-online-risk-child-marriage-and-trafficking-during-pandemic

Schreiber, M. (2022). A fifth of all US child Covid deaths occurred during Omicron surge. *The Guardian.* https://www.theguardian.com/world/2022/mar/11/us-child-covid-deaths-omicron-surge

Shivaram, D. (2021). *Pediatricians say the mental health crisis among kids has become a national emergency.* NPR. https://www.npr.org/2021/10/20/1047624943/ pediatricians-call-mental-health-crisis-among-kids-a-national-emergency

Shukla, M. (2021). *Severely malnourished under-5 children consumed by hunger in the pandemic.* Gaon Connection. https://en.gaonconnection.com/malnutrition-uttar-pradesh-children-hunger-poverty-covid-second-wave-nutrition-icds-healthrural-india/

Sky News. (2021). *Police powers to be strengthened in NSW.* https://www.skynews.com.au/australia-news/crime/police-powers-to-be-strengthened-in-nsw/video/e95f77313894ee6e37278ec53bd61674

Smith-Schoenwalder, C. (2021). CDC director defends not recommending Coronavirus tests in updated isolation, quarantine guidance. *US News*. https://www.usnews.com/news/health-news/articles/2021-12-29/cdc-director-defends-not-recommending-coronavirus-tests-in-updated-isolation-quarantine-guidance

Sorg, A., Hufnagel, M., Doenhardt, M., Diffloth, N., Schroten, H., v. Kries, R., Berner, R., & Armann, J. (2021). Risk of Hospitalization, severe disease, and mortality due to COVID-19 and PIMS-TS in children with SARS-CoV-2 infection in Germany. *medRxiv*, doi: https://doi.org/10.1101/2021.11.30.21267048

Suraksha. P. (2021). Covid-19 lockdowns left kids with speech disorders. *Deccan Herald*. https://www.deccanherald.com/state/top-karnataka-stories/covid-19-lockdowns-left-kids-with-speech-disorders-1018766.html

Sutton, J., & Dominguez, C. (2022). *Judge finds no reason to charge Texas mother who allegedly put her son in the trunk to avoid Covid-19 exposure.* CNN. https://edition.cnn.com/2022/01/10/us/texas-mother-son-trunk-covid-19/index.html

Tareen, S. (2022). *Democrats balance keeping schools open against confronting teachers' unions.* PBS. https://www.pbs.org/newshour/nation/democrats-balance-keeping-schools-open-against-confronting-teachers-unions

The Times of India. (2021). Tamil Nadu: 117 school students test Covid positive since Sep 1. https://timesofindia.indiatimes.com/home/education/news/tamil-nadu-117-school-students-test-covid-positive-since-sep-1/articleshow/86255332.cms

The Daily. (2021). An interview with Dr. Anthony Fauci. *The New York Times*. https://www.nytimes.com/2021/11/12/podcasts/the-daily/anthony-fauci-vaccine-mandates-booster-shots.html

UNESCO. (2021). Total duration of school closures. Retrieved Apr 30, 2022, from https://en.unesco.org/covid19/educationresponse#durationschoolclosures

UNICEF. (2020). UNICEF Executive Director Henrietta Fore's remarks at a press conference on new updated guidance on school-related public health measures in the context of COVID-19. https://www.unicef.org/press-releases/unicef-executive-director-henrietta-fores-remarks-press-conference-new-updated

Viner, R., Russell, S., Saulle, R., Croker, H., Stansfield, C., Packer, J., Nicholls, D., Goddings, A., Bonell, C., Hudson, L., Hope, S., Ward, J., Schwalbe, N., Morgan,

A., & Minozzi, S. (2022, 4). School closures during social lockdown and mental health, health behaviors, and well-being among children and adolescents during the first COVID-19 wave: A systematic review. *JAMA Pediatrics, 176*(4), 400-409. https://doi.org/10.1001/

Vogel, G. (2021). *Critics slam letter in prestigious journal that downplayed COVID-19 risks to Swedish schoolchildren.* Science. https://www.science.org/content/article/critics-slam-letter-prestigious-journal-downplayed-covid-19-risks-swedish

Walderman, K. (2021). *Children's mental health: "The type of self-harm is the worst we have seen".* BBC. https://www.bbc.com/news/uk-england-merseyside-59576669

Ward, J. L., Harwood, R., Smith, C., Kenny, S., Clark, M., Davis, P. J., Draper, E. S., Hargreaves, D., Ladhani, S., Linney, M., Luyt, K., Turner, S., Whittaker, E., Fraser, L. K., & Viner, R. (2022). Risk factors for PICU admission and death among children and young people hospitalized with COVID-19 and PIMS-TS in England during the first pandemic year. *Nature Medicine, 28,* 193-200. https://doi.org/10.1038/s41591-021-01627-9

PART FOUR
Business and Economy

ACTS OF CONGRESS AND COVID-19: A LITERATURE REVIEW ON THE IMPACT OF INCREASED UNEMPLOYMENT INSURANCE BENEFITS AND STIMULUS CHECKS[1]

Elena Falcettoni[2] and Vegard M. Nygaard[3]

Abstract: This chapter provides an overview of economic studies analyzing the impact of the increase in unemployment insurance (UI) benefits and the distribution of stimulus checks prescribed by the CARES Act, which was the first U.S. governmental intervention seeking to provide economic relief from COVID-19 difficulties. A review of the literature shows that, taken together, the increased UI benefits and stimulus checks have been effective at providing stimulus and lowering poverty, which supports the concept of a benevolent government seeking policies that take care of its citizens, especially policies aimed at reducing the hardship of the most vulnerable citizens in the U.S., namely unemployed and low-income citizens. At the same time, we present these findings with an eye on the ethical challenges associated with the implementation of these policies: 1) The trade-off between an increased generosity in UI benefits and its impact on labor market participation, 2) The impact of choosing an equitable distribution of funds rather than pursuing a targeted distribution, and 3) The difficulties associated with reaching the most-marginalized communities in the United States.

Introduction

The sudden arrival of a long-lasting pandemic was a clear shock to any government, and, in particular, to the U.S. government in our example, who suddenly faced both an economic and a health crisis. Such a combined

---

[1] The views expressed in this Chapter are the views of the authors' only and do not represent the views of the colleagues at the Board of Governors or the views of the Federal Reserve System as a whole.
[2] Board of Governors of the Federal Reserve System and Heller-Hurwicz Economics Institute
[3] University of Houston, Department of Economics

crisis led to the Coronavirus Aid, Relief, and Economic Security (CARES) Act first and the following related government interventions, which struck a trade-off for the government between the ethical considerations of protecting its citizens from the pandemic and the economic and ethical consequences of the economic impact of the pandemic on both its citizens and its businesses. To protect its businesses and its economy, the U.S. government included both policies aimed at providing aid and relief for businesses and stimulus components in its policy interventions aimed at boosting consumer spending.

While striking such a trade-off, public health measures were also key components of any decisions. In particular, any local and national rules regarding lockdowns and mask or vaccination mandates were results of both economic and ethical decisions trying to balance economics with personal well-being. In particular, public health measures had direct economic consequences on the U.S. economy, similar to the effects seen in other countries. Pandemic restrictions limited people's movements and, consequently, spending, especially in sectors that benefit from circulation of individuals, such as travel-related businesses. The U.S. government's relief to businesses was a way to counteract the impact of such public health measures on the economy. Similarly, the provision of stimulus payments to individuals was a way to boost spending when spending was sharply decreasing due to the crisis (for example, restaurant spending was immediately affected by the pandemic since individuals were not willing to be in places where one would congregate without masks). While economists have also produced a large COVID-19 literature that discusses such interventions and their results, including papers on health impacts, distancing measures, epidemiological models, pandemic-induced mortality changes, or the impact of other policies, domestic or foreign, we will not focus on these issues. For a more general review of these other topics, please refer to Brodeur et al. (2021).

Instead, our goal for this chapter is to focus on what economists have found regarding the implications of two main components of the CARES Act that directly impacted individuals: the increased UI benefits and the stimulus checks. We present the findings from the literature on these two policies with an eye on the ethical challenges concerning their implementation, hoping to inform potential future governmental interventions. We extend the review in Falcettoni and Nygaard (2021a, 2021b) to this end.

There are three main ethical challenges that this literature review can inform on: First, any increase in unemployment benefit value and duration comes with a discussion on where an increase in generosity leads to individuals' delay in returning to work, which would imply that government funds distort incentives and are misallocated. A review of the literature shows that this increase in generosity did not lead to these perverse incentives but helped its most-vulnerable citizens, who tended to be lower-income and employed in industries that were particularly hit (such as tourism), withstand the crisis. Such a response implies that modeling an automatic increase in unemployment insurance benefits and duration during times of crisis and targeting individuals who are employed in sectors that are particularly affected could be very beneficial for individuals' well-being. Second, a clear ethical challenge lies in the choice on how to distribute funds to individuals and, in particular, whether to follow an equitable distribution (where everyone receives the same amount) or a targeted distribution (where specific groups of individuals receive more funds). The implemented policies imply that the United States followed an equitable distribution of funds, since the increase in generosity of unemployment benefits was independent of the pre-unemployment wage received and the amount of stimulus disbursed was the same for every individual below a given income threshold. A review of the literature highlights that a targeted approach disbursing more funds to the lower-income, the younger, and individuals with children would have been even more effective, as individuals at the very bottom of the low-income distribution were able to use these funds to repay debts and consume, whereas higher-income individuals saved a substantial share of the funds received. Third, funds were not uniformly received to more-marginalized communities. Individuals who were non-tax-return filers had to overcome many difficulties to receive their stimulus checks even if they qualified for them and many of them never received them. Because such individuals tend to be very low-income, the other literature findings imply that they would have benefited substantially from such stimulus and consumed the majority—if not the entirety—of the funds. The difficulties found in the literature imply that limiting these hurdles would make it easier for governments to limit the impact of crises for these marginalized communities as well.

Generally, taken together, the increased UI benefits and stimulus checks have been effective at providing stimulus and lowering poverty, which supports the concept of a benevolent government seeking policies that take care of its citizens, especially policies aimed at reducing the hardship of the most vulnerable citizens in the U.S., namely those that would become unemployed due to the pandemic and low-income citizens. Kaplan et al. (2020) find that the initial UI benefits and stimulus payments boosted aggregate consumption by two percentage points, while Bayer et al. (2020) show that the CARES transfers reduced the output loss due to the pandemic by up to 5 percentage points. By reporting the impact of these two provisions of the CARES Act as found in the literature, we hope to provide readers and practitioners with a summary of both the challenges and successes faced by governments when implementing similar stimulus bills in the future.

For each of the two parts considered, namely UI benefits and stimulus checks, we begin by describing the relevant provisions of the CARES Act before summarizing their impact on different aspects of the economy and citizens' well-being.

Unemployment Insurance Benefits

CARES Act provisions. The CARES Act provisions originally prescribed an additional 13 weeks of federally funded benefits under the Pandemic Emergency Unemployment Compensation (PEUC) program in addition to the standard state-administered UI programs for those currently receiving UI benefits and new applicants. These benefits were then extended for another 13 weeks (and potentially for another seven following those) through the Extended Benefits program. Normal benefits included an additional $600 per week for up to four months, which is a provision that expired on July 31st, 2020. On August 8th, a reduced weekly check of $300 was reinstated for an additional six weeks subject to state application. All states but South Dakota applied for it. Finally, the CARES Act also instituted a new program, the Pandemic Unemployment Assistance (PUA), for individuals who were self-employed, seeking part-time employment, or who otherwise would not qualify for regular UI benefits. The PUA program provided up to 39 weeks of benefit. Importantly, the CARES Act also required states to relax the criterion of actively searching for work to qualify for these benefits to account for illness, quarantine, and movement restrictions.

In normal times, unemployment benefits are always subject to requirements of being actively looking for work. Not unique to the United States, such restrictions are meant to prevent individuals from having an incentive to stay on unemployment without looking for a new job. Note that such conditions never apply to individuals who are unable to work for health reasons, who would instead fall under disability insurance to obtain governmental aid without looking-for-work restrictions. The move away from such restrictions for any type of unemployment, coupled with the increase in both the allowed duration of unemployment and the amount of benefits received, shows the government's interest in protecting its most vulnerable citizens by not only providing them with benefits but also by recognizing that the pandemic could lengthen their unemployment spell and make looking for work not only difficult but potentially dangerous because of the public health crisis.

Impact of COVID-19 on unemployment. The increase in generosity of both the duration and amount of UI benefits is exemplary of the importance of government intervention to protect its most vulnerable citizens. The COVID-19 pandemic impacted employment greatly, especially for lower-pay and nonessential occupations, as shown in Liu and Mai (2020). Over March and April 2020, job losses were larger for these occupations, especially for those with higher physical proximity or lower work-from-home feasibility. Between April and June 2020, the industries that were hit harder also recouped more jobs, but the recovery was far from full. Chetty et al. (2020) showed that high-wage workers experienced a recession that lasted only a few weeks, rarely lost jobs, and quickly faced an almost-back-to-normal market, whereas many low-wage workers lost their job because of the pandemic and experienced a recession that would last for several months. Forsythe et al. (2020a) showed that nearly all industries and occupations saw contraction in postings and spikes in UI claims, with essential jobs taking the smallest hit and leisure and hospitality services the biggest hit. The pandemic-induced increase in unemployment led to the largest rise in UI claims in U.S. history (see, among others, Cajner et al., 2020; Chetty et al., 2020; Goldsmith-Pinkham & Sojourner, 2020; and Kong & Prinz, 2020 for indicators of labor-market changes during this period).

These patterns in the data and in the literature suggest that increases in and extensions of UI benefits in times of crisis can be a key component to protect the most vulnerable individuals in the population. Consequently, ethical considerations regarding the protection of a government's citizens, such as a government's interest in limiting unemployment duration for both high- and low-wage workers and the importance of protecting citizens who work in sectors affected by industry-specific shocks, need to be included when analyzing how to modify such programs in times of crisis relative to the presence of restrictions usually aimed at protecting the government's finances and interests in limiting the duration of unemployment. The relatively fast return-to-normal of jobs that were not as strongly affected suggests that the increase in UI benefits did not lead to individuals remaining unemployed longer by choice, but they guaranteed the protection of the health and financial situation of workers in highly affected occupations. These data patterns suggest that building in adjustments for industry-specific shocks and for sector-specific unemployment duration could benefit a government by both limiting spending for individuals working in sectors that are not as strongly-affected and directing spending to those who might be unemployed for a longer period due to an industry-specific shock that makes it more difficult for them to become employed again in a fast manner.

Effectiveness of UI benefits and difficulty to reach the most marginalized. The effectiveness of the UI benefits has been well-documented. Faria-e-Castro (2021) found that UI benefits are successful at stimulating consumption, leading to an increase in GDP. Han et al. (2020) showed that UI benefits, their expansion, and the stimulus checks led to a decline in poverty during the pandemic, which would have risen in the absence of these programs. Cortes and Forsythe (2020) showed that 49 percent of the UI and CARES benefits went to workers who were in the bottom-third of the earnings distribution before the pandemic happened, which reversed the increase in labor earnings inequality that followed the beginning of the pandemic because of the concentration of job losses among low-paying jobs.

Montenovo et al. (2020) documented the disparities in job losses by occupation and related the pre-pandemic sorting by gender, race, and ethnicity into different occupations and industries to the gaps in unemployment across these categories. Bhutta et al. (2020) used detailed data from the Survey of Consumer Finances to estimate that an additional 38 percent of typical working families would be able to cover six months of expenses after an unexpected income disruption, such as a job loss, under the increased UI benefits implemented with the CARES Act compared to the standard UI benefits alone.

While the literature overwhelmingly found the immediate effectiveness of UI benefits to meet basic needs, analyses of the program also overwhelmingly discovered that reaching the poorest part of the population remained a challenge. For example, Karpman and Acs (2020) and Giannarelli et al. (2020) documented the effectiveness of the increased UI benefits, but also discussed the difficulty to reach the poorest part of the population. Delays in payment of UI benefits, also due to an overwhelmed system, were also documented in Bitler et al. (2020). Parolin et al. (2020) also provided evidence for the challenges involved with reaching the most-marginalized parts of the population and they argued for the need of an expansion of UI benefits to contain poverty. In particular, they showed that minorities were hit particularly hard by the pandemic and that the expiration of the CARES Act benefits led to an increase in poverty which was even higher than pre-pandemic levels. Bell et al. (2020) found that in California alone, communities of concentrated poverty and with a higher share of racial and/or ethnic minorities received UI benefits at such a lower rate than wealthier, Whiter communities that the number of regular UI beneficiaries would have been 23 percent higher if the rate of receipt of UI benefits across the two types of communities had been equalized.

Since it was particularly difficult to reach the individuals in the population who would benefit the most from these programs, this evidence is suggestive of a need for even-greater outreach from the government to the most-marginalized parts of the U.S. population. This fact is even more important in light of the ethical discussion around the ability of a government to use these programs with the goal of protecting its most-vulnerable citizens. Investing in ways to inform the most-marginalized citizens about existing programs and in making these programs as accessible as possible, for example by limiting any hurdles in the application process, could be very beneficial to include more marginalized communities.

Temporary vs. permanent layoffs. While UI benefits were generally effective, a separate strand of this literature analyzed the difference in impact between unemployment types: those who were on temporary layoffs and those who were permanent job losers. The individuals on temporary layoffs were those who were only unemployed on a temporary basis because they had lost their job because of the lockdown but they could expect their unemployment to end as soon as the lockdown ended. The individuals who were permanent job losers were those who had lost their job but who did not expect to resume their job as soon as the lockdown was over.

Barrero et al. (2020) estimated that 42 percent of pandemic-induced layoffs would result in permanent job loss. Carroll et al. (2021) used a consumer model in which individuals are part of three possible employment categories (employment, temporary layoff, permanent job loss) and then estimated the impact of the increased unemployment insurance benefits (as well as the stimulus checks) on consumer spending for consumers of each of these categories. They noted that spending would be lower even without unemployment shocks because restrictive measures to contain the pandemic, such as lockdowns, led to the limited access of goods and services, therefore limiting spending opportunities. The employed, by definition, did not receive any UI benefits. Those individuals who were on temporary layoffs particularly benefited from the CARES Act provisions, which provided them with the means to smooth their consumption throughout their transitory shocks. Their spending recovered fully within a year. For those individuals who were permanent job losers, the authors estimated that regular consumption spending would take three years to recover on average. The impact of UI benefits was high, but the permanent job losers would particularly benefit from an expansion of UI benefits if the lockdown was extended, as their unemployment shock would always be longer than the length of the lockdown itself. We can interpret these results to mean that the permanent job losers would benefit from an extension of the UI benefits as long as any restrictions are in place because their unemployment will be long-lasting even following the end of pandemic-induced restrictions. Gregory et al. (2020) also differentiated between those on temporary layoffs and those who were permanent job losers and found that the lockdown disproportionately disrupted the latter group, because it would take a much-longer period of time for them to find a new job.

Taken together, the difference between a temporary pandemic-induced unemployment and a more permanent job loss is important to inform policy, as discussed in Gallant et al. (2020) and in Forsythe et al. (2020b), who suggested that policies designed to prop up labor demand would be successful. Treating all unemployment losses as equal across any crises could miss out on these important differences and could prevent governmental funds from being optimally allocated.

Generosity of UI benefits and return-to-work decisions. As discussed, the effectiveness of the UI benefits was also due to their generosity: as reported by Ganong et al. (2020), this led to a median replacement rate (the level of total UI benefits divided by the pre-unemployment wage) of 134 percent. They found that around two-thirds of workers had a replacement rate greater than 100 percent (as in, they received higher benefits than the wage they used to receive). This generosity spurred a lot of discussion on whether such high benefits would reduce workers' willingness to go back to work because they suddenly made more than their previous wage (see Barrero et al., 2020).

Both Petrosky-Nadeau (2020) and Boar and Mongey (2020) show that this was not the case because the UI benefits were too small and too short-lived to make it worth it for individuals to give up a return-to-work offer. Their findings were confirmed by data evidence showing that return-to-work and employment rates were not lower in states where the UI benefit expansion was larger (see Altonji et al., 2020; Bartik et al., 2020; Dube, 2021; Marinescu et al., 2020). In the very short term, Fang et al. (2020) found that expanded UI benefits would lead to higher unemployment in the second half of 2020, with larger effects with higher benefits, but that the policy would still enhance well-being for the population as a whole.

All of these findings further support the use of increased UI benefits with fewer restrictions at a time of crisis as a way for the government to fulfill its ethical responsibilities toward its most-vulnerable citizens. In particular, since low-income citizens are more likely to be unemployed and to have fewer savings available to weather a crisis, increased UI benefits are particularly effective at ensuring that low-income individuals are also able to maintain a relatively good level of financial health during times of crisis. The usual counterargument to this enhanced protection is that increased UI benefits make a return-to-work decision less appealing and therefore lead to longer periods of unemployment, which would be detrimental to a government's economy. The observation that individuals did not change their choice to return to work because of the increased benefits suggests that these policies can instead be a key tool for a government to intervene to protect its citizens without fearing long-term repercussions on the labor market.

Optimality of UI benefits. The studies discussed so far analyzed the effectiveness of UI benefits and their impact on return-to-work offers, but they did not focus on whether the policy intervention was optimal. Theoretically, Guerrieri et al. (2020) showed that abundant social insurance is a key ingredient of an optimal policy response in a pandemic (together with a loosening of monetary policy), where such a policy would reallocate income away from workers in sectors not particularly affected to workers in sectors particularly hit by the pandemic. Bredemeier et al. (2020) provided evidence for this result quantitatively. Mitman and Rabinovich (2020) found that the $600/week-policy was close to optimal and that UI benefits should be optimally increased at the start of a crisis but then lowered as the economy reopens to align incentives to return to work. Nevertheless, coupling extended UI benefits with a re-employment bonus would be an even-better option as individuals would receive much-needed help while maintaining all incentives to search for a job. It is worth noting that the previously discussed studies both empirically and quantitatively confirm the finding that return-to-work rates were not significantly affected by increased UI benefits, therefore indicating that this disruption was likely minimal. Birinci et al. (2021) found that the optimal policy would bundle UI benefits with payroll subsidies. Kapička and Rubert (2020) analyzed the optimal policy by including virus transmission and by examining what the optimal labor-market policy would be to save lives and found that it would have been optimal to shut down businesses, impose a quarantine several weeks before the pandemic peak, and move a quarter of workers out of employment to limit transmission. All in all, the studies analyzed found that the policy on UI benefits followed by the U.S. government was close to optimal.

Stimulus Checks

CARES Act provisions. The CARES Act provision prescribed a direct cash payment of $1,200 for each adult with an annual income of $75,000 or less plus $500 for each child. For incomes higher than $75,000, the benefit began to phase out and was nil for any income at or above $99,000. An additional $600 per qualifying adult and dependent was distributed in December 2020. The American Rescue Plan Act prescribed a final round of stimulus checks. Under the American Rescue Plan Act, a direct cash payment of $1,400 was distributed to each adult (and dependent) with an annual income of $75,000 or less. For incomes higher than $75,000, the benefit began to phase out and was nil for any income at or above $80,000. Once again, the provisions focused on providing support to individuals in the lower end of the income distribution, who were hit the hardest by the pandemic and would be more in need of governmental aid to support their consumption.

Impact of stimulus checks on spending. Carroll et al. (2021) used their model to also estimate the impact of the stimulus checks on consumer spending for consumers in each of the three employment categories: those who remained employed, those who were on temporary layoffs, and those who were permanent job losers. The employed were the ones that suffered the least, saved a large share of the stimulus check upon receipt, but increased their spending again immediately as soon as the lockdown ended. The lack of spending choices available during the lockdown induced their higher rate of saving, while spending rebounded once those choices became available again due to those individuals' healthy finances.

For the other two groups, i.e., both for the individuals on temporary layoffs who expected to resume their job once the lockdown ended and for the individuals who were permanent job losers who would not expect to resume their job, the unemployment insurance benefits led to a much bigger impact on their spending because of the larger per-individual amount. For the permanent job losers, the impact of the checks on immediate consumption was particularly small because they knew that they would need to smooth that check over a longer period of time. For the employed, whose spending was only impacted by the stimulus checks (since they did not qualify for any unemployment benefits because they remained employed throughout the period), the authors found that, even without a lockdown, only about 20 percent of the stimulus amount would have been spent immediately. The observation that only 20 percent of the checks would be spent even in the absence of any restrictive measures is indicative of the impact that the pandemic directly had on spending. The pandemic's impact on spending was also evident in household-level bank-account data, as in Bachas et al. (2020) and in weekly state-level data, as in Kobayashi et al. (2020). In aggregate U.S. data, the lower spending due to the pandemic was also verified by the Bureau of Labor Statistics (2020) analysis in April 2020, which showed that aggregate income rose because of the policy interventions despite the output and consumption decline caused by the restriction measures.

Optimality of stimulus checks. The previously discussed papers took government interventions as given. The optimality of these interventions, however, was not examined in those studies. By contrast, Nygaard et al. (2020) analyzed what would be the (constrained-)optimal allocation of the stimulus checks under information that can be observed by the government through the individuals' tax returns, such as the individuals' marital status, age, income, or number of children. To derive the optimal allocation of stimulus checks, they first used a life-cycle consumption-savings model with heterogeneous consumers to predict the consumption responses to $100 increments of cash transfers by age, income, marital status, and number of children. They then compared all feasible allocations of the stimulus checks across households to examine whether the government could have both spent less and achieved more stimulus than what was accomplished under the CARES Act, and derived the allocation that would have led to the highest stimulus effect. They found that the poor and the young, especially those with children, should have received a larger check, which is an allocation that would have allowed for the same stimulus effect at half the cost of the actual allocation. Nygaard et al. (2022) further studied the optimal allocation of the stimulus checks distributed under the American Rescue Plan Act, which distributed an additional $1,400 per qualifying adult (where the income threshold to qualify for such a check was reduced by $10,000).

Taken together, these analyses suggest that directing funds to help individuals at the very bottom of the income distribution would have had the largest impact per dollar spent, but that the government was instead interested in a more-equitable distribution of the funds. In fact, data from the Census surveys estimate that roughly 85 percent of households received at least one stimulus check. The CARES Act stimulus checks, for which more adults were eligible due to the higher income ceiling, was the most equitably spread across families. Such policies, which, at every round, promoted more-equal transfers over targeted distributions, are a signal of the ethical considerations taken into account by the government in the decision-making process: taking care of all its citizens fared above the pursuit of the highest economic impact per dollar spent.

Empirical analysis of spending patterns following stimulus. A separate strand of this large literature used large administrative datasets, such as transaction records, or large-scale surveys (such as Wozniak et al., 2020, among others), to measure how consumption changed following the pandemic. Bhutta et al. (2020) estimated that an additional two percent of typical working families would have been able to cover six months of expenses after an unexpected income disruption, such as a job loss, thanks to the receipt of the stimulus check.

Baker et al. (2020) found that recipients on average spent about a third of the stimulus checks within a few weeks with larger effects for poorer consumers. Coibion et al. (2020) found that individuals reported having spent or planned to spend around 40 percent of the total transfer on average, where the amount was higher for the unemployed, the more financially constrained, those in larger households, the less educated, and those who qualified for smaller transfers. Armantier et al. (2020) found that 29 percent of all stimulus payments was used for consumption, with another 35 percent used to pay down debt and the rest saved. Chetty et al. (2020) found that stimulus payments to low-income households had large effects on their consumption. Karger and Rajan (2020) used transaction-level data during the two weeks before and after the CARES Act stimulus check to analyze the change in credit- and debit-card spending immediately following the stimulus receipt. They found that the poor spent most of their check, while those in better financial health spent 23 percent of their transfer. Sahm et al. (2020) found that poorer individuals spent most of their checks to repay debt and that the richest individuals saved the largest share of the amount received. These data patterns confirm the findings from the optimality literature discussed above, which found that more-targeted distribution toward the poor, the young, and those with children would have led to a higher economic impact per dollar spent. Since the U.S. government chose to maintain an equitable distribution over a targeted one also in the stimulus check distributions following the CARES Act, this choice suggests that the government preferred to pursue policies that did not appear to give a higher weight to a particular group of citizens. However, concentrating more funds at a bottom end of the income distribution and potentially starting the decline in the amount received at a lower income level (effectively, giving less to richer individuals) would have been more effective at stimulating spending for the same total amount.

Misra et al. (2020) used transaction-level data from debit cards and found that about 40 percent of every dollar in stimulus was spent within the first four days from receipt and documented geographical differences in spending. Li et al. (2021) also documented geographical differences by using transaction-level data from debit cards owned by low-income households, but also found that the stimulus payments had a positive and sizable effect on spending for low-income households. They estimated that the positive effect from the stimulus payment was four times as high in absolute value as the negative effect that the lockdown had on spending for the same group. Positive effects on the poverty level were also found by Han et al. (2020). All of these data findings are consistent with the models discussed above: the poor, the young, and those with children were likely to benefit from higher amounts of stimulus as they were (and are) more financially constrained and would have spent a higher amount of the transfer received for any check amount.

All in all, these empirical studies agree that the stimulus checks led to higher spending across all recipients, with the poor, the young, and those with children being the individuals that spent the largest share of the check upon receipt, most likely because they were financially constrained and needed aid the most.

Difficulty to reach the most marginalized. Finally, while the most disadvantaged would have benefitted the most from these stimulus payments, Bitler et al. (2020) discussed how many individuals remained in distress despite the unprecedented policy response due to delays in implementation, the modest payments outside of UI benefits, and statutory requirements that excluded individuals that would have benefitted the most from the payments themselves. In particular, Marr et al. (2020) estimated that 12 million non-tax-return filers who were eligible for the stimulus check did not automatically receive it and had to request it. Because of this extra hurdle, there was a nearly-20-percentage-point difference in the receipt rate of stimulus checks between those eligible individuals below and above the poverty rate, at the expense of the poorer individuals.

Therefore, the papers discussed suggest that while the government sought a very equitable distribution of stimulus checks, difficulties related to the implementation of this policy led to payments not being always disbursed to those who needed them the most. Such an implementation hurt the optimality of the policy as well since payments were made more consistently to those who would spend less of the overall stimulus check amount due to their better financial health. Unlike the policy distributing the 2008 Great Recession stimulus checks, the CARES Act did not require stimulus check recipients to be tax filers. Such policy change was a response to the fact that more-marginalized individuals, who are more likely to be non-tax-return filers and lower-income and yet more in need of stimulus help, were ineligible for stimulus checks in the 2008 crisis. As the literature showed, the very poor were also the individuals who were more likely to use almost the entirety of the stimulus checks for both consumption and debt repayment. In this chapter, we also reviewed that a targeted approach where more funds are allocated to poorer individuals and less to richer individuals would lead to higher economic impact per dollar spent by the government. The delay and often the inability to reach the most-marginalized individuals in the United States is, however, proof that progress is still needed to reduce hurdles associated with the delivery of funds to these communities. Educational resources and research into more-effective ways to disburse funds to individuals who are often unbanked and non-tax-return filers are needed to limit these delays in relief distribution in future crises.

Conclusion

We presented a review of the economics literature analyzing two main components of the CARES Act that directly impacted individuals: the increased UI benefits and the stimulus checks. We presented the findings from the literature on these two policies with an eye on the ethical challenges concerning their implementation. The design of these policies suggest that the U.S. government sought to provide relief to those who needed it the most, in particular the unemployed and the poor. At the same, the large share of households that received at least one stimulus check signals that the U.S. opted for an equitable transfer rather than a targeted one, which is indicative of the government's willingness to protect as many of its citizens as possible instead of pursuing the highest economic impact per dollar spent.

The studies analyzed overwhelmingly found strong positive effects from these government interventions. However, both the papers looking at UI benefits and stimulus checks found that the U.S. government had difficulties distributing these payments to the most-marginalized parts of the U.S. population, i.e., very-low-income individuals and minorities. Because these individuals were the ones that would have benefitted the most from these policies and that needed them the most, delays in payments or the inability to make them altogether suggests that there is room for improvement in the implementation of these policies.

Since low-income individuals also consistently spent a higher share of the payments received than their richer counterparts, the hurdles associated with the receipt of these payments also led to lower economic stimulus altogether, which hurts the optimality of the policy as well. In short, the literature highlights that improvements in the implementation of any future stimulus policies, namely greater outreach and reduction in administrative hurdles, could have strong positive effects for the well-being of both individuals and the economy as a whole.

References

Altonji, J., Contractor, Z., Finamor, L., Haygood, R., Lindenlaub, I., Meghir, C., O'Dea, C., Scott, D., Wang, L. & Washington, E. (2020, July). *Employment effects of unemployment insurance generosity during the pandemic.* https://tobin.yale.edu/sites/default/files/covid-19%20response/CARES-UI_identification_vF(1).pdf

Armantier, O., Goldman, L., Koşar, G., Lu, J., Pomerantz, R., & Van der Klaauw, W. (2020). *How have households used their stimulus payments and how would they spend the next?* (No. 20201013b). Federal Reserve Bank of New York. https://libertystreeteconomics.newyorkfed.org/2020/10/how-have-households-used-their-stimulus-payments-and-how-would-they-spend-the-next/

Baker, S. R., Farrokhnia, R. A., Meyer, S., Pagel, M., & Yannelis, C. (2020). *Income, liquidity, and the consumption response to the 2020 economic stimulus payments* (No. w27097). National Bureau of Economic Research. https://doi.org/10.3386/w27097

Barrero, J. M., Bloom, N. & Davis, S. J. (2020). COVID-19 is also a reallocation shock." *Brookings Papers on Economic Activity,* Summer, 329-371. https://www.brookings.edu/wp-content/uploads/2020/06/SU20_S5_1_Barrero-et-al_-final-paper.pdf

Bartik, A. W., Bertrand, M., Lin, F., Rothstein, J., & Unrath, M. (2020). *Measuring the labor market at the onset of the COVID-19 crisis* (No. w27613). National Bureau of Economic Research. https://doi.org/10.3386/w27613

Bayer, C., Born, B., Luetticke, R., & Müller, G. J. (2020, April). *The coronavirus stimulus package: How large is the transfer multiplier?* (CEPR Discussion Paper No. DP14600). https://ssrn.com/abstract=3594222

Bell, A., Hedin, T. J., Schnorr, G., & Von Wachter, T. (2020). *An analysis of unemployment insurance claims in California during the COVID-19 pandemic.*

California Policy Lab, https://www.capolicylab.org/california-unemployment-insurance-claims-during-the-covid-19-pandemic

Bhutta, N., Blair, J., Dettling, L., & Moore, K. (2020). COVID-19, the CARES Act, and families' financial security. *National Tax Journal, 73*(3), 645-672. https://www.journals.uchicago.edu/doi/abs/10.17310/ntj.2020.3.02

Birinci, S., Karahan, F., Mercan, Y., & See, K. (2021). Labor market policies during an epidemic. *Journal of Public Economics, 194*, 104348. https://doi.org/10.1016/j.jpubeco.2020.104348

Bitler, M., Hoynes, H. W., & Schanzenbach, D. W. (2020). *The social safety net in the wake of COVID-19* (No. w27796). National Bureau of Economic Research. https://doi.org/10.3386/w27796

Boar, C., & Mongey, S. (2020). *Dynamic trade-offs and labor supply under the CARES Act* (No. w27727). National Bureau of Economic Research. https://doi.org/10.3386/w27727

Bredemeier, C., Juessen, F., & Winkler, R. (2020, June). Bringing back the jobs lost to Covid-19: The role of fiscal policy. *Covid Economics Vetted Real Time Papers, 29*, 99-140. https://cepr.org/file/9156/download?token=Uh_6nkID

Brodeur, A., Gray, D., Islam, A., & Bhuiyan, S. (2021). A literature review of the economics of COVID-19. *Journal of Economic Surveys, 35*(4), 1007-1044. https://doi.org/10.1111/joes.12423

Bureau of Economic Analysis (2020). *Personal income and outlays: April 2020*. BEA 20−24. Bureau of Economic Analysis, Washington, DC.

Cajner, T., Figura, A., Price, B. M., Ratner, D., & Weingarden, A. (2020). Reconciling unemployment claims with job losses in the first months of the COVID-19 crisis. (No. 2020-55). FEDS Working Paper. https://dx.doi.org/10.17016/FEDS.2020.055

Carroll, C. D., Crawley, E., Slacalek, J., & White, M. N. (2021). Modeling the consumption response to the CARES Act. *International Journal of Central Banking, 17*(1), 107-141.

Chetty, R., Friedman, J. N., Hendren, N., & Stepner, M. (2020). *The economic impacts of COVID-19: Evidence from a new public database built using private sector data* (No. w27431). National Bureau of Economic Research. https://doi.org/10.3386/w27431

Coibion, O., Gorodnichenko, Y., & Weber, M. (2020). *How did US consumers use their stimulus payments?* (No. w27693). National Bureau of Economic Research. https://doi.org/10.3386/w27693

Cortes, G. M. & Forsythe, E. (2020). *Impacts of the COVID-19 pandemic and the CARES Act on earnings and inequality.* (No. 20-332). Upjohn Institute Working Paper. http://dx.doi.org/10.2139/ssrn.3689187

Cox, N., Ganong, P., Noel, P., Vavra, J., Wong, A., Farrell, D., Greig, F., & Deadman, E. (2020). Initial impacts of the pandemic on consumer behavior: Evidence from linked income, spending, and savings data. *Brookings Papers on Economic Activity, 2020*(2), 35-82. https://doi.org/10.1353/eca.2020.0006

Dube, A. (2021). *Aggregate employment effects of unemployment benefits during deep downturns: Evidence from the expiration of the Federal Pandemic Unemployment Compensation* (No. w28470). National Bureau of Economic Research. https://doi.org/10.3386/w28470

Falcettoni, E., & Nygaard, V. M. (2021a). A literature review on the impact of increased unemployment insurance benefits and stimulus checks in the United States. *Covid Economics, 64,* 186-201. https://cepr.org/file/10211/download?token=ZZzuKAeJ

Falcettoni, E., & Nygaard, V. M. (2021b). Acts of Congress and COVID-19: A literature review on the impact of increased unemployment insurance benefits and stimulus checks. *FEDS Notes.* Washington: Board of Governors of the Federal Reserve System. https://doi.org/10.17016/2380-7172.2848.

Fang, L., Nie, J., & Xie, Z. (2020). *Unemployment insurance during a pandemic.* (No. 20-07). Federal Reserve Bank of Kansas City Working Paper. https://dx.doi.org/10.2139/ssrn.3673321

Faria-e-Castro, M. (2021). Fiscal policy during a pandemic. *Journal of Economic Dynamics and Control, 125,* 104088. https://doi.org/10.1016/j.jedc.2021.104088

Forsythe, E., Kahn, L. B., Lange, F., & Wiczer, D. (2020a). Labor demand in the time of COVID-19: Evidence from vacancy postings and UI claims. *Journal of Public Economics, 189,* 104238. https://doi.org/10.1016/j.jpubeco.2020.104238

Forsythe, E., Kahn, L. B., Lange, F., & Wiczer, D. G. (2020b). *Searching, recalls, and tightness: An interim report on the covid labor market* (No. w28083). National Bureau of Economic Research. https://doi.org/10.3386/w28083

Gallant, J., Kroft, K., Lange, F., & Notowidigdo, M. J. (2020). *Temporary unemployment and labor market dynamics during the COVID-19 recession* (No. w27924). National Bureau of Economic Research. https://doi.org/10.3386/w27924

Ganong, P., Noel, P., & Vavra, J. (2020). US unemployment insurance replacement rates during the pandemic. *Journal of Public Economics, 191,* 104273. https://doi.org/10.1016/j.jpubeco.2020.104273

Giannarelli, L., Wheaton, L., & Acs, G. (2020). *2020 Poverty Projections.* Washington, DC: Urban Institute. https://www.urban.org/sites/default/files/publication/102521/2020-poverty-projections.pdf

Goldsmith-Pinkham, P., & Sojourner, A. (2020). Predicting initial unemployment insurance claims using Google Trends. In *Technical Report.* Yale School of Management. https://paulgp.github.io/GoogleTrendsUINowcast/google_trends_UI.html

Gregory, V., Menzio, G., & Wiczer, D. G. (2020). *Pandemic recession: L or V-shaped?* (No. w27105). National Bureau of Economic Research. https://doi.org/10.3386/w27105

Guerrieri, V., Lorenzoni, G., Straub, L., & Werning, I. (2020). *Macroeconomic implications of COVID-19: Can negative supply shocks cause demand shortages?* (No. w26918). National Bureau of Economic Research. https://doi.org/10.3386/w26918

Han, J., Meyer, B. D., & Sullivan, J. X. (2020). *Income and poverty in the COVID-19 pandemic* (No. w27729). National Bureau of Economic Research. https://doi.org/10.3386/w27729

Kapicka, M., & Rupert, P. (2020). Labor markets during pandemics. *Manuscript, UC Santa Barbara.* http://www.covid-19-research-conduit.org/wp-content/uploads/2020/04/Kapi%C4%8Dka_Rupert_Epidemics_latest.pdf

Kaplan, G., Moll, B., & Violante, G. L. (2020). *The great lockdown and the big stimulus: Tracing the pandemic possibility frontier for the US* (No. w27794). National Bureau of Economic Research. https://doi.org/10.3386/w27794

Karger, E., & Rajan, A. (2020). Heterogeneity in the marginal propensity to consume: Evidence from Covid-19 stimulus payments. (No. 2020-15). Federal

Reserve Bank of Chicago Working Paper. https://dx.doi.org/10.2139/ssrn.3612828

Karpman, M., & Acs, G. (2020). *Unemployment insurance and economic impact payments associated with reduced hardship following CARES Act.* Washington, DC: Urban Institute. https://www.urban.org/sites/default/files/publication/102486/unemployment-insurance-and-economic-impact-payments-associated-with-reduced-hardship-following-cares-act.pdf

Kong, E., & Prinz, D. (2020). The impact of shutdown policies on unemployment during a pandemic. *Covid Economics, 17*(13), 24-72. https://iris.unitn.it/retrieve/handle/11572/284873/395182/CovidEconomics17.pdf#page=33

Li K., Foutz N. Z., Cai Y., Liang Y, Gao S. (2021). Impacts of COVID-19 lockdowns and stimulus payments on low-income population's spending in the United States. *PLoS ONE 16*(9): e0256407. https://doi.org/10.1371/journal.pone.0256407

Liu, O., & Mai, T. (2020). *Employment during the COVID-19 pandemic: Collapse and early recovery.* (No. 3682369). SSRN. https://dx.doi.org/10.2139/ssrn.3682369

Marinescu, I. E., Skandalis, D., & Zhao, D. (2020). Job search, job posting and unemployment insurance during the COVID-19 crisis. *Job posting and unemployment insurance during the COVID-19 crisis.* https://dx.doi.org/10.2139/ssrn.3664265

Marr, C., Cox, K., Bryant, K., Dean, S., Caines, R., & Sherman, A. (2020). *Aggressive state outreach can help reach the 12 million non-filers eligible for stimulus payments.* Center on Budget and Policy Priorities. https://www.cbpp.org/sites/default/files/atoms/files/6-11-20tax.pdf

Misra, K., Singh, V., & Zhang, Q. (2020). *Impact of the CARES Act stimulus payments on consumption.* UC San Diego.

Mitman, K., & Rabinovich, S. (2020). *Optimal unemployment benefits in the pandemic.* (No. 3638019). SSRN. https://ssrn.com/abstract=3638019

Montenovo, L., Jiang, X., Rojas, F. L., Schmutte, I. M., Simon, K. I., Weinberg, B. A., & Wing, C. (2020). *Determinants of disparities in COVID-19 job losses* (No. w27132). National Bureau of Economic Research. https://doi.org/10.3386/w27132

Nygaard, V. M., Sørensen, B. E., & Wang, F. (2020). *Optimal allocation of the COVID-19 stimulus checks.* (No. 3691091). SSRN. http://dx.doi.org/10.2139/ssrn.3691091

Nygaard, V. M., Sørensen, B. E., & Wang, F. (2022). Optimal allocations to heterogeneous agents with an application to stimulus checks. *Journal of Economic Dynamics and Control*, 104352. https://doi.org/10.1016/j.jedc.2022.104352

Sahm, C., Shapiro, M., & Slemrod, J. (2020). *Consumer response to the coronavirus stimulus programs*. Slides.

Parolin, Z., Curran, M., Matsudaira, J., Waldfogel, J., & Wimer, C. (2020). Monthly poverty rates in the United States during the COVID-19 pandemic. *Poverty and social policy working paper, center on poverty & social policy*. https://www.povertycenter.columbia.edu/s/COVID-Projecting-Poverty-Monthly-CPSP-2020.pdf

Petrosky-Nadeau, N. (2020). *Reservation Benefits: Assessing job acceptance impacts of increased UI payments*. (No. 2020-28). Federal Reserve Bank of San Francisco Working Paper. https://doi.org/10.24148/wp2020-28

Satoshi, K., Kaori, K., Takemasa, T., & Yoichi, U. (2020). The impact of COVID-19 on US consumer spending: Quantitative analysis using high-frequency state-level data. *Bank of Japan Review*. https://www.boj.or.jp/en/research/wps_rev/rev_2020/rev20e07.htm/

Wozniak, A., Willey, J., Benz, J., & Hart, N. (2020). *COVID impact survey: Version 1* [dataset]. National Opinion Research Center. https://www.covid-impact.org

ETHICAL CONSIDERATIONS OF BUSINESS CSR DURING THE COVID-19 PANDEMIC

Terri Herron[1] and Tim Manuel[2]

Abstract: The pandemic required businesses to face rapidly evolving business and ethical challenges. Managers suddenly faced existential challenges to the firm's survival as governments mandated closures and customers and employees modified behaviors that could lead to exposure to the COVID-19 virus. Even as profitability and earnings fell, the need for firms to take actions to help society dramatically increased. Moreover, public scrutiny of firm choices to maintain profitability or focus on their responsibility to employee and external stakeholders increased dramatically. This left managers with many ethical challenges in choosing between short-term profitability and acting to meet society's needs. To survive and keep their employees and customers safe, many firms increased philanthropic donations, modified their business models, changed their working environments, and/or assisted employees. Businesses engaged in more extensive and targeted corporate social responsibility (CSR) programs in response to the pandemic. This chapter summarizes some of these CSR responses and evaluates how ethics plays a role in them.

Introduction

Coronavirus Disease 2019 (COVID-19) swiftly reached pandemic proportions in the United States in early 2020. The severity of the virus' impact became apparent very quickly, but the means of viral transmission were not well understood and there was little agreement on methods to contain the spread of the virus. As a result, many businesses were forced to shut down by local governments or had to close because of necessity. Some firms were also forced to modify their business models and working environments in response. Many firm managers faced ethical choices to prioritize business profits in a challenging environment or responding to

---

[1] Faculty Fellow, University of Montana, Missoula, Montana, USA

[2] Professor, University of Montana, Missoula, Montana, USA

society's needs engendered by the pandemic, even at the expense of firm profits. Numerous businesses chose to engage in additional outreach and philanthropy to communities adversely affected by the disease. The speed of the pandemic spread, and the uncertainties associated with the disease required a swift response from businesses and brought ethical considerations to the forefront. The public expected firms to respond to pandemic needs and not proceed with the usual primary focus on profits. EY's Global Integrity Report (2020) states, "COVID-19 is a test for business integrity. Those who pass will differentiate themselves as seldom before. Those who fail are likely to be held accountable after the crisis has passed..." (p. 2).

Managers have an explicit responsibility to shareholders to act as stewards of shareholder-supplied funds and provide a return to shareholders commensurate with the risk of the business. Businesses operate within an implicit social contract to provide goods and services to individuals who interact with the business in various roles. Other entities are still impacted by business activity. Thus, business managers have responsibilities to many stakeholders. Broadly speaking, a stakeholder is anyone who is impacted by the firm's activities. These potential impacts of the firm's actions create a moral responsibility to many stakeholders other than stockholders. As a result of this responsibility, many businesses engage in corporate social responsibility (CSR) activities. CSR activities occur when a business "consciously and deliberately acts to enhance the social well-being of those whose lives are affected by the firm's economic operations" (Frederick, 2018). CSR activities are actions that help businesses be accountable to themselves, their stakeholders, and the public (Fernando, 2021).

Even before the pandemic, CSR was clearly important to a diverse set of constituents. A 2014 study of 30,000 consumers in 60 countries found that 67% prefer to work for socially responsible companies, and 55% would pay extra for goods and services sold by companies committed to positive environmental and social impacts (Nielsen, 2014). A follow up survey in 2015 showed the willingness to pay extra had grown to 66% in just one year (NielsenIQ, 2015). CSR activities before the pandemic were quite diverse. These activities encompassed a wide range of practices and programs related to the environment, human rights, employment practices, community programs, and more. When the pandemic hit, CSR activities became more focused on responding to societal needs caused by the crisis at hand.

A public health crisis such as a pandemic sharpens public focus on managers' ethical choices of acting to sustain the business' profitability during the crisis versus focusing on the welfare of non-owner stakeholders. Some managers may respond to a crisis in an egoistic manner to preserve their own position and self-interests by engaging in price gouging of scarce products or overstating the health benefits of their products (Udell, 2020). The EY Global Integrity Report (2020) cited above and surveys by (Edelman 2020a, 2020b) indicate that firms that prioritize profitability over social responsibility may pay a long-term price in the form of reputation and customer loss. The public expected that the pandemic would elevate the priority of stakeholder concerns over business and managers' economic interests (Manuel & Herron, 2020). In this chapter, we review specific business responses in the area of CSR undertaken in the pandemic environment, how those CSR responses may have been motivated, and the role that ethics plays.

Instrumental, Deontological, and Virtue Motives for Ethical Actions

If ethics requires managers to consider more than the bottom-line impact on their firm's profits, how should they evaluate the impact of their decisions on various stakeholders in an ethical manner? In other words, when business managers and employees are faced with ethical choices, what framework should they use to make their decisions? Many firms' charters claim managers will make decisions to benefit a variety of stakeholders, including stockholders, employees, customers, creditors, the community in which the firm operates, and even society. How does a firm choose between competing interests of various stakeholders when their interests are not aligned? For instance, providing a reasonable return to shareholders may require laying off employees when the firm could not operate during the pandemic, even though doing so would harm employees and the local community. There are various ethics traditions or approaches to problem-solving that can help managers think through these situations. For instance, deontological thinking uses a duty-based approach to making decisions that is focused on upholding the underlying principle of ethical action. This thought process focuses on doing what is right or following a moral code regardless of the result (Jeanes, 2019). An application of deontological thinking may be to apply a principle such as protecting employees and the local community during the shutdown by continuing to pay employees such as NBA teams, Wal-Mart and other firms who chose to pay employees even when they couldn't work, or were being asked to work in hazardous conditions. Other firms increased donations to help those in need even when the firm's profits were being hurt by the pandemic. Examples would include Marriott, British Airways, United Airlines, and many others as noted below.

John Rawls deepened our understanding of what constitutes ethical decision-making by incorporating the ideas of justice and fairness in the decision process. Rawls argued that to be moral or just, ethical choices must not harm the least well-off or the most vulnerable (Rawls, 1958). Decisions must lead to fair outcomes and employ a fair process such that an impartial observer would agree with the ethics of the process or outcome. Thus, when examining consequences or applying principles, the analysis must consider whether the decision is fair to more vulnerable groups such as low-income individuals, minorities, or women. The MacKenzie Scott donation mentioned below falls in this category.

Virtue ethics was developed by Aristotle several millennia ago. In this thinking, the ethics of an action stems from the virtue and intention of the decision-maker rather than from examining consequences or following rules or principles. For instance, a truly virtuous manager will pursue ethical actions because of the manager's character (Velasquez et al., 1988). There is no self-interest in the decision process, and business decisions would be completely altruistic in intent. The altruistic intent (or lack thereof) is not directly observable and perhaps the best we can do is to infer the intent from the firm's actions over time (Godfrey, 2005, 2006). Some firm's CSR actions led to profit declines and reduction in firm value which indicates an altruistic intent. One study of hospitality firms' CSR during the pandemic found that strategic CSR was related to *lower* firm value (Shin et al., 2021). Some firms switched product lines entirely to meet societal needs. One such example was LVMH's switch from cosmetics to hand sanitizer, which was then donated to hospitals and health care workers. On the other hand, some managers simply looked out for themselves and their firms. This is called ethical *egoism and* is focused on making decisions with positive outcomes for the decision maker, with little consideration for impacts on others (Burgess-Jackson, 2013; Cummiskey, 1989). For example, Congress created Paycheck Protection Plan (PPP) loans so that small businesses could continue to employ workers at firms hurt by the shutdowns (Coronavirus Aid, Relief and Economic Security Act, 2020). Several banks however initially only made PPP loans available to existing bank customers and turned away many small businesses who would otherwise quality because they were not bank customers (Leatherby, 2020). Because many minority- and women-owned small businesses are less likely to use banking services than businesses owned by White men, this meant the program was not made available to many minority-owned firms, contrary to the will of Congress.

Ethics-Driven Examples of Business CSR Activities

CSR activities fall into three categories, philanthropic, improved operations, and transformed business models (Rangan et al., 2015). Most early CSR pandemic responses were philanthropic or transformative. Manuel and Herron (2020) list many examples of both philanthropic and transformative CSR responses from early in the pandemic (examples of participating companies are listed in parentheses). Employee safety and well-being requirements emerged in the pandemic that led to a third category that we term employee care responses.

Philanthropic Responses

Corporate philanthropic disaster responses (CPDRs) are most often related to natural disasters, yet COVID-19 had impacts similar to a natural disaster in many respects (e.g., resource scarcity and threats to health). Health care workers were the beneficiary of many philanthropic responses. Hotels donated millions of rooms and meals, as evidenced by 20 separate initiatives announced between April and July 2020 (Shin et al., 2021). Airlines donated vacation packages (American Airlines); communications companies donated phone chargers and internet service (AT&T) and reduced cost cellular service (Verizon). Companies made financial or product donations to support food banks, which saw significant increases in demand (Walmart, Carrier Transicold, Pepsico, Land o'Lakes). Medical companies donated to programs supporting people with diabetes who lost their medical insurance due to unemployment (Medtronic). Companies supported education by donating computers (Amazon) and providing free technology classes to children learning from home (Best Buy). Restaurants and food companies offered free or at-cost meals or food to nonprofits and food banks (Nestle') to meet higher demand resulting from soaring unemployment (Guillaume-Grabisch, 2020). Restaurants donated millions of meals to healthcare workers and first responders (McDonalds) and later donated scholarships, grants, and contracts to farmers hurt by the plummeting demand from the hard-hit restaurant industry (Chipotle) (Ou et al., 2021).

Many nonprofits were hurt by the pandemic. One study found that more than one-third of U.S. nonprofits were at risk of closing within two years due to the pandemic's financial effects even though corporations gave $9.4 billion in cash and in-kind donations to nonprofits in 2020 (Candid & The Center for Disaster Philanthropy, 2021). The largest such gift was $400 million to reduce or eliminate processing fees for small businesses impacted by COVID-19 and to fund community development finance institutions supporting small businesses owned by African Americans (Wells Fargo). Individual actors within corporations in industries disproportionately affected also responded philanthropically by taking significant base pay cuts (Lyft, Marriott, British Airways, United Airlines, Disney, Comcast). Individuals whose wealth was rooted in corporate profits made significant donations, such as MacKenzie Scott's $4 billion donation for COVID-19 aid for nonprofits working in areas of high poverty and low access to capital (Candid & The Center for Disaster Philanthropy, 2021).

Transformational Responses

Some businesses transformed their business models to accommodate pandemic-specific needs (Manuel & Herron, 2020). General Motors and Ford both revamped their production process to produce ventilators in the early months of the pandemic.[3] Both companies indicated they would not profit from the production. In fact, the ventilator unit cost was projected to be nearly $10,000 less than a previous federal contract (Wayland, 2020). Ford also produced and donated 120 million respirators and masks for schools, higher education, state, and local governments, first responders, and nonprofits (Ford Motor Company Fund, n.d.), and other companies did the same (Whirlpool, in partnership with Dow and Reynolds). The Armani fashion company converted its four Italian apparel plants to manufacture single-use overalls for medical professionals (Yahoo!News, 2020). Companies repurposed large buildings into food distribution centers (United Airlines). Cosmetic companies converted their production facilities to make hand sanitizer (LVMH). These are examples of fundamental changes to how companies used their assets and expertise to meet societal needs during the pandemic.

Many business-to-consumer firms transformed their processes. Healthcare providers turned to telemedicine and used in-car waiting to reduce contact in waiting rooms. Grocers and other retailers created specific shopping hours for older and at-risk customers, as well as curbside pickup and delivery where they had not done this previously (Manuel & Herron, 2020). Many large retailers and restaurants changed their policies and procedures to allow for contactless card payment (Walmart, Burger King, UPS).

Employee Care Responses

Ethical responses to the pandemic include socially responsible policies related to how companies treat their employees. The pandemic threatened employee health and job security and heightened the need for employee-centered assistance, and this need was widespread rather than localized like other natural disasters. Airbnb established a $250 million relief fund for certain hosts to recapture fees they pay to Airbnb on cancelled reservations. The work-from-home mandates introduced hardships for

---

[3] Both companies initiated production preparations before President Trump invoked the Defense Production Act. The Act avoids patent issues and gives the President power to mandate such production.

many employees who lacked proper space and equipment to do so effectively. Companies such as Shopify, Google, and Twitter provided $1,000 stipends to employees to set up a home office (Nova, 2020). Other companies, such as Feather, provided stipends for a weekly meal that may have otherwise been provided in the office. Childcare challenges were heightened with children attending at-home school or losing access to daycare. Companies such as Zillow granted caregiver days off to provide flexibility for parents in this situation (Liu, 2020). Retailers such as Kroger, Amazon, and Walmart who remained open to provide essential services provided hazard pay in the initial months, but they were later criticized for cessation of those programs despite robust profits (Bhattarai & Ingraham, 2020). Many companies granted special sick pay policies for COVID-19 illness. For example, Verizon updated its leave of absence policy to include eight weeks of 100% paid sick leave, followed by 16 weeks of 60% paid sick leave. Employees who are diagnosed with COVID-19 are entitled to up to 26 weeks of paid sick leave (Verizon, 2022). While many companies paid employees only on a short-term basis when the first stay-at-home orders forced their closure, others extended this policy. Event-based employers who were unable to hold events paid venue workers as if the events had taken place. Examples include many NHL and NBA teams who own their venues (Hadden, 2020).

Analysis and Conclusion

CSR activities are business decisions to act beyond shareholder interest that improve the lives of stakeholders, society, or the environment. CSR activities may be philanthropic in nature, or they may be designed to improve operations or transform the firm's business model to improve the well-being of employees and other stakeholders or the environment. The pandemic increased the demand for business CSR and raised awareness that businesses are expected to be involved in improving society. From a deontological perspective, business has a moral obligation to use its resources to benefit society in times of crisis. Virtuous managers will desire to do so because it is in their character. Managers concerned with justice may focus on benefiting more vulnerable or marginalized constituents as their resources and skill allow.

Many firms began or increased philanthropic activity such as donations of money, products, or services to help those hurt by the pandemic. Some even changed their business model to produce items needed such as masks, ventilators, hand sanitizer, and other personal protective equipment. In many cases these items were donated by the firms. Companies quickly introduced new employee assistance to support their workforce facing loss of childcare/school, furloughs, reduced hours, and other hardships such as caring for themselves or others who had COVID-19.

Businesses increased investment in socially responsible actions during COVID-19 for a variety of reasons. The pandemic has elevated investors,' customers,' and other external stakeholders' desire for CSR activities (He & Harris, 2020). The pandemic emphasized the need for businesses to help customers, employers, and the public to manage both economic and health risks (Edelman, 2020a). In choosing these policies, managers may choose CSR activities to gain short-term profit improvements, meet stakeholders' expectations, and/or the good of society, or a combination of all three (Aguilera et al., 2007). It is very difficult to disentangle and identify specific motivations, but many businesses appeared to take actions designed to benefit society more than profitability during the pandemic.

Questions remain whether the increased demand for CSR activities will continue as the pandemic wanes. We believe it is likely that the demand for corporate philanthropy will probably fall, but firms are likely to be expected to remain active or increase their activity in climate amelioration, reducing inequality, employee assistance, and justice concerns. The popularity of environmental, social and governance (ESG)[4] bonds and the increasing move to standardize firms' ESG reporting indicate that CSR activities remain very important to investors (Wirz, 2020a, 2020b). ESG is becoming more important to capital markets, as evidenced by a recent Securities and Exchange Commission (SEC) proposal to improve and regulate disclosures for funds and advisors purporting an ESG focus (SEC,

---

[4] CSR and ESG are closely related. CSR is a business model for companies to operate in a way aligned with CSR values, while ESG is the criteria that investors use to assess how companies are impacting the environment and relationships with whom they operate, including the business governance tactics (Cook, 2021).

2022). Allan Murray, Chief Executive Officer (CEO) of Forbes, reports that many other CEOs now believe that firms must continue to make a broader positive impact on society in areas ranging from ameliorating climate change effects, improving social justice, and many more. These activities are now expected as part of the implicit contract between business and society (Narisetti, 2022). We believe that most firms will be expected to maintain or increase their corporate social responsibility actions even long after the concerns of the pandemic fade.

References

Aguilera, R., Rupp, D., Williams, C., & Ganapathi, J. (2007). Putting the S back in corporate social responsibility: A multilevel theory of social change in organizations. *Academy of Management Review 33*(3), 836-863. https://doi.org/10.5465/amr.2007.25275678

Bhattarai, A. & Ingraham, C. (2020, November 23). Workers call on Walmart, Amazon, and other retailers to bring back hazard pay ahead of holiday rush. *The Washington Post.* https://www.washingtonpost.com/business/2020/11/23/retail-workers-pandemic-pay/

Burgess-Jackson, K. (2013). Taking egoism seriously. *Ethical Theory and Moral Practice, 16,* 529–542. https://doi.org/10.1007/s10677-012-9372-5

Candid & The Center for Disaster Philanthropy. (2021). Philanthropy and COVID-19: Measuring one year of giving. https://www.issuelab.org/resources/38039/38039.pdf

Cook, J. (2021, September 2). What is the difference between ESG and CSR? *Business Leader.* https://www.businessleader.co.uk/what-is-the-difference-between-esg-and-csr/

Coronavirus Aid, Relief, and Economic Security Act, Public Law 116–136. (2020). https://assets.documentcloud.org/documents/20059055/final-final-cares-act.pdf

Cummiskey, D. (1989). Consequentialism, egoism, and the moral law. *Philosophical Studies: An International Journal for Philosophy in the Analytic Tradition, 57,* 111–134. www.jstor.org/stable/4320067

Edelman. (2020a, March 16). Edelman trust barometer special report on COVID-19 demonstrates essential role of the private sector. https://www.edelman.com/r

esearch/edelman-trust-barometer-special-report-covid-19-demonstrates-essential-role-private-sector

Edelman. (2020b, March 30). Edelman trust barometer special report: Brand trust and the coronavirus pandemic. https://www.edelman.com/research/covid-19-brand-trust-report

EY. (2020). *Global Integrity Report*. EYGM Limited. https://www.ey.com/en_us/legal-statement

Fernando, J. (2021). *Corporate social responsibility (CSR)?* Investopedia. https://www.investopedia.com/terms/c/corp-social-responsibility.asp

Ford Motor Company Fund. (n.d.). *120 million mask donations*. https://www.fordfund.org/masks

Frederick, W. (2018). Corporate social responsibility: From founders to millennials. In J. Weber & D. Wasieleski (Eds.), *Corporate Social Responsibility* (pp. 3-38). Emerald Publishing Limited.

Godfrey, P. C. (2005). The relationship between corporate philanthropy and shareholder wealth: A risk management perspective. *The Academy of Management Review, 30*, 777–798.

Godfrey, P. C. (2006). A reply to bright: Virtuousness and the virtues of the market. *The Academy of Management Review, 31*(3), 754–756. https://doi.org/10.2307/20159241

Guillaume-Grabisch, B. (2020). *How Nestle' is helping feed the hungry during the pandemic*. https://www.nestle.com/stories/nestle-donations-help-feed-hungry-during-pandemic-covid

Hadden, J. (2020, March 27). Here are the ways Walmart, Uber, and other major companies are taking care of their employees in the US who have been told not to work in light of the coronavirus pandemic so far. *Business Insider*. https://www.businessinsider.com/how-companies-are-taking-care-of-employees-because-of-the-coronavirus-2020?utm_source=copy-link&utm_medium=referral&utm_content=topbar

He, H., & Harris, L. (2020). The impact of COVID-19 pandemic on corporate social responsibility and marketing philosophy. *Journal of Business Research, 116*, 176-182. https://doi.org/10.1016/j.jbusres.2020.05.030

Jeanes, E. (2019). *A dictionary of organizational behaviour*. Oxford University Press. https://www.oxfordreference.com.weblib.lib.umt.edu:2443/view/10.1093/acref/9780191843273.001.0001/acref-9780191843273

Leatherby, L. (2020). Coronavirus is hitting black business owners hardest. *The New York Times*. https://nyti.ms/2UWhYH1

Liu, J. (2020, August 25). *How companies are preparing employees for long-term work-from-home*. CNBC.com. https://www.cnbc.com/2020/08/25/how-companies-are-supporting-work-from-home-until-2021or-forever.html

Manuel, T. & Herron, T. (2020). An ethical perspective of business CSR and the COVID-19 pandemic. *Society and Business Review, 15*(3), 235-253. https://doi.org/10.1108/SBR-06-2020-0086

Narisetti, R. (2022, May 5). Author Talks: Tomorrow's capitalist is socially conscious: Interview with Allan Murray. McKinsey & Company. https://www.mckinsey.com/featured-insights/mckinsey-on-books/author-talks-tomorrows-capitalist-is-socially-conscious

Nielsen. (2014). Doing well by doing good (Nielsen Global Survey of Corporate Social Responsibility). Nielsen. https://www.nielsen.com/wp-content/uploads/sites/3/2019/04/global-corporate-social-responsibility-report-june-2014.pdf

NielsenIQ. (2015, October 12). The sustainability imperative. https://nielseniq.com/global/en/insights/analysis/2015/the-sustainability-imperative-2/

Nova, A. (2020, June 3). *Working from home? You might be able to expense a new desk*. CNBC.com. https://www.cnbc.com/2020/06/03/companies-are-paying-for-their-workers-home-offices.html

Ou, J., Wong, I. A., & Huang, G. I. (2021). The coevolutionary process of restaurant CSR in the time of mega disruption. *International Journal of Hospitality Management, 92*, 102684. https://doi.org/10.1016/j.ijhm.2020.102684

Rangan, V., Chase, L., & Karim, S. (2015). The truth about CSR, *Harvard Business Review, 93*(1/2), 40-49. https://hbr.org/2015/01/the-truth-about-csr

Rawls, J. (1958). Justice as fairness. *The Philosophical Review, 67*(2), 164-194. https://doi.org/10.2307/2182612

Securities and Exchange Commission (SEC). (2022, May 25). SEC proposes to enhance disclosures by certain investment advisors and investment companies about ESC investment practices [press release]. https://www.sec.gov/news/press-release/2022-92

Shin, H., Sharma, A., Nicolau, J. L., & Kang, J. (2021). The impact of hotel CSR for strategic philanthropy on booking behavior and hotel performance during the COVID-19 pandemic. *Tourism Management, 85*, 104322. https://doi.org/10.1016/j.tourman.2021.104322

Udell, J., Ahalt, K., & Armas, J. (2020). DOJ launches COVID-19-related fraud and price gouging cases. *Law.Com.* 14 May. Available at: www.law.com/newyorklawjournal/2020/05/14/doj-launches-covid-19-related-fraud-and-price-gouging-cases/?slreturn=20200514145541 (accessed 14 June 2020).

Velasquez, M., Andre, C., Thomas Shanks, S.J., and Meyer, M. (1988, January 1). Ethics and Virtue. Markkula Center for Applied Ethics. Originally appeared in *Issues in Ethics 1*(3), Spring 1988. https://www.scu.edu/ethics/ethics-resources/ethical-decision-making/ethics-and-virtue/

Verizon. (2022). *COVID-19 employee information.* https://www.verizon.com/about/news/covid-19-employee-information#absencepolicy

Wayland, M. (2020, April 16). *GE, Ford sign $336 million federal contract to make ventilators for coronavirus outbreak.* CNBC.com. https://www.cnbc.com/2020/04/16/ge-ford-sign-336-million-federal-contract-for-ventilator-production.html

Wirz, M. (2020a, February 10). Green bonds branch out with record sale, by Matt Wirz, *The Wall Street Journal.* https://www.wsj.com/articles/green-bonds-branch-out-with-record-sale-11581353864

Wirz, M. (2020b, December 17). Why going green saves bond borrowers' money, *The Wall Street Journal.* https://www.wsj.com/articles/why-going-green-saves-bond-borrowers-money-11608201002

Yahoo!News. (2020, March 26). *Armani's Italian factories to make medical overalls.* https://news.yahoo.com/armanis-italain-factories-medical-overalls-180204465.html?soc_src=social-sh&soc_trk=ma

TWO CONTRASTING ETHICAL PERSPECTIVES ON LEADERSHIP AND THE COVID-19 "RETURN TO WORK" DILEMMA: KANT'S CATEGORICAL IMPERATIVE AND GILLIGAN'S ETHIC OF CARE

Jeff Youngquist[1]

Abstract: The following chapter explores the ethical aspects of the "return to work" decision that many organizational leaders have had to make during the COVID-19 pandemic. This exploration is done from two different and potentially contrasting ethical perspectives, that of Immanuel Kant's categorical imperative and Carol Gilligan's ethic of care. Making this decision is an ethical dilemma because the outcome of the decision has the potential to impact the health and well-being of employees and there are strong arguments that both ethical perspectives can lead to a "right," albeit very different, decision. Examples are provided where the decisions of actual organizational leaders are reflective of these two ethical perspectives. The author argues that Gilligan's ethic of care assumes the higher moral ground and may be more palatable to organizational employees, while also recognizing that there are many contextual variables and situations related to the pandemic that prohibit the application of one moral or ethical perspective to all leaders and organizations. The author also argues that even though Kant's categorical imperative and Gilligan's ethic of care seem fundamentally opposed to one another in this ethical dilemma, they may be able to coexist with the ethic of care essentially acting as a categorical imperative.

Introduction

Since the beginning of the pandemic, leaders throughout the world have been presented with myriad ethical dilemmas related to the COVID-19 pandemic. One of the most prominent dilemmas has been the decision of whether employees should return to work in the office, rather than working remotely. Because the virus was still spreading and not all people were

---

[1] Associate Professor, Oakland University, Oakland County, Michigan, USA

vaccinated, this decision of whether employees should return to work became an ethical dilemma. An ethical dilemma is when two core values conflict with one another (Kidder, 1995), typically leaving the individual with unclear guidance on how to act or what decision to make. Prior to the development of a COVID-19 vaccine, leaders of organizations across the globe responded to the pandemic by instructing their organizational members to conduct their work remotely rather than face-to-face. Once a vaccine was developed, these same leaders were confronted with the ethical dilemma of whether to instruct their organizational members to return to a face-to-face manner of conducting their work even though the pandemic still raged and not all people had received the vaccine. At a minimum, this decision on returning to work had the potential to affect an employee's health, and possibly affect it quite seriously. Organizational leaders who made such decisions were essentially asking themselves "is this the right thing to do?" Is it right to instruct employees to return to work with the virus still in existence? As the number of people infected by the virus declines, at what point is it arguably "right" to expect people to return to work? Or, is it ever right, as a leader, to make a decision that puts individuals at risk for the sake of meeting organizational goals, regardless of how small that risk actually is? Should leaders impose their will on followers regarding whether to return to work, or is it "right" to allow the individual to make this decision themselves, especially when it has been shown that the organizations can function and exist with workers working remotely?

This chapter briefly explores the "return to work" ethical dilemma in more detail as it relates to organizational leadership. Any expression of "return to work" in this chapter simply means returning to work in an office in a face-to-face manner. The chapter then presents two relevant but contrasting ethical perspectives including: (1) Immanuel Kant's categorical imperative, an absolutist perspective with no regard for context or circumstance, and (2) Carol Gilligan's ethic of care, a more situational or contextual perspective. Real world examples of organizational decision-making that are reflective of these ethical perspectives are also presented, and a possible resolution to the ethical dilemma is proposed. In the conclusion, it is argued that the ethic of care is both a more palatable resolution to this ethical dilemma and it claims the higher moral ground. However, it is also suggested in the conclusion that these two seemingly mutually exclusive ethical perspectives can actually coexist. The comparison of Kant's categorical imperative and Gilligan's ethic of care in this chapter is not intended to be an ethical guideline for leaders looking to resolve the "return to work" dilemma. Rather, when leaders make decisions regarding the "return to work" dilemma, their thoughts and actions may be reflective of the ideological contrast described in the following pages.

The "Return to Work" Ethical Dilemma and Leadership

Ethics, in its most basic sense, is the study or consideration of what are the right and wrong actions to take in life, or what are the good and bad ends to pursue (Deigh, 2010). When deciding how to act in an ethical dilemma, the decision is typically not clear cut, not easy, and the decision-maker seldom feels great confidence that he or she did, indeed, make the right decision.

Most organizational leaders, of course, will not consult with readings on ethics tucked away in their libraries when deciding whether or not their organizations will return to work. At best, they'll consciously reflect on the ethical lessons they studied in their days as a student. At worst, they'll make their decisions by focusing exclusively on the bottom-line with no concern whatsoever for the ethical aspects of the situation and with no concern regarding the impact their decision will have on their followers. Nonetheless, organizational leaders have had to make these decisions regarding whether or not employees should return to work, and they've done so while considering a complex web of concerns, needs, desires, impulses, instincts, advice, market constraints, labor negotiations, and innumerable other factors. Amongst the many variables often considered when determining whether to implement "return to work" policies are things such as how it will affect the spread of COVID-19, the economic impacts, the social effects, the developmental effects, and restrictions on personal liberties (Bernstein et al., 2019). In many cases, organizational leaders have no say in whether employees return to work as the issue is controlled by national or local laws and regulations. Nonetheless, even with the many other factors that can influence a leader's decision, there will still be the lingering question, "what is the right thing to do?" This is no different from most ethical decisions where the individual must sort through myriad influential forces while striving to find the "right" path. At its core, returning to work is an ethical decision for organizational leaders that directly affects the people in the organization and the people in the surrounding communities.

The global experience of managing the "return to work" ethical dilemma seems to reflect two distinctly different perspectives on ethics. On the one hand, the COVID ethical dilemma is sometimes seemingly addressed by leaders from a position that is detached, distant, and authoritative. With such an approach, a leader makes a decision that impacts all of his or her followers as if they were the same person and in the same situation. The decision-maker's primary focus may be on the common good (i.e., determining if returning to work functions to further exacerbate the pandemic) and is guided by logic and reason. The idea of acting towards a common good is a fluid concept that can be difficult to define and can shift over time. But, for the sake of the arguments presented in this chapter, acting towards the common good is something that benefits all of society (McManus et al., 2018). On the other hand, some leaders resolve the dilemma by focusing on the unique individuals who are their followers and the varied and changing contexts within which the individuals exist. Both of these disparate ways of thinking regarding the COVID "return to work" dilemma are interestingly reflective of two different ethical philosophies: Immanuel Kant's categorical imperative and Carol Gilligan's ethic of care.

Kant's Categorical Imperative

Immanuel Kant's categorical imperative stands out as an exemplar of absolutism which is where there are no exceptions (Tangwa, 2004). Kant expresses the absolutism of the categorical imperative in the following:

> Unless we want to deny to the concept of morality any truth and any relation to some possible object, we cannot dispute that its law is so extensive in its import that it must hold not only for human beings but for all rational beings as such, not merely under contingent conditions and with exceptions but with absolute necessity. (as cited in Cholbi, 2016, p. 19)

For Kant, universal moral laws were "objectively valid for all rational beings" (Acton, 1970, p. 21) and should, through rational will, be followed by everyone at all times.

Important to understanding Kant's categorical imperative is understanding that the supreme principle of morality must only be known through *a priori* reasoning. This means that the principle cannot be derived from, or connected to, circumstances or sensory experiences (Cholbi, 2016). The supreme principle of morality must, essentially, be generated from factors other than context and other than our unique lived experiences and our moment in time. Kant's categorical imperative, his supreme principle of morality:

> ...must not be sought in the nature of the human being or in the circumstances of the world in which he is placed, but a priori simply in concepts of pure reason; and that any other precept, which is based on principles of mere experience – even if it is universal in a certain respect – insofar as it rests in the least part on empirical grounds. . .can indeed be called a practical rule, but never a moral law. (as cited in Cholbi, 2016, p. 22)

Because of this, the categorical imperative functions similarly to mathematics. The moral principles that are derived from this imperative are inescapable and inevitable (Acton, 1970). Moral laws, then, become known through human reason and are universal, impersonal, and objective. They are valid for all people and applicable at all times and in every way. Kant was a rigorist and he believed that there were no exceptions to any fundamental moral laws as he understood them.

Kant's categorical imperative, then, is absolute without exception and is derived purely through reason. Additionally, Kant's supreme principle of morality is non-consequentialist. This means that the rightness or wrongness of actions are not connected to the outcomes of those actions (Cholbi, 2016). Instead, it is the individual's motive that is important. The individual's motive "is morally worthy if it is sanctioned by reason" (Kim, 2015, p. 61) and if it is applicable to all people. It is morally worthy if it can be embraced by everyone, and everyone can take actions that are guided by it.

Cholbi (2016) identifies a critique of Kant's categorical imperative which is particularly relevant to this discussion. He says that "one might worry that Kant appears committed to defending a theory of morality that is very remote from human concerns" (p. 34) and that "We might worry that Kant divorces morality from human concerns – from our particular ends, we might say – that it may seem to have no point at all" (p. 34). This is, indeed, a notable critique and worthy of significant attention.

Kant's categorical imperative is less a specific moral law, and more a set of criteria for what a (or *the*) moral law should be, and guidelines on how to discover it. As Acton (1970) aptly expresses regarding Kant's philosophy, "He may well be right in saying that duty and the good will are basic to morality, but it is a pity that he has so little to say about ideals of conduct" (p. 63). In essence, the categorical imperative and any resulting supreme principle of morality is infallibly absolutist and becomes known to us through reason. Its most prominent characteristic that is tied to its absolutist nature is its subsequent disregard for circumstance, context, or cultural factors (McManus et al., 2018).

With a leader that approaches "return to work" ethical dilemmas with a similar frame of mind, the decision that is made will also be absolutist in effect. That is, there can be no exception to this decision; there can be no deviation or variation. If a leader determines that workers should return to work, they all return to work. If a leader determines that workers should not return to work, then no worker returns to work. Such a leader would determine, based on his or reasoning and with little concern for the context, that returning to work is the "right" thing to do. Such a leader's intention would be to derive the right course of action in a universal sense. This leader would make a decision that would influence all followers with little input (or, more likely, no input) from these followers. In making a decision in this manner, the leader will have resolved the ethical dilemma of whether followers should return to work while the pandemic is still in effect.

Gilligan's Ethic of Care

Carol Gilligan is credited with originating and developing what is called the ethic of care. Gilligan's work was built off of the problems she identified in the work of her mentor, Lawrence Kohlberg, and his ethic of justice (Simola, 2003). However, in this chapter, Gilligan's ethic of care is compared to the much earlier work of Immanuel Kant as his philosophy seems to embody the detachment that so fundamentally contrasts with Gilligan's work.

Gilligan's early work found that men and women followed different paths in their moral decision-making. But, because the dominant paradigm and the research at that time focused primarily on men, the women who typically followed different paths of moral decision-making were seen as morally deficient (Simola, 2003). How were women different in their moral decision-making? Women were "more likely to be ambivalent about acting in ways that reflected the separation and autonomy needed to make 'fair' decisions, and more organized around maintaining connections and nurturing the web of relationships within which they were embedded" (p. 354). Women were found to be more interested in care of themselves, care of others, and caring for both themselves *and* others. Women did not approach situations that demand moral decision-making as if they were problems to be solved. They did not use abstract reasoning when thinking through these moral issues. Instead, they approached these situations as actual, real, human experiences that impacted human lives, and which must be approached with these lives clearly in mind (Noddings, 1984).

With the development of the ethic of care, Gilligan emphasized caring for others rather than caring about others. Caring for others is accomplished through actual relationships whereas caring about others can be accomplished without these relationships. Through relationships, we become aware of, and responsive to, each individual's unique feelings and concerns. We become aware of the context within which each individual exists and the circumstances they are experiencing. It means developing empathy which is accomplished through an understanding of the real needs of each individual and which is tailored to the unique circumstances of those individuals (Simola, 2003). Gilligan's (1995) writings contrast the ethic of care with more disassociated perspectives (e.g., Kant's categorical imperative). To be detached and disassociated is to not see, speak to, or listen to others, to not know others, and to not care about our real, human, living world. Gilligan (1995) makes it very clear that the ethic of care is a feminist ethic that is founded on connection. Connection is fundamental in human life and "human lives are interwoven in a myriad of subtle and not so subtle ways" (p. 122).

In many ways, Gilligan's ethical perspective contrasts sharply with Kant's categorical imperative. Gilligan (1995), in describing the feminist foundation of her ethic of care, alludes to the detached and rational voice prevalent in Kant's philosophy. She says:

> From this standpoint, the conception of a separate self appears intrinsically problematic, conjuring up the image of a rational man, acting out of relationship with the inner and outer world. Such autonomy, rather than being the bedrock for solving psychological and moral problems itself becomes the problem, signifying a disconnection from emotions and a blindness to relationships which set the stage for psychological and political trouble. (p. 122)

The self in the ethic of care is not autonomous and detached. Instead, the self is interconnected and exists in relation to others. Decision-making and addressing moral dilemmas are not accomplished through the use of formal logic. Instead, the ethic of care focuses on the real and unique needs of others and on their subjective experiences. This sometimes demands a creative effort to fulfill moral responsibilities that may be in conflict with one another (Simola, 2015). Kant's perspective on ethics is disengaged and views the self as separated from others, whereas the ethic of care emphasizes community harmony and recognizes the interconnectedness of self and others (French & Weis, 2000). Morally, the needs and welfare of individuals may be more important than adherence to an ethic that may be logical and rational but is also detached, uncaring, and void of empathy (Lo, 2000). Nonetheless, there may be a way that these two disparate ethical and philosophical perspectives can coexist. This possibility is discussed in the conclusion of this chapter.

"Return to Work" Examples During the COVID-19 Pandemic

Leaders in most organizations have struggled with the dilemma of whether employees should return to working in the office and struggled with how to make this happen. As described in the paragraphs above, this is an ethical dilemma because leaders must determine the "right" path to follow. This is potentially problematic for organizational leaders because there are equally compelling yet conflicting ethical arguments for mandating that employees return to work (or don't return to work), or giving employees the power to decide for themselves, individually, whether they should return to work. There have been many approaches to resolving this dilemma, but most of them seem to exhibit reasoning that is reflective of either Kant's categorical imperative, or Gilligan's ethic of care, or some hybrid approach. A few examples of each of these approaches are included in the paragraphs below.

Many organizational leaders have approached this ethical dilemma from a patriarchal standpoint resembling an absolutist ethical perspective, much like Kant's categorical imperative. It could be argued that this has been the dominant approach to resolving the return-to-work dilemma. Some examples of such companies include American Express, Meta Platforms, and Cisco Systems. These companies are exemplars of decision-making where the decision to "return to work" is made with a broad application, with seemingly little regard for the unique individual or the varied contexts, and sometimes with an obscured or poorly explained rationale. For instance, a Cisco executive described this decision-making process as "we're looking for moments" and had identified March 1 as "a moment when our employees can come in" (Cutter, 2022). By "moments," the Cisco executive appears to have meant at a time when the rate of COVID infections had declined significantly such that the decision-makers felt it was safe (or reasonable) for employees to return to work, though this rationale is certainly not clear.

Of course, for some occupations, working face-to-face has been unavoidable (e.g., many health care jobs). But, throughout the pandemic, it has also been shown that many occupations do not actually need to be conducted face-to-face and can be conducted remotely. Working remotely demands change, and these changes are accompanied by new problems that need to be managed and/or overcome, but a simple resistance to change is not a valid reason to prevent people from working remotely. Nonetheless, some of these organizations where at least some of the jobs can be conducted remotely have been pushing for employees – all employees – to return to work. Banking firms such as Goldman Sachs and JP Morgan have been strong proponents of trying to get employees, en masse, back to work in the office. The result, in the case of Goldman Sachs, was that employees threatened to quit if they were forced to return to the office five days a week. Management had indicated that employees had the choice of whether or not to return to working in the office, but then ominously tracked those who attended the office and those who did not. The Goldman Sachs CEO, David Solomon, described working from home as an "aberration" and said, "It's an aberration that we're going to correct as quickly as possible." Solomon's explanation for why this was an aberration was it "is not ideal for us, and it's not a new normal." One employee posted "It's f**cking bulls**t from top management saying they are people first" (Bunyan, 2022). With a similar attitude, Bank of America has described itself as a "work-from-work company" (Kelly, 2022).

The leadership attitude expressed above extends much further than these few examples. In a survey of 10,000 employees in the summer of 2021 by the group Future Forum, it found that 66% of executives surveyed reported that "they are designing post-pandemic workforce policies with little to no direct input from employees" (Kelly, 2022).

Not surprisingly, the decision-making described above has led to anger and discontent from significant numbers of employees in these organizations. These leaders have attempted to make decisions that appear, at least initially, to be devoid of concern for the individual, the situation, and the context. Instead, these decisions are apparently driven by logic and reason alone. Leaders make these decisions poised between two contrasting perspectives, both of which can be seen as the "right" perspective. Should the leader make the decision for the employees, on behalf of the employees, and from a perspective that is authoritative and seemingly from a higher level of knowledge and understanding? Or, should the leader make this decision with, and through, the employees? In those situations where the decision is distilled to these two contrasting perspectives, it becomes an ethical dilemma. Both are potentially "right," but which approach is the best approach? In some organizations, allowing employees to work remotely may actually put the organization at risk and, consequently, may potentially sacrifice the jobs of all employees in the organization. But, even then, this becomes an ethical dilemma for the leader, especially in the context of a pandemic. Is the best decision to risk the health and welfare of a few for the success and viability of the organization? Should this decision be made for all employees, or, alternatively, through and with all employees? Even when the logic of the decision-makers in the previous paragraphs are laid bare, the followers have become unsettled and unhappy because management seems to be disconnected and the employees' unique situations and lives are ignored. However, these are not the only ways that leaders of organizations have attempted to resolve the "return to work" dilemma. Some organizational leaders have addressed this ethical dilemma with what appears to be a hybrid between an absolutist patriarchal approach and a feminist ethic of care approach.

Google and Apple have both taken this hybrid approach. Early in the pandemic, Google allowed employees to voluntarily work from home. However, as COVID cases declined, Google shifted to a hybrid model where employees were allowed to work where they pleased for a portion of the week, but they were also required to work in the organization's offices for the remainder of the week (Abdel-Baqui, 2022). Apple has followed a similar model where employees are initially required to work one day a week from the office to be followed later by a requirement to work three days a week from the office (Reichert, 2022). At this point, these organizations appear to be following these hybrid strategies with little resistance or conflict. However, considering that these hybrids simultaneously exhibit a controlling patriarchal perspective along with a feminist focus on individual needs, it is unlikely that they will last long without some form of conflict occurring, and neither of these organizations see this as a long-term resolution.

Another exemplar of the conflict between the two ethical perspectives described in this chapter occurred at Activision Blizzard, the maker of the popular video game *Call of Duty*. Decision-making regarding returning to the office at this organization has been driven by upper management which seemingly paid lip service to the concerns and desires of the individuals within the organization. Initially, Activision Blizzard mandated the vaccine for those employees working in the office, and then later officially lifted this vaccine mandate. The initial vaccine mandate was the result of management conducting polls and feedback sessions with employees, but the repeal of the mandate was *not* made in consultation with employees. Per a Supreme Court ruling, the U.S. government does not have the authority to impose a far-reaching vaccine mandate (Japsen, 2022), but individual organizations have not been restricted from imposing their own vaccine mandates (Iafolla, 2022). The result of this is that employees threatened to walk out (as of the writing of this chapter) and A Better ABK, an organization that advocates for better working conditions at Activision Blizzard, published demands which included "The decision to work remote or in office should be made by each individual employee" (Peters, 2022).

Unlike the controlling patriarchal examples and hybrid examples described above, some organizations have tried, in various ways, to be attentive to the unique situation or context of the individual employee. These approaches are most reflective of Gilligan's ethic of care and Twitter is one well known organization where the leadership exhibited such an approach. Twitter told its employees that as of March 15, 2022, they could work from wherever they wanted. Twitter's CEO, Parag Agrawal, said "Wherever you feel most productive and creative is where you will work, and that includes working from home full time forever" (Reichert, 2022). Of course, some organizations like Twitter are naturally more able to give employees the power to determine which approach works best for themselves – face-to-face, remote, or some hybrid. Conversely, some organizations are more aligned with a face-to-face approach to work (e.g., emergency room health care workers). But the pandemic has shown that many occupations can be conducted, either partially or completely, in a remote manner. With this in mind, and with the premise that leaders should be concerned about the human needs of their employees and not just with identifying the most effective, efficient, or profitable way to do a job, organizational leaders are presented with an ethical dilemma. They are positioned to make a decision that directly impacts the welfare, safety, and health of their employees. They can make this decision in a knowing and authoritative manner that affects all employees equally, or they can make this decision by working with and through their individual employees to discover and determine multiple paths forward.

As chair of a large academic department at a university in Michigan, I had to work through my own "return to work" ethical dilemma. At the onset of the initial surge in COVID cases which was halfway through spring semester of 2020, my university mandated that all classes shift from a face-to-face format to an online format. As with most academic institutions, our faculty were ill-prepared for this abrupt transition but responded admirably and, in the end, effectively. In subsequent semesters, the university allowed classes to return to a face-to-face format if students and faculty followed strict COVID guidelines. The scheduling authority, however, was left in the hands of the department chairs. Department chairs, then, could make the decision to return all classes to a face-to-face format (no chairs made such a decision, to my knowledge), or keep all classes in an online format (which some did), or come up with some other approach. As with similar "return to work" decisions made outside of the academic context, this decision involved many more variables than the simple preference of the department chair.

For me, I had no desire to assume the singular authority and impose my will upon the faculty in my department. Prior to the pandemic, I had always tried to be very conscientious of each of our faculties' unique concerns, desires, and wants with regards to setting up their teaching schedules. Doing this demanded that I develop an understanding of who they were and what they wanted, and this could only be done by developing a relationship with each of them and giving their preferences very high priority. With this in mind, I delegated the authority of deciding whether to teach online or face-to-face to each individual faculty. By doing this, I tried to recognize and acknowledge their fears and their concerns (or lack of them) regarding the pandemic. This delegation of authority was something that I took very seriously, even when such decisions sometimes caused other scheduling problems. At no point did I deny, or even consider denying, the desires of our faculty. I even made the commitment (to myself) to resist our upper-level administration when they started gently pushing to move more and more classes back to a face-to-face format. If someone was going to tell a professor that she or he had to teach a face-to-face class when they did not want to because of their fears of the pandemic, that person was not going to be me. On the surface, this can be seen as an issue of compliance. However, ethical decisions must be made by responsible leaders at all levels of an organization, not just those at the top, and sometimes this may mean resisting compliance. Such resistance is often the product of a decision which has been shaped by ethical considerations.

An organization that mirrored my approach to the return-to-work dilemma was Minnesota-based 3M. This organization understood the stresses that organizational members had been experiencing, directly and indirectly, as a result of the pandemic. Instead of issuing a company-wide policy mandating a return to the office, 3M instead gave workers the authority to decide for themselves where they wanted to work (at home or in the office) and their work schedules. The only requirement was that they fulfilled their work duties and responsibilities, and this empowerment was met by 3M employees with relief (DePass, 2022).

Kelly (2022), in an article in *Forbes Magazine* that addressed the general disconnect between management and employees regarding pandemic policies, suggested that "Leaders who listen, are genuine and authentic, will craft policies that suit the individual needs of people. This will make team members feel wanted and appreciated." This advice connects directly and eloquently with Gilligan's ethic of care.

As can be seen from these examples, organizational leaders are approaching the "return to work" ethical dilemma from a variety of directions, with varying levels of success and acceptance. Leaders that have mandated that employees return to work en masse are approaching the problem from a direction that most resembles Kant's categorical imperative. They are making decisions from a patriarchal perspective, with no allowances for deviations or exceptions, and with no concern for the individual and their unique context and situation. Some leaders, on the other hand, have been attempting to do nearly the opposite. They are attentive to their individual followers and are finding ways to address the unique situation of each employee as it relates to the pandemic. These leaders are approaching this dilemma from a direction that most resembles Gilligan's ethic of care. In addition to these two extremes, there are also leaders of organizations that are trying to find some middle ground, or some hybrid approach.

Resolving the Ethical Dilemma

History would suggest that humans have a *tendency* to seek out, or at least value, universal moral laws that transcend all human experience and are derived from some higher plain. Kant was generous enough to at least credit our human capacity to reason as an important factor in this process.

However, many moral principles that we adopt as guides for our actions are, at best, connected to reasoning that is shrouded in the distant past and that sometimes barely connects with our actual lives in the modern world. These higher principles certainly do not take into account the individual human and her or his actual lived experiences, and there are some very real problems that can occur when this happens. For instance, when only considering the dichotomy of returning to work or working remotely, it ignores the potential negative impact this may have on some marginalized groups. Some may not have the necessary skills, such as the technological skills, to work remotely whereas some may actually work better either remotely *or* in-person. Similarly, some may not have the resources such as computers, software, or wireless connections to work at home. Conversely, some may have their personal resources taxed by working from an office by such things as rising fuel costs, daycare costs, or car ownership (Spur, 2022). And, of course, actions that compel employees to return to work (e.g. mandatory vaccines) are regarded by some as ethically questionable (Pennings & Symons, 2021).

The "return to work" decision could be as simple as instructing all employees to return to work, or instructing all employees to continue to work from home. Or, the decision may be a more nuanced version of the same dichotomous choice where various criteria are put in place to dictate which individuals within an organization will return to work and which individuals will continue to work from home (e.g., the "essential workers" mandate). As framed here, these decision options are top-down decisions that are typically organizationally driven and not reflective of the concerns and thoughts of the individual members.

Resolving the "return to work" dilemma using absolutist ethical perspectives will likely be problematic for organizational members who would then be expected to enact the decision and who also experience the consequences of the decision. If an employee is instructed to return to work in the midst of a pandemic, vaccinated or not, they run the risk of harm to themselves and/or harm to others because of the contagious nature of the virus and a vaccine that is not 100% effective. Conversely, if the decision is made for all employees to continue to work remotely, those organizational members who feel dissatisfied with remote work or who feel unable to do their job to the best of their ability may also feel unhappy with the leader's decision. Regardless, leaders with an ethical perspective similar to Kant's categorical imperative will not be influenced by the feelings and experiences of those who are impacted by their ethical decisions.

Conversely, if an ethic of care is applied by a leader to the COVID-19 "return to work" dilemma, this leader will likely attempt to take into account the unique context of each individual worker and the unique needs and concerns of each follower. Leaders who cultivate a strong relationship with their followers will better understand these differences, have a stronger sense of empathy, and will be less likely to make a "return to work" decision that is universal in nature. In larger organizations, of course, this would be difficult and such a leader is likely to conclude that she or he can meet the spirit of the ethic of care by allowing individuals to determine for themselves whether or not to return to work. This option respects each individual and gives them the power and authority to chart their own course and determine their own future. The ethic of care is concerned with, and is evaluated by, its effects (Lawrence & Maitlis, 2012) and giving organizational members the freedom of choice in whether or not to return to work will likely lead to more satisfied followers who feel both empowered and respected. Nonetheless, making decisions in a manner that reflects the ethic of care is complicated by the cognitive framework that is currently prevalent. That is, we have a tendency to polarize issues into "good or bad", or "right or wrong", or "this or that" and this tendency fits nicely with a Kantian perspective on ethics where the ultimate goal is to search for and find a categorical imperative.

There is a moral flaw in absolutist ethical perspectives that completely disregard the individual, the circumstances, and the context. Decision-making under such perspectives starts and ends with the leader and shows little regard for the individual follower or the organizational member. One decision is made for all. Because of this, these ethical perspectives function to perpetuate highly centralized power structures. Decision-making based on the ethic of care, in contrast, considers the followers and organizational members and may lead to shared decision-making and shared power. It is no surprise, when viewed in this way, that the ethic of care is grounded in feminist thought. In a way, the ethic of care is on morally higher ground because it *is* what Kant's categorical imperative *is not*.

Conclusion

As stated in the introduction, the comparison of Kant's categorical imperative and Gilligan's ethic of care in this chapter is not intended to be an ethical guideline for leaders looking to resolve the "return to work" dilemma. Rather, it is a comparison between a particularly patriarchal way of thinking and decision-making in the Kantian categorical imperative and a particularly feminist way of thinking and decision-making in Gilligan's ethic of care. The thoughts and actions of leaders who make decisions regarding whether their employees should return to work during the pandemic may be reflective of the ideological contrast described in this chapter.

This comparison of Kant's categorical imperative and Gilligan's ethic of care is, on the surface, a conflict between absolutism or universalism and what may seem like relativism. Kant's categorical imperative is absolutist and does not allow for deviations. The ethic of care, on the other hand, demands openness to deviations through consideration of context. Is the ethic of care, then, pure relativism? No, it is always relative but also always bound by a deeper universal, possibly absolute, ethic.

Instead, the ethic of care is a blend of universalism and relativism. In fact, it actually exhibits some aspects of Kant's categorical imperative. For instance, the ethic of care allows us to have a choice on how to act just as Kant's categorical imperative demands. The ethic of care reflects what we already know as does Kant's categorical imperative. As in, we intuitively know that it is important to place high value on relationships and to never completely neglect the unique concerns and needs of each individual. The ethic of care can be expressed as a "rationally necessary command" or a categorical imperative (Cholbi, 2016, p. 14-15) which we must adopt. The continued existence of our *humanity* may be dependent on our willingness (or not) to accept Gilligan's premise. But Gilligan's ethic of care veers sharply away from Kant's categorical imperative and other such ethical perspectives with her concern for the unique individual along with the contexts and situations within which each individual exists. Leaders who are thinking about the "return to work" dilemma would do well to avoid the allure of being the all-powerful figure who makes one decision for all followers based purely on reason and that is detached from the worlds which each of us live in. Instead, leaders should take steps to learn about the many unique individuals that are their followers, to develop real and meaningful relationships with them, and to discover how they are experiencing the pandemic. This will provide such leaders with a solid foundation, not for making one decision regarding returning to work, but for collaborating with followers to make many such decisions.

References

Abdel-Baqui, O. (2022, March 2). Google sets its return to office plans for April 4. *Wall Street Journal,* https://www.wsj.com/articles/google-sets-its-return-to-office-plans-for-april-4-11646249204

Acton, H. B. (1970). *Kant's moral philosophy.* MacMillan.

Bernstein, J., Hutler, B., Reider, T., Faden, R., Han, H., & Barnhill, A. (2020, May 27). *An ethics framework for the COVID-19 reopening process* [working paper]. Johns Hopkins Berman Institute of Bioethics. http://bioethics.jhu.edu/wp-content/uploads/2019/10/FINAL-SF-Agora-Covid-19.pdf

Bunyan, R. (2022, March 31). Junior Goldman Sachs bankers whose salaries start at $110k threaten to quit over demands they return to the office five days a week. *DailyMail.com.* https://www.dailymail.co.uk/news/article-10672645/Junior-Goldman-Sachs-bankers-threaten-quit-demands-return-office-five-days-week.html

Cholbi, M. (2016). *Understanding Kant's ethics.* Cambridge University Press.

Ciulla, J. B. (2009). Leadership and the ethics of care. *Journal of Business Ethics, 88*(1), 3-4.

Cutter, C. (2022, March 1). Companies seize on March as a moment to reopen the office. *Wall Street Journal,* https://www.wsj.com/articles/companies-see-an-opening-for-office-reopening-11646130602?mod=article_inline

Deigh, J. (2010). *An introduction to ethics.* Cambridge University Press.

DePass, D. (2022, April 2). Stress mounts for Minnesota workers returning to the office. *Star Tribune*. https://www.startribune.com/stress-mounts-for-minnesota-workers-returning-to-the-office/600161625/

French, W., & Weis, A. (2000). An ethics of care or an ethics of justice. *Journal of Business Ethics, 27*(1/2), 125-136.

Gilligan, C. (1995). Hearing the difference: Theorizing connection. *Hypatia, 10*(2), 120-127.

Gilligan, C. (1982). *In a different voice: Psychological theory and women's development.* Harvard University Press.

Iafolla, R. (2022, May 4). Vaccine mandates at work part of 'new normal,' employers say. *Bloomberg Law*. https://news.bloomberglaw.com/daily-labor-report/vaccine-mandates-at-work-part-of-new-normal-employers-say

Japsen, B. (2022, February 2). Despite Supreme Court ruling, most employers implemented COVID vaccine mandates. *Forbes*. https://www.forbes.com/sites/brucejapsen/2022/02/02/despite-supreme-court-ruling-most-employers-forging-ahead-with-covid-vaccine-mandates/?sh=56d9042871af

Kelly, J. (2022, April 2). The great disconnect between bosses and workers. *Forbes*. https://www.forbes.com/sites/jackkelly/2022/04/02/the-great-disconnect-between-bosses-and-workers/?sh=79952c591411

Kidder, R. M. (1995). *How good people make tough choices.* William Morrow and Company.

Kim, H. (2015). *Kant and the foundations of morality.* Lexington Books.

Lawrence, T. B., & Maitlis, S. (2012). Care and possibility: Enacting an ethic of care through narrative practice. *Academy of Management Review, 37*(4), 641-663.

Lo, B. (2000). *Resolving ethical dilemmas: A guide for clinicians.* Lippincott Williams & Wilkins.

McCleskey, J. A. (2016). Emotional intelligence and the ethic of care. *Journal of Applied Management and Entrepreneurship, 21,* 118-132.

McManus, R. M., Ward, S. J., & Perry, A. K. (2018). *Ethical leadership: A primer.* Edward Elgar Publishing.

Noddings, N. (1984). *Caring: A feminine approach to ethics and moral education.* University of California Press.

Pennings, S., & Symons, X. (2021). Persuasion, not coercion or incentivisation, is the best means of promoting COVID-19 vaccination. *Journal of Medical Ethics, 47*(10), 709-711.

Peters, J. (2022, April 1). Activision Blizzard confirms vaccine mandate is over, employees will walk out April 4th. *The Verge.* https://www.theverge.com/2022/4/1/23007115/activision-blizzard-workers-walkout-vaccine-mandate-a-better-abk

Reichert, C. (2022, March 4). Google, Apple, Twitter reveal return to office policies. *C|Net Tech.* https://www.cnet.com/tech/google-apple-twitter-reveal-return-to-office-policies/

Simola, S. (2015). Understanding moral courage through a feminist and developmental ethic of care. *Journal of Business Ethics, 130*(1), 29-44.

Simola, S. (2003). Ethics of justice and care in corporate crisis management. *Journal of Business Ethics, 46*(4), 351-361.

Spur, B. (2022, March 13). Friction over the return to work is settling on a hated aspect of office life: Getting there. *Toronto Star.* https://www.thestar.com/news/gta/2022/03/13/friction-over-the-return-to-work-is-settling-on-a-hated-aspect-of-office-life-getting-there.html

Tangwa, G. B. (2004). Between universalism and relativism: A conceptual exploration of problems in formulating and applying international biomedical ethical guidelines. *Journal of Medical Ethics, 30,* 63-67.

EMPATHETIC OR DESTRUCTIVE? – IMPACT OF LEADERSHIP BEHAVIOR DURING A PANDEMIC AND ETHICS OF CARE

Karen Perham-Lippman[1] and Jimmy Payne[2]

Abstract: Leadership behaviors become amplified during any crisis and even more so when they are at a level like the COVID-19 global pandemic. Typically, greater focus is given to leaders at the apex of any crisis, and this is often true regardless of whether those crises are internal or external because considerable emotional and cognitive challenges must be faced (König et al., 2018). Furthermore, organizational culture and behavior generally start at the highest levels of leadership and conventionally flow outward, influencing other leaders within the organization. Throughout this chapter, we focus on both destructive and empathetic leadership behaviors at the highest levels of organizations and their impact on both followers and organizations during the COVID-19 pandemic. While the examples provided in this chapter include executives leading organizations, our discussion could be inferred to all levels of leadership. We focus on the behaviors of leaders with the understanding that leaders at all levels can have a profound impact on others during crises.

Introduction

With a total of 81,814,169 cases reported and 1,008,007 deaths in the United States (CDC, 2022) as well as 490,527,831 cases and 6,172,945 deaths worldwide (Worldometer, 2022) at the time of this writing, the recent COVID-19 pandemic certainly qualifies as a crisis on an expansive scale. Leaders in organizations everywhere had to adjust quickly to keep their followers as safe as possible and to ensure their organizations remained operational. With this in mind, we explore leader behaviors within organizations. In some cases, these behaviors led to damaging

---

[1] Adjunct Professor, Community College of Denver, Denver, Colorado, USA

[2] Program Manager for the Naval Sea Systems Command, Washington, DC, USA

effects, which we will discuss further in this chapter. König et al. (2018) suggest that leaders with empathy express emotional behavioral tendencies initiated by the distress others experience in a crisis. As such, Spatoula et al. (2019) asserted that leaders with empathy have the "capacity to understand or feel what another person is experiencing from within their frame of reference" (p. 902). This idea of empathy stemmed from Rothschild's (2006) discussion of how one's whole self-interacts with the phenomenon of empathy to further our understanding of what empathy actually is and how it affects all individuals involved. Behaviors such as empathy are essential skills that put leaders in others' shoes to thoroughly examine and realize their goals, motivations, fears, and priorities within their organization. Tran et al. (2020) summed it up this way, "how organizations treat employees during crises communicates the value they have for those they employ, with their actions potentially leaving lasting impressions that persist beyond the events" (p. 39). Leaders engaged in empathy do more than understand their followers; they ask why they feel the way they do about their experience. Leaders who display empathy display more relations-oriented behaviors versus task-oriented behaviors (Mahsud et al., 2010). As the pandemic has negatively impacted a global community, deep concern for the welfare of others expressed as protection alongside a desire to understand, develop and empower others is an essential value of ethical leaders (Mahsud et al., 2010). Values and behaviors can become amplified in some instances, and if this amplification occurs in a positive manner, then the better it is for everyone involved.

Ethics and empathy should work hand in hand daily, but if they do not, during a crisis specifically, the consequences may be felt negatively long after that crisis has passed. Vardarlier (2016) stated, "Since organizations cannot escape crises, they should be well prepared to reduce the effects" (p. 469). Ethical leaders pay close attention to how others are being, not just doing by developing and maintaining employee-centered environments within their organizations. Employers' treatment of individuals as professionals provokes a sense of loyalty and commitment to the group. The COVID pandemic presented a real test to many organizations' existing culture and climate, especially concerning the employer-employee relationships. When a leader implements a more humanistic Human Resource Management (HRM) practice, individuals feel more respected and calmer, thereby promoting an environment where they are less stressed and worried. Humanistic HRM focuses on the social well-being of individuals, their values, and needs; it is centered on how they can be made to feel more integrated into their organization. Arnaud and Wasieleski (2013) related this by describing a workplace that allows autonomy, stimulation, and trustworthiness and in which there is a focus on individuals as humans. Conveying empathy is representative of effective leadership which expresses sensitivity to employee burnout, creates a climate of support, and fosters successful performance outcomes (Gentry et al., 2016).

In contrast, severely limited empathetic behavior permits crises to escalate without preemptive action, facilitating negative outcomes. Furthermore, when destructive leadership is present within organizations, it adversely impacts members' well-being, leading to many issues such as health problems, emotional trauma, and psychological stress for individuals. Research shows that destructive leaders pursue personal goals through the control and coercion of others causing adverse effects on both individuals and organizations (Camgöz & Ekmecki, 2021; Northouse, 2021). Camgöz and Ekmecki (2021) point out that leaders who use negative means to serve themselves, despite positive intention to further performance, engage in coercive behaviors that may lead to destructive outcomes.

The pandemic has elucidated representative examples of empathetic and destructive leadership behaviors, highlighting how critical it is to explore and understand their individual implications. Leadership behaviors exhibiting empathy will be underscored in this chapter, along with comparative examples of destructive leader behaviors. This comparison will focus on how empathetic leaders develop and maintain employee-centered environments within their organizations during a crisis, leading to the treatment of individuals as professionals and provoking a sense of loyalty and commitment to the group. Conversely, examples of destructive leadership behaviors will illustrate how the devastating impacts of crises like the COVID-19 pandemic are further exacerbated.

The Complex Interaction Between Leadership and Crisis Management

A complex crisis such as the COVID-19 pandemic is an extremely dynamic event that has impeded normal functioning within organizations leading to unexpected and disruptive outcomes with profound implications. As the pandemic has transitioned from an acute phase to a steady multi-year march across the globe, its impacts remind us of the critical role that leaders play in dealing with unexpected crises. Leaders' position of influence and their success under crises is largely dependent upon their ability to be adaptive in their response, effectively managing followers' expectations and alleviating anxiety (Bundy et al., 2016). Crises present a tremendous challenge that reveals leader efficacy through their readiness to learn from others while simultaneously pursuing self-improvement (Chiu et al., 2016). Bauman's (2011) evaluation of ethical approaches to crisis leadership argues that an ethics of care approach most effectively guides leaders' ability to reduce the impact of harm on others due to its emphasis on deepening relationships. Centered on the formation of relationships and the fostering of their development, the ethics of care approach places value "upon the connections that bind us to other people" (Linsley & Slack, 2013, p. 286). Gilligan (1995) asserts that its origin is a feminine ethic of care that "begins with connection, theorized as primary and seen as fundamental in human life" such that recognizing the interdependence of our lives is critical (p. 122). The application of this approach is not only an awareness of the necessity for maintaining connection but also the conscientiousness that one's actions have an impact on how others feel (Bauman, 2011; Linsley & Slack, 2013). Empathy is the emotional reaction elicited when we are oriented toward others' needs (Batson et al., 2002) and Held (2006) suggests that this emotion is cohered with an ethic of care. Furthermore, Slote (2007) argues that empathy "plays a determinative role" in the development of an ethics of care approach (p. 12). Bauman (2011) posited that this approach is most suited for managing crises as it "requires leaders to manage the complexity and human relationships that are part of a crisis" (p. 288). In the case of the COVID-19 pandemic, there are examples of leader behaviors toward followers or employees that illustrate both an empathetic approach and a destructive approach and these will be explored in the context of an ethic of care.

Employee Retention in the COVID-19 Crisis

The environmental disruptions organizations have faced, given the economic and social turbulence caused by the pandemic, have catalyzed the necessity for change at an organizational and individual level. Leaders who propel the commitment of organizational members through a focus on culture and values that are relationship-centered will simultaneously redefine organizational success in the future. As such leaders at all levels must reimagine their role within organizations amid the turmoil of the pandemic in order to rethink a multitude of strategies, including effective human resource management that considers the impact that environmental trends have on both the individuals and organizations going forward. The practice of human resource management has evolved from a focus on specific functions such as selection, appraisal, compensation, and training to better understand how these elements may collectively enable strategic management (Wright & Snell, 1991). Boselie et al.'s (2005) research highlighted the relevance of human resource management in relation to the resource-based view (RBV) theoretical framework in which it complements internal systems responding effectively to organizational environments. Despite many insights gained by Boselie et al. (2005), they were quick to point out that while human resource management is understood as activities related to the management of employees there is a rich diversity of interpretations of the practice in general. Difficulties in identifying the consistent application of human resource management historically still exist, which Lucas and Grant (2018) suggest is due to underestimation of its complexity owing to competition exerting pressure for performance with fewer resources and a consistently evolving workforce. McGuire et al. (2021) argue that moving past a resource-based view to focus on employee-centered Human Resource Development (HRD) practice with an ethics of care approach in post-pandemic workplaces provides the foundation for addressing the complexity of individual needs within organizations. Effective human resource management recognizes that the most essential element for success within organizations is the people.

While some employers are actively recruiting amidst the pandemic's disruption, others are reducing the workforce. This concept is particularly relevant as employers consider methods to improve and reinvent the way employees work and their human resource strategies for attraction, selection, and retention. More than 81% of current candidates in the job market are seeking employers focused on company culture and value (Ryan, 2020). With the increased complexity of the COVID-19 crisis, being intentional about demonstrating understanding and care as an organizational value is not only the right thing to do but also a business imperative. Post-COVID workplaces that encourage transformation rather than reform as a reevaluation of their HRD must adopt an ethics of care approach that considers employees' individual well-being needs within organizations (McGuire et al., 2021). While organizations continue to address challenges in identifying and hiring the right talent through this crisis, having effective retention measures is equally important. "Beyond the cost of hiring and training replacements, turnover hurts performance because newcomers' lack of experience, skills and local knowledge increases errors and reduces efficiency" (Kacmar et al., 2006, as cited in Bolman & Deal, 2017, p. 140).

Maintaining a relationship with employees that ensures the retention of talent during change is critically important. A recent McKinsey study surveying employee experience during the coronavirus pandemic found that employees with remote work options felt greater trust and affiliation towards their organizations when companies were perceived as responding effectively with attention to their safety and security needs (Emmett et al., 2020). Furthermore, a recent survey of nearly 900 US-based employees across industries during COVID-19 utilizing the relational empathy (CARE) measure (Mercer et al., 2004) showed that empathetic leadership was found to contribute to both inclusive workplace experiences and employee retention (Bommel, 2021). Bommel's (2021) research found that the presence of senior leaders modeling empathy predicted reduced employee intent to leave due to their greater visibility in organizations. Emmet et al. (2020) suggest building on the trust employers have earned by continuing empathy and communication, embedding change management plans beyond crisis intervention, and personalizing the employee experience journey. A leadership culture that communicates well-being across all levels of the organization centered on fostering empathy for employees will contribute to successful retention goals. In this chapter, we make an argument for reducing destructive leadership behaviors and fostering empathetic leadership behaviors to improve organizational retention outcomes during crises like the global pandemic.

Destructive Leadership and Ethics of Care in a Crisis

Destructive leadership has increasingly been referred to as a hypernym for toxic, abusive, unethical, and bad (Northouse, 2021; Thoroughgood, 2021). More recently, it has been defined as a process in which goals are pursued by an individual through the control and coercion of others for personal gain regardless of potentially negative impact on the organization or its individuals (Northouse, 2021). Destructive leadership has been shown to consistently result in detrimental outcomes for which unethical behaviors such as dishonesty, lack of accountability or transparency, misuse of power, and a focus on self-interest are integral (Camgöz & Ekmekci, 2021). While not all destructive leaders are necessarily unethical, the two often work in concert with each other. Zheng et al. (2021) identified a moderating effect of unethical leadership on individuals' feelings of empowerment and behavior. Behavior that is aggressive, narcissistic, and overbearing is characteristic of destructive leaders, though not all leaders exhibit these same behaviors all the time. Given the turmoil and stress that crises create for both organizations and individuals, the presence of destructive leadership only serves to exacerbate existing challenges. According to the Society of Human Resource Management failed leadership has resulted in workplace toxicity and high turnover, leading to over $223 billion in costs due to the loss of 20% of U.S. workers in the past five years (*Purpose. People. Progress. Insights on Culture in a Time of Uncertainty*, 2020). This is extremely concerning given the increase in the prevalence of toxic leadership. Matos (2017) research surveying 1,000 college-educated U.S. employees found that 56% of participants reported their leader is toxic and 73% of employees that worked for highly toxic leaders expressed the intent to leave.

Within the ethic of care framework, Giacalone and Promislo (2013) define ethical behavior as actions that foster the well-being of others through caring while simultaneously preventing undue harm. Furthermore, they point out that ethics of care stands in stark contrast to self-focused behaviors. During crises, internal and external expectations that leaders mitigate associated harms increase exponentially. Nevertheless, research indicates that conditions characterized by extreme stress contribute to leadership behavior that is destructive (Brandebo, 2020). Research by Sull, Sull, & Zweig (2022) to determine attrition predictors associated with the pandemic's Great Resignation, reviewed 34 million online employee profiles identifying a sample of nearly 25% of employees from U.S. for-profit based companies and found that 22% of employees left their jobs due to organizational culture. Furthermore, outcomes indicated that white-collar and blue-collar sectors were equally affected with toxic culture, such that it was 10 times more powerful than compensation at predicting employee turnover (Sull, Sull, & Zweig, 2022). The primary elements contributing to organizational toxic culture included unethical behavior, employees feeling disrespected, and a lack of diversity, equity, and inclusion. In their follow up research Sull, Sull, Cipolli, et al. (2022) analyzed 1.3 million company reviews on Glassdoor given by U.S. employees across 40 different industries finding that disrespectful, non-inclusive, unethical, cutthroat, and abusive management are the primary attributes of toxic culture leading to employee attrition during the Great Resignation. In the case of abusive management, leaders described as engaging in bullying, disparaging and hostile behaviors contributed to perceptions of toxic workplace culture (Sull, Sull, Cipolli, et al., 2022).

During the pandemic, April Koh, the CEO, and co-founder of Spring Health, a 2-billion-dollar startup, has been described as having destroyed her employees' mental health by driving a culture of workaholism and fear (Russell, 2021a). Ironically, employees at Spring Health were providing mental health services to their client companies during the pandemic while experiencing both systemic and detrimental burnout themselves. Schmid et al. (2019) define leaders prioritizing their needs over others through self-interest as a construct of destructive leadership termed exploitative. In the case of Spring Health, Koh's intense selfish ambition to move fast in meeting customer demand during the pandemic crisis was described as deceitful by her employees. Especially given that employees were coaching clients on burnout while being forced to work innumerable hours (Russell, 2021a). Negative outcomes of Koh's destructive behavior towards employees during the COVID-19 crisis resulted in dozens of employees quitting due to an organizational environment in which they felt pressured to work even when they were personally sick with coronavirus (Russell, 2021b). Reina et al. (2017) found that leaders who use pressure as an influence tactic reduce resource availability thereby inducing stress which leads to increased employee turnover. Self-interest that incites manipulative influence pressure and the overburdening of already overloaded employees is exemplative of exploitative leadership behaviors (Schmid et al., 2019). According to Lipman-Blumen (2007) manipulation, unethical behaviors, and lack of empathy typify behaviors of toxic leaders. Koh's zealous growth at any cost approach to leadership at Spring Health manifested in a sense of urgency such that she prioritized her goals over that of her employees. Overly goal-focused leaders manifested over-controlling leadership, a behavior that followers perceived as destructive (Brandebo, 2020). In the case of Koh's destructive leadership behaviors, she later acknowledged her behavior, which was followed by an apology along with a pledge to take action to develop a "people philosophy" framework that now measures how company policies will affect employees before adoption (Russell, 2021b).

Empathetic Leadership and Ethics of Care in a Crisis

Empathetic leaders display behaviors that are more people-oriented, and as such, they generally take time to connect more deeply with organizational members (König et al., 2018). Furthermore, leaders who engage in empathy express understanding for employees' thoughts, perspectives, and emotions through care and concern (Clark et al., 2019). Batson (2017) argues that when we experience altruistic motivation, we "positively value a person's welfare" (p. 167). This empathetic concern is consistent with placing value on how different events affect others (Batson, 2017). Mahsud et al. (2010) identify the behavior of altruism as a key component of ethical leadership. While all leaders must face the challenges of being both ethical and effective in their role, this has never been more relevant than during the coronavirus pandemic. Ciulla (2009) suggests that leaders who place emphasis on their attention to duty by being a source of comfort are engaged in ethics of care. As such, leader empathy may also be considered key to effective ethical leadership.

As the coronavirus pandemic was becoming a global crisis, Slack's CEO, Stewart Butterfield, transitioned in-person events for global offices to a virtual format in early March 2020 and implemented company-wide travel restrictions (Butterfield, 2020). Butterfield also quickly closed more than 16 office locations in nine countries, shifting all employees to remote work (Butterfield, 2020). Employee webinars and virtual consultations were launched for remote workers with a focus on employee health and safety. Within a few short weeks, the employees at Slack were prepared for the potential impact of COVID-19 by developing a collective sense of purpose, and a shared vision and objectives for their work which drove the collaboration necessary to weather pandemic associated challenges (Butterfield, 2020). In the face of a crisis such as the pandemic, this expands on the vision of the organization which states "[Slack] is a world where organizational agility is easy to achieve regardless of an institution's size and that agility is what we aim for ourselves" (Butterfield, 2020, p. 30). As employees established new norms for their availability, Butterfield (2020) praised Slack's acceptance of the workplace changes forced upon companies due to COVID-19's impact through acknowledgment of children, pets, and families appearing in the background of virtual leadership and employee meetings. Butterfield's empathetic approach to doing business and its core principle of focusing on feedback from employees played a role in its evolution of success amidst the pandemic's global health crisis. In 2021, Slack was acquired by Salesforce, led by CEO Marc Benioff, who similarly reports leading his organization with a focus on empathy and understanding the needs of employees. Corker (2020) describes Salesforce leadership as "audience-centric" or putting the "audience at the heart of everything" by understanding who the audience is, which requires empathy.

Leaders who are understanding and empathetic to the challenges individuals face exemplify a more humanistic approach to human resources management. Zenger and Folkman (2016) refer to the contagious nature of leader behaviors as catalyzing a "trickle-down effect of both good and bad leadership" across organizational management levels. Suppose leaders discount the humanistic approach to employee management, their followers will likely discount the approach in an equivalent manner. Furthermore, empathy generates interest in, and appreciation of, others. It paves the way to more productive working relationships. Therefore, empathy is more than just a tool of management to be learned alongside other techniques for the ethical leader. It is a significant way of being and acting; it helps leaders work across organizational and cultural boundaries. Empathy helps one better understand people with different perspectives and experiences. Crises such as the pandemic have highlighted the critical need for empathy to facilitate adaptation and organizational change.

Implications for Practice and Future Research

Predictably destructive leaders are often perceived as reassuring in the face of crises, especially if followers pledge allegiance to them. Regardless of the mounting evidence that illustrates profoundly negative outcomes, there continue to be destructive leaders engaged in behaviors that destroy both employees and the organizational climate. Brandebo (2020) describes several archetypes of the destructive leader in crises management, which include the perfect commander, or one who is believed by their followers to be a "hero that saves the situation" (p. 569). Lipman-Blumen (2007) refers to these toxic leaders as those that we believe will slay dragons ensuring that we may sleep peacefully once again. Our fatal attraction to these leaders is based on the human desire to feel a sense of belonging which inherently drives our willingness to forgo our freedom by engaging in unwavering followership (Lipman-Blumen, 2007). Even though employees in Matos' (2017) study reported experiencing destructive leaders engaged in manipulative, demoralizing, and sabotaging behaviors, a significant percentage of those working for these leaders were still highly engaged. Matos (2017) suggested that this may be the case because "highly toxic leaders quickly reduce engagement for those who are not intrinsically devoted to their jobs and disengaged employees then turnover rapidly, leaving behind their more intrinsically motivated counterparts" (p. 11). This may have been the case for those employees who remained with Koh serving under her leadership despite so many other employees that made the choice to leave. Matos (2017) points out that if we don't speak more openly about the nature and impact of toxic culture in our workplaces employees will be left to wonder if their individual "experiences qualified as toxic behavior worthy of intervention" (p. 17). For Koh, the detrimental impact on her followers and her organization led her to express regret. According to Lipman-Blumen (2017) crises produce ideal environments for leaders who may under any other circumstance be sensible and nontoxic to then become toxic. Research has shown positive correlations between unethical and destructive leaders and the followers' emotional exhaustion, thereby negatively affecting organizational performance (Narjes & Mohsen, 2019). Expanding on this research through both qualitative and longitudinal studies could help to elucidate the nature of follower engagement and disengagement towards destructive leaders over time. It could also promote increased understanding of leader behaviors that seem constructive under normal conditions and destructive during crises.

Addressing destructive leaders and toxic cultures will not be solved overnight and may be especially challenging in the midst of the existing turmoil found during crises as in short-term engagements destructive leaders are often successful (Matos, 2017). This may be further exacerbated by the fact that destructive leaders cluster followers that are supportive, thereby reducing the potential for replacements within organizational talent pipelines. Mitigation efforts to address destructive leadership can improve employee retention outcomes during crises. Matos (2017) recommends being honest about the existing culture that may be driving or tolerating toxic behaviors, conducting a third-party analysis to assess existing culture and leadership performance, and improving succession planning to address the gaps created by burnt-out followers that leave.

In practical application, ethical leadership conducted in an empathetic manner during a crisis can aid in the retention of an organization's people. Conducting operations in this manner makes people feel seen and heard, and therefore they feel integral to the organization's goals and mission. Leadership development with a focus on ethics, empathy, and crisis management should be implemented to aid in dealing with existing and future crises. Improved leader enablement for dealing with the problems that arise should include expanded learning and development focused on empathy for all organizational levels. This development would benefit those impacted both internally and externally. Reinforcement of empathetic behaviors with long-term checks incorporated into reward structures that promote employee well-being and encourage upward feedback would foster a more positive empathetic organizational culture (Matos, 2017).

Gentry et al. (2016) apply the concept that "empathy can be learned" (p. 7), allowing ethical leaders, or any leader for that matter, the ability to grow. Expanding on the idea of leaders learning empathy through ethics of care, Bauman (2011) points out that leaders can ease the damage of a crisis by following "the AAA strategy: Acknowledge, Apologize, and Act" (p. 290). Putting this into practice could aid organizations in dealing with future crises. While often the apology portion of the AAA strategy might seem out of place, in situations such as COVID-19, where an organizational leader might not be the cause of the crisis, it may aid the leader's expression of empathy for their followers through acknowledgment of their experiences. Though not crucial in the middle of a crisis, the more learned behaviors a leader has in their repertoire, the better they will be able to manage a given situation.

Conclusion

Empathetic leaders remain flexible in times of crisis and exhibit behaviors that create an environment for all involved to remain willing to engage in and contribute to the mission. Doing this in a supportive versus destructive means only benefits everyone involved. Vardarlier (2016) suggests that an increase in training and professional development might aid in retaining employees even during a crisis. Maak et al. (2021) purported that this pandemic uncovered the idea that responsible leadership during a crisis requires sustained engagement, and a willingness to change, from leaders everywhere. Furthermore, crisis response requires leaders to understand followers' emotional needs. Failure to reduce destructive leadership behaviors and a failure to "foster ties that bind social groups together and enable them to endure crises" will also lead to failure in preventing the "catastrophic loss of human life" (Maak et al., 2021, p. 25). Leaders can instill hope and create human moments in affected areas, helping to establish a relational foundation for widespread support for crisis countermeasures.

The examples presented in this chapter illustrate the need for an ethics of care approach with the enablement of empathetic leader behaviors and mitigation of destructive leader behaviors to address negative outcomes during crises. Both empathetic and destructive leadership within the literature require continued research and understanding. Organizational crises are inevitable, yet those on the scale of the COVID-19 pandemic are uncommon. However, in this case, it will have a profound impact on our global community for decades to come. The nature of the pandemic we are currently living through teaches us that a crisis can erupt at any moment and have a profound global impact even in relatively remote areas. Since organizations cannot escape this potential, they must be better prepared to reduce the potential negative effects caused by crises to ensure the best possible outcomes for their people. Leaders who recognize that crises are unavoidable occurrences and adapt accordingly to engage in, or attempt to learn, empathetic leadership behaviors take positive steps towards retaining and valuing their greatest resource, their people.

References

Arnaud, S., & Wasieleski, D. M. (2013). Corporate humanistic responsibility: Social performance through managerial discretion of the HRM. *Journal of Business Ethics, 120*(3), 313-334. https://doi.org/10.1007/s10551-013-1652-z

Batson, C. D., Ahmad, N., Lishner, D. A., & Tsang, J.-A. (2002). Empathy and altruism. In C. R. Snyder & S. J. Lopez (Eds.), *Handbook of Positive Psychology* (pp. 1–829). Oxford University Press.

Batson, C. D. (2017). Empathy and altruism. In K. W. Brown & M. R. Leary (Eds.), *The Oxford handbook of hypo-egoic phenomena* (pp. 1–318). Oxford University Press.

Bauman, D. C. (2011). Evaluating ethical approaches to crisis leadership: Insights from unintentional harm research. *Journal of Business Ethics*, *98*(2), 281–295. https://doi.org/10.1007/s10551-010-0549-3

Bolman, L. G., & Deal, T. E. (2017). *Reframing organizations: Artistry, choice, and leadership* (6th ed.). Jossey-Bass.

Bommel, T. V. (2021). *The power of empathy in times of crisis and beyond (Report)*. Catalyst. https://www.catalyst.org/reports/empathy-work-strategy-crisis/

Boselie, P., Dietz, G., & Boon, C. (2005). Commonalities and contradictions in HRM and performance research. *Human Resource Management Journal, 15*(3), 67–94. https://doi.org/10.1111/j.1748-8583.2005.tb00154.x

Brandebo, M. F. (2020). Destructive leadership in crisis management. *Leadership & Organization Development Journal, 41*(4), 567–580. https://doi.org/10.1108/lodj-02-2019-0089

Bundy, J., Pfarrer, M. D., Short, C. E., & Coombs, W. T. (2016). Crises and crisis management: Integration, interpretation, and research development. *Journal of Management, 43*(6), 1661–1692. https://doi.org/10.1177/0149206316680030

Butterfield, S. (2020). The CEO of Slack on adapting in response to a global crisis. *Harvard Business Review, 98*(4), 30-35.

Camgöz, S. M., & Ekmekci, O. T. (Eds.). (2021). *Destructive leadership and management hypocrisy: Advances in theory and practice*. Emerald Publishing.

CDC. (2022, February 9). *COVID data tracker weekly review*. Centers for Disease Control and Prevention. https://www.cdc.gov/coronavirus/2019-ncov/covid-data/covidview/index.html

Chiu, C.-Y. C., Owens, B. P., & Tesluk, P. E. (2016). Initiating and utilizing shared leadership in teams: The role of leader humility, team proactive personality, and team performance capability. *Journal of Applied Psychology, 101*(12), 1705–1720. https://doi.org/10.1037/apl0000159

Ciulla, J. B. (2009). Leadership and the ethics of care. *Journal of Business Ethics, 88*(1), 3–4. https://doi.org/10.1007/s10551-009-0105-1

Clark, M. A., Robertson, M. M., & Young, S. (2019). "I feel your pain": A critical review of organizational research on empathy. *Journal of Organizational Behavior, 40*(2), 166–192. https://doi.org/10.1002/job.2348

Corker, J. (2020, December 18). *Why empathy matters*. Salesforce Blog; Salesforce.com. https://www.salesforce.com/eu/blog/2020/12/why-empathy-matters.html

Emmett, J., Schrah, G., Schrimper, M., & Wood, A. (2020). COVID-19 and the employee experience: How leaders can seize the moment. *Organization Practice*.

Gentry, W. A., Weber, T. J., & Sadri, G. (2016). *Empathy in the workplace a tool for effective leadership* (p. 1–14). Center for Creative Leadership.

Giacalone, R., & Promislo, M. (2013). Broken when entering: The stigmatization of goodness and business ethics education. *Academy of Management Learning & Education, 12*(1), 86–101. https://doi.org/http://dx.doi.org/10.5465/amle.2011.0005

Gilligan, C. (1995). Hearing the difference: Theorizing Connection. *Hypatia, 10*(2), 120–127. https://doi.org/10.1111/j.1527-2001.1995.tb01373.x

Gorgenyi-Hegyes, E., Nathan, R. J., & Fekete-Farkas, M. (2021). Workplace health promotion, employee well-being and loyalty during COVID-19 pandemic— large scale empirical evidence from Hungary. *Economies, 9*(2), 55. https://doi.org/10.3390/economies9020055

Held, V. (2006). *The ethics of care: Personal, political, and global* (pp. 1–222). Oxford University Press.

König, A. S., Graf-Vlachy, L., Bundy, J. N., & Little, L. (2018). A blessing and a curse: How CEOs' empathy affects their management of organizational crises. *Academy of Management Review, 45*(1), 130-153. https://doi.org/10.5465/amr.2017.0387

Linsley, P. M., & Slack, R. E. (2013). Crisis Management and an ethic of care: The case of Northern Rock Bank. *Journal of Business Ethics, 113*(2), 285–295. https://doi.org/10.1007/s10551-012-1304-8

Lipman-Blumen, J. (2007). *The allure of toxic leaders: Why we follow destructive bosses and corrupt politicians--and how we can survive them*. Oxford University Press.

Lucas, M., & Grant, J. (2018). *Strategic human resource management: Perspectives, implementation and challenges*. Hauppauge: Nova Science Publishers, Inc.

Maak, T., Pless, N. M., & Wohlgezogen, F. (2021). The fault lines of leadership: Lessons from the global COVID-19 crisis. *Journal of Change Management, 21*(1), 1–21. https://doi.org/10.1080/14697017.2021.1861724

Mahsud, R., Yukl, G., & Prussia, G. (2010). Leader empathy, ethical leadership, and relations-oriented behaviors as antecedents of leader-member exchange quality. *Journal of Managerial Psychology, 25*(6), 561-577. https://doi.org/10.1108/02683941011056932

Matos, K. (2017). *Toxic leadership: Detoxifying your culture and encouraging more mindful leadership*. 15Be.

McGuire, D., Germain, M.-L., & Reynolds, K. (2021). Reshaping HRD in light of the COVID-19 Pandemic: An ethics of care approach. *Advances in Developing Human Resources, 23*(1), 152342232097342. https://doi.org/10.1177/1523422320973426

Narjes, A., & Mohsen, G. (2019). Relationship between unethical and destructive leadership with emotional exhaustion and job performance. *Ethics in Science & Technology, 14*(3), 63–70.

Northouse, P. G. (2021). *Introduction to leadership: Concepts and practice* (5th ed.). SAGE Publications, Inc.

Purpose. People. Progress. Insights on culture in a time of uncertainty. (2020). Association of Executive Search and Leadership Consultants.

Reina, C. S., Rogers, K. M., Peterson, S. J., Byron, K., & Hom, P. W. (2017). Quitting the boss? The role of manager influence tactics and employee emotional engagement in voluntary turnover. *Journal of Leadership & Organizational Studies, 25*(1), 5–18. https://doi.org/10.1177/1548051817709007

Rothschild, B. (2006). *Help for the helper: The psychophysiology of compassion fatigue and vicarious trauma.* WW Norton & Company.

Russell, M. (2021a, November 22). April Koh built a $2 billion mental-health startup by age 29. Current and former employees say she led a fast-paced culture that created panic and fear. *Business Insider.* https://www.businessinsider.com/spring-health-april-koh-mental-health-startup-culture-burnout-quitting-2021-11

Russell, M. (2021b, December 7). After dozens of employees quit, Spring Health CEO April Koh says she's now focused on harmonizing hypergrowth with mental health. *Business Insider.* https://www.businessinsider.com/spring-health-ceo-april-koh-slush-interview-startup-culture-2021-12

Ryan, R. (2020, May 27). How the coronavirus is changing hiring and recruiting going forward. *Forbes.* https://www.forbes.com/sites/robinryan/2020/05/27/how-the-coronavirus-is-changing-hiring-and-recruiting-going-forward/#4434dda15ce4

Schmid, E. A., Pircher Verdorfer, A., & Peus, C. V. (2014). Shedding light on leaders' self-interest: Theory and measurement of exploitative leadership. *Academy of Management Annual Meeting Proceedings, 2014*(1), 1.

Slote, M. (2007). *The ethics of care and empathy*. Routledge.

Spatoula, V., Panagopoulou, E., & Montgomery, A. (2019). Does empathy change during undergraduate medical education? – A meta-analysis. *Medical Teacher*, *41*(8), 895–904. https://doi.org/10.1080/0142159x.2019.1584275

Sull, D., Sull, C., & Zweig, B. (2022, January 11). Toxic culture is driving the great resignation. *MIT Sloan Management Review*. https://sloanreview.mit.edu/article/toxic-culture-is-driving-the-great-resignation/

Sull, D., Sull, C., Cipolli, W., & Brighenti, C. (2022, March 16). Why every leader needs to worry about toxic culture. *MIT Sloan Management Review*. https://sloanreview.mit.edu/article/why-every-leader-needs-to-worry-about-toxic-culture/

Thoroughgood, C. (2021). Destructive leadership: Explaining, critiquing, and moving beyond leader-centric perspectives. In S. M. Camgoz & O. T. Ekmekci (Eds.), *Destructive Leadership and Management Hypocrisy* (pp. 1–286). Emerald Publishing.

Tran, H., Hardie, S., & Cunningham, K. M. (2020). Leading with empathy and humanity: Why talent-centered education leadership is especially critical amidst the pandemic crisis. *International Studies in Educational Administration (Commonwealth Council for Educational Administration & Management [CCEAM])*, *48*(1), 39-45.

Vardarlier, P. (2016). Strategic approach to human resources management during crisis. *Procedia, Social and Behavioral Sciences, 235*, 463-472.

Worldometer. (2022, February 12). *Coronavirus toll update: Cases & deaths by country*. Worldometers. https://www.worldometers.info/coronavirus/

Wright, P. M., & Snell, S. A. (1991). Toward an integrative view of strategic human resource management. *Human Resource Management Review, 1*(3), 203–225. https://doi.org/10.1016/1053-4822(91)90015-5

Zenger, J., & Folkman, J. (2016, January 14). The trickle-down effect of good (and bad) leadership. *Harvard Business Review*. https://hbr.org/2016/01/the-trickle-down-effect-of-good-and-bad-leadership

Zheng, F., Khan, N. A., & Khan, M. W. A. (2021). Unethical leadership and employee extra-role behavior in information technology sector: A moderated mediation analysis. *Frontiers in Psychology, 12,* 708016-708016. https://doi.org/ 10.3389/fpsyg.2021.708016

CONTRIBUTOR BIOGRAPHIES

Janis Balda, J.D., Ph.D., is Senior Lecturer in International Business at the Robert C. Vackar College of Business and Entrepreneurship, University of Texas Rio Grande Valley where she also teaches international law and global leadership and sustainability. With a broad background in international law, she has worked on legal issues in over 20 countries addressing a variety of matters related to human resources, international development, contract management, intellectual property, organizational structure, and real property law. She has addressed concerns as both a practitioner and an educator, seeking to examine alternative perspectives for problem solving and dispute resolution. In her twenty-year career as a professor, she developed business school programs and taught in Brazil, the Caribbean, South Texas, and rural Maine. Her degrees include law degrees from both Loyola University, Los Angeles, and Cambridge University, U.K., as well as a master's degree in management (studying under Peter F. Drucker), and doctoral degree from Claremont Graduate University, CA. Janis is a member of the International Leadership Association (ILA) Board of Directors and serves as its Vice-Chair. From addressing logistics of the drought in Ethiopia to facilitating human resource negotiations in the Philippines, she has advanced her understanding of ways to navigate the tensions inherent in resource-constrained communities.

Dr. Islam Borinca is a Lecturer/Assistant Professor in the School of Psychology, University College Dublin (Ireland). He obtained his doctorate degree in Social Psychology from the Universities of Geneva and Lausanne (Switzerland) as a Ph.D. Scholarship Excellence Recipient on an individual Ph.D. project sponsored by the Swiss Federal Commission for Scholarships for Foreign Students. Afterward, he worked as a teaching/research assistant at the Center Emile Bernheim, Université Libre de Bruxelles (Belgium). Following that, he conducted his postdoctoral research at the University of Limerick (Ireland). His research focuses on intergroup relations, specifically examining help, contact, and group norms, with an emphasis on emotions, empathy, dehumanization, meta-dehumanization, intergroup apologies, prejudice, and discrimination in hostile and non-hostile contexts. He also investigates gender norms, gender roles, and behaviors. In addition, his research examines intragroup processes regarding threats, expectations, and health.

Zamumtima Chijere, Ph.D., has been a noteworthy leader, educator, and a social entrepreneur in Malawi for over 15 years. He is a co-founder and Executive Director of RiseMalawi Ministries, an organization that works on improving the plight of marginalized young people and children in Malawi. He is also a college professor at African Bible Colleges where he is the Director of Graduate Studies. He also heads the Quality Assurance department at the College. Dr. Chijere graduated salutatorian from African Bible College, Malawi in 2007. He holds a MSc. in Leadership and Change Management from Leeds Metropolitan University (UK) under Leeds School of Business and Law. He obtained a Ph.D. in Organizational Leadership from Eastern University (USA). He grew up in the capital city of Malawi, but currently he does most of his work in the rural villages in the central part of Malawi. His aspiration is to see more educated young men and women from rural communities in Malawi where poverty and injustice is so high. Dr. Chijere has founded a high school for the underprivileged and is in the process of establishing a vocational training school for high school graduates in rural Malawi.

James F. Childress is University Professor Emeritus at the University of Virginia where he was the John Allen Hollingsworth Professor of Ethics, Professor of Religious Studies, Professor of Public Policy, and Professor of Research in Medical Education in the School of Medicine. He is currently a member of the core faculty of the Center for Health Humanities and Ethics in the School of Medicine. Professor Childress was the founding director of the Institute for Practical Ethics and Public Life and is the author of numerous articles and several books in biomedical ethics and in other areas of ethics. His books in biomedical ethics include Principles of Biomedical Ethics (with Tom L. Beauchamp), now in its 8th edition and translated into several languages; Priorities in Biomedical Ethics; Who Should Decide? Paternalism in Health Care; and Practical Reasoning in Bioethics. He is also co-editor of Belmont Revisited: Ethical Principles for Biomedical Research (with Eric Meslin and Harold Shapiro), and Organ Donation: Opportunities for Action (with Catharyn Liverman). He received his B.A. from Guilford

College, his B.D. from Yale Divinity School, and his M.A. and Ph.D. from Yale University.

Bethany Huxford Davis, Ph.D. serves as dean of academic operations and teaches in the College of Business & Leadership at Point University in Georgia. Her research interests include workplace faith integration and work-life balance equations. She brings 20 years of experience in nonprofit and higher education administration to her research lens and believes her best writing is done with a dog sitting near her desk.

Elena Falcettoni, Ph.D., is an Economist at the Board of Governors of the Federal Reserve System in Washington, DC and she sits on the Board of Directors of the Federal Reserve Federal Credit Union. Dr. Falcettoni is also an Affiliate Scholar at the Heller-Hurwicz Economics Institute (HHEI). She collaborates with HHEI on policy briefs and she is one of the mentors for the Women in Economics program in collaboration with the Department of Economics at the University of Minnesota. Dr. Falcettoni researches topics in health economics, affordable housing, and inequality across the United States. Her work has been presented in several conferences and seminars around the world and featured in the media multiple times. For her policy work at the Board, Dr. Falcettoni leads data collections and analyzes industry trends in the debit card industry to provide key insights which inform policy-making decisions. She also participates in some international work groups, including one of the groups working on the G20 roadmap for enhancing cross-border payments. Prior to joining the Federal Reserve, Dr. Falcettoni earned her Ph.D. in Economics at the University of Minnesota, where she also obtained her M.A. in Economics. From 2016 to 2019, she worked at the Federal Reserve Bank of Minneapolis. She also holds an M.Sc. and B.Sc. in Finance from Bocconi University (Milan, Italy), where she graduated at the top of her class.

Helene D. Gayle, MD, MPH, president of Spelman College, previously served as president and CEO of The Chicago Community Trust, one of the nation's leading community foundations. Under her leadership, the Trust adopted a new strategic focus on closing the racial and ethnic wealth gap in the Chicago region. Dr. Gayle was president and CEO of CARE, a leading international humanitarian organization. An expert on global development, humanitarian, and health issues, she spent 20 years with the Centers for Disease Control, working primarily on HIV/AIDS. She worked at the Bill & Melinda Gates Foundation, directing programs on HIV/AIDS and other global health issues. Dr. Gayle serves on public company and nonprofit boards, including The Coca-Cola Company, Organon, Palo Alto Networks, Brookings Institution, Center for Strategic and International Studies, New America, ONE Campaign, Federal Reserve Bank of Chicago, and Economic Club of Chicago. She is a member of the American Academy of Arts and Sciences, Council on Foreign Relations, Alpha Omega Alpha Medical Honor Society, National Academy of Medicine, American Public Health Association, National Medical Association, and American Academy of Pediatrics. She was awarded the Chicago Mayor's Medal of Honor for her work on Chicago's COVID relief and recovery. Named one of Forbes' "100 Most Powerful Women" and one of NonProfit Times "Power and Influence Top 50," she authored numerous articles on global and domestic public health issues, poverty alleviation, gender equality, and social justice. Born and raised in Buffalo, NY, Dr. Gayle earned a BA in psychology at Barnard College, an MD at the University of Pennsylvania and an MPH at Johns Hopkins University. She received 18 honorary degrees and holds faculty appointments at the University of Washington and Emory University.

Mariuche Gomides, Ph.D., is a Postdoctoral Researcher at the University College Dublin (UCD) School of Psychology (Ireland). She holds a Ph.D. in Psychology, a master's degree in Neuroscience, and a BA in Psychology from the Federal University of Minas Gerais, Brazil. Her research interests concern the underlying cognitive mechanisms of mathematical development. Currently, she is investigating if digital game-based interventions improve mathematical performance and alleviate math anxiety.

Terri Herron, Ph.D. is the Paul and Betty Haack Distinguished Faculty Fellow in Accounting at the University of Montana. She holds Ph.D. and a Master's degree in accounting from the University of Texas at Arlington, and a BS degree from Baylor University. Dr. Herron researches auditor regulation, ethics, judgement, and education issues. She has published her research in a wide range of accounting, ethics, and business journals, including Society and Business Review, Business Ethics Quarterly, Auditing: A Journal of Practice & Theory, Current Issues in Auditing, and Journal of Accountancy. Her recent paper with Dr. Tim Manuel in Society and Business Review won that journal's Literati Award for Best Paper. Dr. Herron has provided numerous professional education seminars on ethics for Montana CPAs. She has been at the University of Montana for 26 years, most recently teaching auditing and financial accounting. She is a licensed CPA and a member of the Montana Society of CPAs, where she is vice-chair of the Ethics Committee.

Steve Jeantet, Ph.D. is the principal of Radical Greatness Leadership Consulting and an experienced nonprofit executive in Sarasota, Florida. His doctoral research focused on the relationship between spiritual maturity and ethical decision-making. As an Appreciative Inquiry certified facilitator, Steve's work focuses on the flourishing of nonprofits. Steve serves as an adjunct at multiple universities teaching courses on nonprofit management and leadership. His writings have been featured in the Journal of Management, Spirituality and Religion and the Journal of Applied Christian Leadership. When not writing or thinking about helping nonprofits thrive, Steve can often be found coaching his sons' baseball teams.

Tim Manuel, Ph.D., is a professor of finance and is the Rudyard B. Goode Professorship honoree at the College of Business at the University of Montana. Dr. Manuel holds a Ph.D. in Business from the University of South Carolina and MBA and BS degrees from Virginia Tech. His areas of expertise include asymmetric information, announcement effects, capital structure, dividend policy, international finance and ethics. His teaching interests include markets and institutions, derivative securities, valuation, international finance, ethics and investments. Dr. Manuel has been recognized with numerous teaching awards over the years for excellence in the classroom; most recently he received the 2019-2020 Outstanding Faculty Award from Beta Alpha Psi. Dr. Manuel's academic work has been published in some of the leading business journals in the country including the Journal of Business, Journal of Financial Economics, Journal of Financial Research, Society and Business Review, Business and Society Review, and others. In recognition of their recent paper in the Society and Business

Review, Emerald Publishing honored Dr. Manuel and coauthor Dr. Terri Herron with an Emerald Literati Award for "Outstanding Paper."

Max Alexander Matthey M.A. is the Director of Communication at Incentives for Global Health and a member of the Green Impact Fund for Technology of the Yale Global Justice Programme. Working on his Ph.D. in economics, he analyses the potential of Impact Funds in both Global Pharma Research and Global Green Technologies. A paramedic by training, his research focuses on Neglected Tropical Diseases and the Diffusion of Green Technologies in LMICs.

Haley McDevitt earned a Bachelor of Arts in Marketing with a Minor in Civic and Professional Leadership from West Chester University of Pennsylvania (WCU). While studying, Haley served as a Leadership Studies Fellow for the Honors College, an academic leadership position in which she facilitated student discussion and learning about visions of "life worth living." She applies her skills of marketing and leadership by serving as a Marketing Director in addition to leading her own photography business. Haley is an active alumni volunteer in the Leadership Studies Program at WCU.

Sevim Mustafa, Ph.D., is a Professor of Psychology at the AAB College in Kosovo. In her research, she examines the characteristics of gifted children in relation to self-esteem and family dynamics. Moreover, she investigates the relationship between self-esteem and academic achievement among adolescents. In addition to this, her research examines the impact that the COVID-19 pandemic has on individuals suffering from mental illness.

Vegard Mokleiv Nygaard, Ph.D., is an Assistant Professor in the Department of Economics at the University of Houston in Houston, Texas. Dr. Nygaard is a macroeconomist interested in topics related to inequality, health economics, and public finance. His work has been published in several top-tier peer-reviewed journals and presented in several seminars and conferences world-wide. He has also contributed to an e-book chapter and several policy briefs. At the University of Houston, he also advises several doctoral students and teaches both undergraduate and graduate classes in his topics of expertise. Prior to joining University of Houston, Dr.

Nygaard earned his Ph.D. in Economics at the University of Minnesota, where he was also a research assistant for Prof. Tim Kehoe. During his Ph.D., he also visited the T. H. Chan School of Public Health at Harvard University and he was awarded the Doctoral Dissertation Fellowship at the University of Minnesota in 2018. He joined the Ph.D. program after a year at the Central Bank of Norway. He also holds an M.A. and B.A. from the University of Oslo (Oslo, Norway).

Mark F. Olaf, DO, FACEP is Vice Chair of Education for Emergency Medicine and an Associate Regional Dean for the Geisinger Commonwealth School of Medicine (GCSOM) where he is an Associate Professor of Emergency Medicine. He is an Emergency Physician at Geisinger Health System in Danville, PA. A Diplomate of the American Board of Emergency Medicine, and a Fellow of the American College of Emergency Physicians (FACEP), Dr. Olaf is also a distinguished fellow of the ACEP Teaching Fellowship. Dr. Olaf is a graduate of the Philadelphia College of Osteopathic Medicine in Philadelphia, Pennsylvania. He completed emergency medicine residency training at the Geisinger Health System in Danville, Pennsylvania, where he served as Chief Resident. Dr. Olaf has demonstrated expertise in advising and mentoring emergency medicine bound students. He has published numerous peer reviewed articles and collaborated with colleagues from across the country to further knowledge and share information related to emergency medicine education and advising in medical school. Dr. Olaf has lectured extensively within his institution and in multiple venues across the United States. He has been awarded multiple institutional awards for mentoring and advising students. His ongoing academic and education research interests include evidence-based advising, medical student transitions to residency, and curriculum development for emergency medicine education. Dr. Olaf is a previous Co-Chair of the Advising Students Committee of the Council of Residency Directors in EM (CORD-EM). He currently is leading work groups to provide and publish evidence based advising to emergency medicine interested students across the country. He is also a member of the Clerkship Directors of Emergency Medicine (CDEM) Academy of the Society for Academic Emergency Medicine (SAEM). He is a member of the American College of Emergency Physicians (ACEP) and the Pennsylvania College of Emergency Physicians (PACEP), having served on the wellness committee, and having been awarded the PACEP Leadership Scholarship Award.

Jimmy Payne, Jr., Ph.D., a recent Regent University graduate, has conducted research on destructive leadership, ethics, and failed organizations. He was involved with youth development for 14 years and taught youth leadership development for over ten years with Scouts, BSA. Additionally, he is qualified as a leadership development trainer through the Alpha Phi Omega, LEADS program and is currently completing his Certified Nonprofit Professional (CNP) credential. Through Mr. Payne's educational background in Business Administration, Technical Management, and Organizational Leadership, he has applied team building, budget management, and program execution in action, including many different elements of ethical training. In his current role, as a Program Manager for the Naval Sea Systems Command (NAVSEA), he oversees 22 teams and is responsible for overseeing the life cycle maintenance for the same number of Guided Missile Cruisers in the Navy's current inventory and has been hand-selected to fill the same position with the newest frigate class of ships expected to be delivered in 2025. Additionally, he has developed new communication processes and deliverable review and submission methods to address the needs of his teams during the pandemic.

Karen Perham-Lippman, MS, CDP, CAGS is a dynamic executive and mission-driven business strategist with nearly fifteen years of demonstrated strategic and processing thinking results in diversity, equity and inclusion, corporate social responsibility, community outreach and employee engagement. As a practitioner with consultancy experience, she has worked with nonprofit, business, state government, and municipal clients. Ms. Perham-Lippman leads supplier diversity and ESG with Xcel Energy and is an Adjunct Professor with the Community College of Denver's Center for Business, Industry, Technology & Public Service. She received her Certified Diversity Professional credentials from Cornell University and is a Ph.D. candidate at Eastern University. Ms. Perham-Lippman's dissertation work is focused on exploring destructive leadership, followers, and conducive environments as a group process with a particular focus on the technology sector. Her research focus also includes Women and Leadership, for which she is a co-author of a SAGE Publishing business case study, Employee Workload and Retention in an Environment of Unpaid Labor: Acknowledging and Supporting "Women's Work" (2022). Ms. Perham-Lippman has been recognized with numerous awards for her leadership contributions and service to nonprofits and public schools, and for dedication to serving youth and families in poverty. She serves her local community with Girls Inc. of Metro Denver and the National Association for Multi-ethnicity in Communication's Denver chapter. Nationally, she serves on DisabilityIN's Mental Wellness Executive Committee and co-chairs their Substance Use Disorder subcommittee. In 2021 she was appointed to the State of Colorado's Business Experiential Learning Commission by Governor Polis.

Bhaskaran Raman is a Professor in the Department of Computer Science and Engineering at the Indian Institute of Technology at Bombay. He has been following data and statistics related to COVID-19 since the declaration of the pandemic. He is a working committee member of the Universal Health Organization (UHO): https://uho.org.in/. Toward the end of 2021, he launched the "Happy 2022, Happy for Kids Too" initiative, to work toward a normal and enjoyable childhood as deserved by each child: https://happy22kids.org/. He maintains the "Understand, Unclog, Unpanic, Unscare, Unlock (U5) India" website at https://tinyurl.com/u5india

Benjamin Roth M.mel. is a research associate at the Center for Health Ethics in Hannover (Germany) and a member of the doctoral research group "Human Rights and Ethics in Medicine for the Elderly" of the Institute of Medical Ethics (Friedrich-Alexander University Erlangen-Nuremberg). His Ph.D. topic is the problem of polypharmacy in the treatment of elderly patients. His research interests are in global health-, public health- and pharmaceutical ethics. In these contexts, he is particularly interested in the effects and normative implications of financial incentives.

Joanna Stanberry, M.A., is a doctoral student engaged in the Initiative for Leadership and Sustainability (IFLAS) at the University of Cumbria, United Kingdom. Previously she assisted with international legal issues both at Cravath, Swaine, and Moore, LLC, and for Tiger Management in New York City. As a founding member of the Center for the Study of the Holocaust and Human Rights under the philosopher John Roth at Claremont McKenna

College, she researched significant concerns of global justice. She has worked alongside local leaders actively building community solidarity in the Global South. Her current research explores pathways to developing sustainability leadership at the intersection of cross-sector partnerships to accomplish the Sustainable Development Goals and includes applications for adult moral development for citizenship and local flourishing. In her nonprofit role as Director of Communications at Project Renewal, New York's largest agency serving the unhoused, she experienced the significance of individual stories that impact societal transformation and their power for change. Joanna taught at the MacArthur School of Leadership at Palm Beach Atlantic University in Florida. She received the M.A. in Leadership from Eastern University in Pennsylvania.

Michael Tomlinson, FGIA, FCG, Ph.D., is an independent Higher Education Governance and Quality Consultant. He was formerly a Director at Australia's Tertiary Education Quality and Standards Agency (TEQSA), where he led case teams to conduct assessments of all registered providers and was decision maker for all their course applications. Before TEQSA, he worked for twenty years in Australian universities, for the last fifteen of these in senior positions at Swinburne University of Technology. Dr. Tomlinson is a Fellow of the Governance Institute of Australia and of the (international) Chartered Governance Institute. He has been an expert panel member or chair for a number of offshore reviews for the national accreditation agency in Timor Leste; the Fiji Higher Education Commission (re the University of the South Pacific); and the Department of Higher Education, Research, Science and Technology of Papua New Guinea. Dr. Tomlinson is Chair of the Human Research Ethics Committee at Australia's National Institute of Integrative Medicine. He also holds a number of other positions at Australian institutes and universities: Chair of the Academic Board, Nan Tien Institute of Higher Education; Member of the Board at Australian College of the Arts Pty Ltd ('Collarts'); Member of the Academic Board at Victorian Institute of Technology; and Honorary (Principal) Fellow, LH Martin Institute at The University of Melbourne.

Samuel White is an Adjunct Research Fellow at the University of New England, Associate Researcher at the Research Unit for Military Law and Ethics, Adjunct Lecturer and Ph.D. Candidate at the University of

Adelaide. In 2021, he was recognised by the International Committee of the Red Cross as an 'Emerging Voices' for his scholarship in international humanitarian law. He holds a Bachelor of Arts and Bachelor of Laws (Hons) from the University of Queensland; a Master of Laws (Hons I) from the University of Melbourne; and a Master of War Studies from the University of New South Wales. In 2018, he served as Associate to the Honourable Justice John Logan of the Federal Court of Australia, Supreme & National Courts of Papua New Guinea, and President of the Defence Force Discipline Appeals Tribunal.

Zachary C. Wooten, Ph.D., serves as an Instructor of Leadership Studies at West Chester University for the Honors College and Minor in Civic and Professional Leadership, teaching courses in leadership theory, self-awareness, decision-making, public discourse, ethics, leadership development, interfaith leadership, and religious studies. After earning a Bachelor of Arts in Communication Studies from West Chester University of Pennsylvania (WCU), Zachary obtained a Master of Divinity from Princeton Theological Seminary. Dr. Wooten earned his Ph.D. at Alvernia University researching spirituality and philosophies of leadership education. As a scholar, he is an active member of the Association of Leadership Educators (ALE) and the International Leadership Association (ILA).

Jeff Youngquist (Ph.D., Wayne State University) is an Associate Professor in the Department of Communication, Journalism, and Public Relations at Oakland University. His research and writing focus on various facets of academic and organizational leadership as they relate to decision-making, creativity, adaptability, and ethics. He has been published in journals such as The Department Chair, Communication Studies, and Communication Teacher. He regularly attends leadership conferences across the globe and is especially fond of the International Leadership Association conference. He teaches both undergraduate and graduate communication courses that focus on leadership, organizational communication, organizational theory, and communication ethics. He has also taught courses in Oakland University's Executive MBA program including Executive Communications and Bargaining, Negotiations, and Communications. Dr. Youngquist was the department chair at Oakland University for 6 years and this was an experience that he considers one of his most challenging and most rewarding. In addition to being the department chair, he has held numerous other leadership positions all of which have been exceptional environments for learning about the complexities of leadership and discovering how to be a better leader. Dr. Youngquist is an avid traveler and enjoys seeing and experiencing as much of this diverse and wonderful world as he possibly can. One of his current projects is developing a study-abroad class titled Communication and Leadership in Taiwan.

Anne Zimmerman, JD, MS, CIPP-US, Founder, Modern Bioethics; Chair, New York City Bar Association Bioethical Issues Committee; Editor-in-Chief, Voices in Bioethics (Columbia University journal and podcast); Consultant, MyBioethics technology-based bioethics learning tool; Co-Founder and Co-Chair, Bioethics Forum in partnership with the Collaborative for Palliative Care. Her prior experience includes corporate governance, criminal justice reform, and nutrition with a focus on policy surrounding access to a healthy food supply.